Office-Based Surgery
of the
Head and Neck

Office-Based Surgery of the Head and Neck

Editor

Yosef P. Krespi, M.D.

Director
Department of Otolaryngology
Head and Neck Surgery
St. Luke's/Roosevelt Hospital Center
Professor
Columbia University
New York, New York

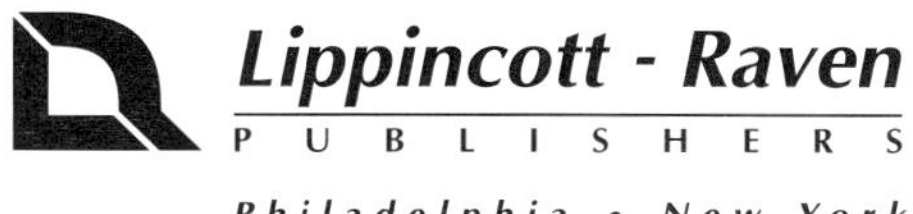

Lippincott - Raven

PUBLISHERS

Philadelphia • New York

Acquisitions Editor: Danette Knopp
Developmental Editor: Emilie Linkins
Manufacturing Manager: Dennis Teston
Production Manager: Jodi Borgenicht
Production Editor: Kimberly Monroe
Cover Designer: Marsha Cohen
Indexer: Keith T. Shostak
Compositor: Lippincott–Raven Electronic Production
Printer: Quebecor Kingsport

Printed in the United States of America

9 8 7 6 5 4 3 2 1

Library of Congress Cataloging-in-Publication Data

Office-based surgery of the head and neck / editor, Yosef P. Krespi.
    p.   cm.
    Includes bibliographical references and index.
    ISBN 0-397-51590-1
    1. Otolaryngology, Operative. 2. Ambulatory surgery. 3. Face—Surgery. I. Krespi, Yosef P.
[DNLM: 1. Head—surgery. 2. Neck—surgery. 3. Laser Surgery—methods. 4. Ambulatory
Surgery—methods. WE 705 032 1998]
RF51.038   1998
617.5′1—dc21
DNLM/DLC
For Library of Congress

Contents

CONTENTS

Contributing Authors

Jeffrey M. Ahn, M.D.
Assistant Professor
Department of Otolaryngology–
  Head and Neck Surgery
Columbia University
16 East 60th Street, Suite 360
New York, New York 10022

William J. Binder, M.D., F.A.C.S.
Assistant Clinical Professor
Department of Head and Neck Surgery
  UCLA School of Medicine
9201 West Sunset Boulevard (S.809)
Los Angeles, California 90069

Andrew Blitzer, M.D., D.D.S.
Professor of Clinical Otolaryngology
Director, New York Center for
  Voice and Swallowing Disorders
Columbia University
425 West 59th Street
New York, New York 10019

Mitchell F. Brin, M.D.
Associate Professor of Neurology
Director of Movement Disorders
The Mount Sinai Medical Center
One Gustave L. Levy Place
New York, New York 10029

Brian B. Burkey, M.D.
Assistant Professor of Otolaryngology
Department of Otolaryngology
Vanderbilt University School of Medicine
S-2100 MCN
Nashville, Tennessee 37232

Daniel I. Choo, M.D.
Neurotology Branch
National Institute on Deafness and Other
  Communicative Disorders
10 Center Drive, Building 10, Room 5055
Bethesda, Maryland 20892

Niall J. Daly, B.Sc, F.R.C.S.I.
Clinical Fellow
Department of Otolaryngology
Addenbrooke's Hospital
Hills Road, Cambridge, CB2 2QQ
United Kingdom

Cindi L. Davis, B.S.N., R.N.
Nurse Clinician
The Mount Sinai Nasal Sinus Center
26900 Cedar Road
Beachwood, Ohio 44122

Peter D. M. Ellis, M.A., F.R.C.S.
Department of Otolaryngology
Addenbrooke's Hospital
Hill's Road, Cambridge, CB2 2QQ
United Kingdom

Monica Elman, M.D.
Specialist in Dermatology
A.M.A. Medical Service Ltd.
11 Tarzav Street, Holon 58312
Tel-Aviv, Israel

C. Gaelyn Garrett, M.D.
Assistant Professor of Otolaryngology
Vanderbilt Department of Otolaryngology
Vanderbilt University Hospital
Vanderbilt Voice Center
2700 The Village at Vanderbilt
1500 21st Avenue, South
Nashville, Tennessee 37212

Philip T. Ho, M.D.
Department of Otolaryngology–
  Head and Neck Surgery
Columbia-Presbyterian Medical Center
180 Fort Washington, Harkness Pavilion, 8th Floor
New York, New York 10032

Anthony F. Jahn, M.D.
Professor of Clinical Otolaryngology
Columbia University College of
  Physicians and Surgeons
425 West 59th Street, Suite 4E
New York, New York 10019

Matthew E. Karen, M.D.
Post-Doc Residency Fellow
Department of Otolaryngology–
  Head and Neck Surgery
Columbia University, St. Luke's/
  Roosevelt Hospital Center
425 West 59th Street
New York, New York 10019

Anat Keidar, M.A., CCC-SLP, Ph.D.
Director
Voice Laboratory
Head and Neck Surgery Group
St. Luke's/Roosevelt Hospital Center
425 West 59th Street, Suite 4E
New York, New York 10019

M. Morad Khosh, M.D.
Clinical Instructor
Department of Otolaryngology–
    Head and Neck Surgery
University of Washington
3505A East Olive Street
Seattle, Washington 98122

Eric M. Kitain, M.D.
Clinical Assistant Professor of Anesthesia
Department of Anesthesiology
Columbia University College of
    Physicians and Surgeons
425 West 59th Street
New York, New York 10019

Yosef P. Krespi, M.D.
Director
Department of Otolaryngology–
    Head and Neck Surgery
St. Luke's/Roosevelt Hospital Center
Professor
Columbia University
425 West 59th Street
New York, New York 10019

Jeffery J. Kuhn, M.D.
Assistant Professor of Clinical Otolaryngology
Department of Otolaryngology–
    Head and Neck Surgery
Naval Medical Center Portsmouth
620 John Paul Jones Circle
Portsmouth, Virginia 23708

Daniel B. Kuriloff, M.D., F.A.C.S.
Assistant Professor
Department of Otolaryngology–
    Head and Neck Surgery
Columbia University College of
    Physicians and Surgeons
425 West 59th Street
New York, New York 10019

Wayne F. Larrabee, Jr., M.D., M.S.Hyg.
Clinical Professor of Otolaryngology–
    Head and Neck Surgery
University of Washington at Seattle
600 Broadway
Seattle, Washington 98122

William Lawson, M.D.
Professor of Otolaryngology
Department of Otolaryngology
The Mount Sinai Medical Center
One Gustave L. Levy Place
New York, New York 10029

Howard L. Levine, M.D.
Director
The Mount Sinai Nasal Sinus Center
Cleveland Ear, Nose, and Throat Center
The Mount Sinai Medical Center
26900 Cedar Road, Suite 22N
Cleveland, Ohio 44122

Z. Paul Lorenc, M.D.
Assistant Professor of Plastic Surgery
Department of Plastic Surgery
New York University School of Medicine
124 East 65th Street
New York, New York 10021

Michael Mayer, M.D.
Department of Otolaryngology
St. Luke's/Roosevelt Hospital Center
425 West 59th Street
New York, New York 10019

Gary J. Nishioka, M.D., D.M.D.
Private Practice
600 Broadway, Suite 280
Seattle, Washington 98122

David S. Orentreich, M.D.
Assistant Clinical Professor
Department of Dermatology
Mount Sinai School of Medicne
New York, New York 10029

Robert H. Ossoff, D.M.D., M.D.
Guy M. Maness Professor and Chairman
Department of Otolaryngology
Vanderbilt University Medical Center
21st and Garland Avenue
Nashville, Tennessee 37232

Steven J. Pearlman, M.D., F.A.C.S.
Assistant Professor of Clinical Otolaryngology
Department of Otolaryngology
St. Luke's/Roosevelt Hospital Center
425 West 59th Street
New York, New York 10019

S. James Quinn, M.B.B.S., F.R.C.S.
Senior Registrar
Department of Otolaryngology
Guy's Hospital
London SE1 9RT
United Kingdom

Anthony J. Reino, M.D., M.Sc.
Assistant Clinical Professor
Department of Otolaryngology
The Mount Sinai Medical Center
One Gustave L. Levy Place
New York, New York 10029

Seth I. Rosenberg, M.D., F.A.C.S.
Clinical Assistant Professor
Department of Otorhinolaryngology–
* Head and Neck Surgery*
University of Pennsylvania School of Medicine
Philadelphia, Pennsylvana 19104
Vice President
Ear Research Foundation and
* Florida Ear and Sinus Center*
Sarasota, Florida 34239

Zvi Rozenberg, Ph.D.
Physics Department
Laser Industries
Neve Sharett, PO Box 13135
Tel Aviv, Israel 61131

Herbert Silverstein, M.D., F.A.C.S.
Clinical Professor
Department of Otorhinolaryngology–
* Head and Neck Surgery*
University of Pennsylvania School of Medicine
Philadelphia, Pennsylvania 19104
Clinical Professor of Surgery
Division of Otolaryngology
University of South Florida
Tampa, Florida 33612
President
Ear Research Foundation and
* Florida Ear and Sinus Center*
Sarasota, Florida 34239

Michael Slatkine, Ph.D.
Vice President
Development of New Applications
Sharplan Lasers, Inc,
1 Pearl Court
Allendale, New Jersey 07401

Kurian Thomas, M.D.
Assistant Professor
Department of Anesthesiology
St. Luke's/Roosevelt Hospital Center/
* Columbia University*
1000 10th Avenue
New York, New York 10019

Amir Waldman, Ph.D.
Sharplan Lasers, Inc.
1 Pearl Court
Allendale, New Jersey 07401

Lynn Weatherby, Ph.D.
Nicolet Biomedical Incorporated
5225 Verona Road
Madison, Wisconsin 53711

Gary K. Zammit, Ph.D.
Director
Sleep Disorders Institute
Clinical Associate Professor of Psychology
* (in Psychiatry)*
Columbia University College of
* Physicians and Surgeons*
1090 Amsterdam Avenue
New York, New York 10025

Preface

Significant data were collected in Maryland from 1989 to 1992 reporting surgical statistics in otolaryngology–head and neck surgery. These data showed an annual average decrease in inpatient surgical procedures of 5.2% and a corresponding increase in outpatient otolaryngologic surgeries of 5.1% (1).

Office-based surgery in the 1990s underwent significant changes due to the development and use of new technology that allows physicians to perform safe, cost-effective, and rapid office procedures with equivalent, if not better, clinical outcomes. Educated and well-informed patients prefer the high-tech environment that can be offered in an office setting. The time loss and inconvenience of hospital and ambulatory surgery centers is not usually preferred by patients and physicians.

Effective marketing of a practice does not consist of contracting a public relations consultant and getting brochures and a snappy logo. It means taking extraordinary care of patients. One can do that simply and economically by establishing an office-based surgical environment. An office-based surgical suite provides a convenient set-up for physicians. They can operate in a comfortable, familiar environment and their schedule is not dictated by an institution. The surgeon can work with a familiar staff that has been specially trained on the equipment for that office procedure. In this way, better care is facilitated.

Advances with endoscopic equipment provide access to deep anatomic regions and cavities, as well as excellent illumination, visualization, and magnification. Video cameras can be attached to the endoscope and allow observation of the surgical procedure on a television screen. Laser fibers and accessories that have been developed in the past 10 years allow the surgeon a safe and effective method for treating conditions involving organs such as the soft palate, tongue base, oral cavity, tonsils, turbinates, nasopharynx, and tympanic membrane. These new methods will be developed further to increase the surgical application of endoscopes, lasers, and other tools in office-based surgery.

Patient selection has been an important element in successful surgical outcomes. Medically unstable patients and those with other general medical problems will continue to have medical care in a hospital setting. However, the majority of minor and elective surgeries will be shifted from an ambulatory surgical setting to an office or clinic setting.

Office-Based Surgery of the Head and Neck will familiarize the otolaryngologist, head and neck surgeon, and facial plastic surgeon with current surgical procedures that can be performed in an office/clinic setting. I predict that these surgical methods will be developed further and used widely in the field of otolaryngology–head and neck surgery.

Yosef P. Krespi, M.D.

REFERENCE

1. Manoukian, MD et al: Recent trends in utilization of procedures in otolaryngology-head and neck surgery. *Laryngoscope* 107:472–477, 1997.

Office-Based Surgery of the Head and Neck

PART 1

Introduction

Office-Based Surgery of the Head and Neck
Edited by Yosef P. Krespi, MD
Lippincott–Raven Publishers, Philadelphia © 1998

1

Laser Safety in Office-Based Ambulatory Surgery

Daniel B. Kuriloff

In 1954, a team of physicists at Columbia University, headed by Charles H. Townes, laid the groundwork in quantum electronics that produced the first microwave laser or "MASER," an acronym for microwave amplification by stimulated emission of radiation. Townes was awarded the Nobel Prize in physics in 1964 (1). The first visible light laser (a synthetic ruby crystal) was developed in 1960 by Theodore Maiman from Hughs Research Laboratories. It produced visible red light lasting a few microseconds and was used for photocoagulation of retinal vessels by the mid-1960s (2). Other industrial and medical applications for laser energy rapidly followed with an ensuing explosion in technologic refinements. Along with a several-fold increase in site-specific applications throughout medicine, the number of different lasers (Argon, KTP/532, CO_2, Neodymium:YAG, Erbium:YAG, Homium:YAG, THC:YAG, Excimer, Gold Vapor, Copper Vapor, Mercury Vapor, Pulsed Dye, Tunable Dye, Homium, Diode, Q-Switched Lasers, and Free Electron Lasers) has proliferated over the last decade along with new delivery systems (optical fibers, wave guides, and contact tips), and new beam distribution technology (SwiftLase, Silk-Touch, UltraPulse, and Flash Scan). Specialized laser instrumentation has also evolved to improve smoke evacuation, permit endoscopic application, and protect adjacent non-target structures.

The unique properties of laser energy (monochromatic, coherent) allow it to be concentrated into a small target area from a dis-tance and its biologic effect controlled by varying the energy density and delivery rate of the beam. The biologic response to a specific energy density causes an immediate physical effect that ranges from warming and blanching to complete vaporization. The laser-tissue interaction is also dependent on both the specific wavelength of the energy and the tissue composition (eg, pigmentation, water content, and vascularity). The mechanisms of laser-tissue interaction involve photochemical, photothermal, and photomechanical effects. The ultimate biologic response is determined by the summation of these effects on cellular and subcellular tissue components, the inflammatory response, and long-term healing (3).

Because of its hemostatic properties, controlled precision, deliverability to previously inaccessible regions of the body, and ability to cut through muscle without electrical stimulation, the laser has gained widespread use in surgery. In the last decade, its use has increased in the ambulatory surgery environment, and more recently the laser has become a standard piece of equipment in the office setting.

The hemostatic properties of the laser are especially advantageous in upper aerodigestive tract surgery, which in the past required endotracheal intubation to protect the airway from bleeding and obstruction. "Bloodless" surgery in this region of the head and neck can now be performed safely on an awake patient in an ambulatory setting. With the popularization of laser-assisted office-based procedures, such as laser-assisted uvulopalatoplasty, intranasal surgery, endoscopic laryngeal surgery, and laser-assisted skin resurfacing, both the number of physicians using laser technology and the number of procedures performed are expected to increase dramatically.

Despite its many excellent attributes as a surgical tool, no other medical device or technology in the history of medicine has had as great a potential to cause catastrophic harm to both patients and support personnel. Because of the laser beam's ability to travel some distance from the patient and the freehand aiming of the laser aperture, unaware bystanders are also at risk for potential injury. Although hospitals and most outpatient facilities have adopted strict guidelines and administrative controls to ensure the enforcement of safety issues and to facilitate reporting potential problems or complications related to the use of the laser, it is unclear to what extent laser safety guidelines are enforced in the private sector. Although it is expected that prior to the purchase and use of an office laser, physicians have already received their credentials by taking laser courses (with specific didactic and hands-on instruction in safety issues), credentialing for laser use outside of the hospital setting is not required by the companies selling lasers or by local or state regulatory agencies (Table 1).

TABLE 1. *American National Standard for the Safe Use of Lasers (ANSI Z136.3) Guidelines for Physician Credentialing*

Physician training
  Mandatory laser course attendance (8–10 hours)
    Basic laser physics
    Laser tissue interaction
    Discussion of specific clinical applications
      (specialty)
    Hands-on experience
  Consultation with experienced laser physician
    6–8 hours of observation/hands-on experience or
      accredited residency training that includes
      laser use
Laser-safety training
    Potential hazards
    Requirements for laser safety
    Standard operating procedures

Medical practices are currently subject to the Occupational Safety and Health Administration (OSHA) Hazard Communications Standard of 1987 and the Blood Borne Pathogen Standard 29 CFR 1910.1030 (copies available from the US Department of Labor). Both of these standards require written policy manuals and formal training with documentation. Failure to display proper warning signs alerting the public and office staff of potentially hazardous energy (x-ray, laser, magnetic, electrical) or not protecting staff from blood-borne pathogens by providing adequate protection from exposure to smoke or body fluids gives OSHA the authority to fine violators from as little as $100 for minor violations to as much as $70,000 for "willful" violations (4).

The potential for disaster and the likelihood of litigation when the laser is used by inexperienced or careless individuals in the office should not be underestimated. It is essential that every member of the surgical team, including the patient, be educated and informed about the surgical procedure for which the laser is to be used. The patient should understand the specific benefits of the laser over other existing technology and it should not be used unless those benefits have been well documented through clinical trials and peer review. The patient must also understand the unique risks associated with the use of laser energy and the potential for injury away from the operative field. This information should be included in the process of informed consent. This chapter highlights the major potential health risks in laser surgery and details specific steps that should be taken to ensure laser safety in an office setting.

SAFETY GUIDELINES AND CREDENTIALING

Early recognition of potential disasters during industrial use of the laser led to the publication of safety guidelines in 1930 by the American National Standards Institute (ANSI), the "American National Standard for the Safe Use of Lasers (ANSI Z136.1)" (5). In 1988, safety standards for laser use in medicine were first outlined in a subsequent ANSI report, "Laser Safety in the Health Care Environment" (ANSI Z136.3), which was based on the prior, more general and comprehensive ANSI publication (6). The latter standard itself outlines specific procedural and administrative controls necessary to ensure the safety of patients and healthcare professionals working with lasers. Both standards are intended as guides to aid the manufacturer, the consumer, and the general public. Although the ANSI reports have defined the current standard of care for the safe use of lasers in the healthcare environment, compliance in general is voluntary unless required by a specific organization (eg, hospital or ambulatory facility).

Administrative controls in the healthcare environment include the establishment of a laser-safety committee and appointment of a laser-safety officer. The laser-safety committee is generally a multidisciplinary group that includes physicians, nurses, biomedical engineers, hospital administrators, and so forth, who meet on a regular basis to establish and enforce adequate protective measures against laser-induced injury and provide in-service training for the management of laser-induced catastrophes (eg, fires, burns, and explosions).

Credentialing procedures must be set up and monitored by the committee for physicians, anesthesiology staff, nurses, technical support staff, and other healthcare personnel. Educational programs of at least 16–20 hours with 50% of the time dedicated to hands-on experience have been suggested as a minimal requirement for credentialing (7). The program must include exposure to all of the specific wavelengths of energy that will be used as well as comprehensive training in all aspects of laser biophysics and safety. As new wavelengths of laser energy are introduced, specific additional hands-on training would also be required.

The laser-safety officer must ensure continuing surveillance and enforcement of safety regulations and credentialing require-

ments. Any laser-related complications or problems are documented and reported directly to the committee for review and appropriate corrective action. New laser installations require inspection by the laser-safety officer in conjunction with the manufacturer and biomedical engineer. The inspection should include assessment of other special considerations, such as electrical, fire, and explosion hazards; eye exposure risks; laser smoke evacuation; and the flammability of anesthetic agents and drapes.

The incidence of serious laser-related injuries at institutions adhering to the ANSI guidelines remains astonishingly low despite an increase in laser use across surgical subspecialties (6,8). Healy et al. (9) reviewed >4000 carbon dioxide (CO_2) laser procedures and found a complication rate of only 0.2%. Ossoff (7) retrospectively reviewed 204 CO_2 laser procedures and found a complication rate of 4%. Accidents occurring during laser surgery are almost always related to breaches in safety protocol or to surgical accidents. Brodmahn et al. (10) recently reviewed operating room personnel morbidity in a teaching hospital environment from CO_2 laser use during resident supervised surgery. Despite extensive training requirements before use of the laser, complications still occurred in 9% of all procedures reviewed during 1 year and were primarily due to surgeons' technical errors. Morbidity included major and minor burns (both operator and patient). In one case, the operator's gown ignited and in another the anesthesia screen ignited. None of the complications could be attributed to equipment malfunction. The authors suggested that laser-resistant drapes be developed and that a laser technician run the laser control panel at all times with a CO_2 fire extinguisher readily available. They stressed the importance of experience and education in preventing laser injuries.

If laser-related complications are to remain low in the office setting, it is incumbent on physicians in solo practice or the office manager or other responsible person in a group practice to appoint an individual to be a laser-safety officer and establish a specific safety protocol for office-based laser surgery. Safety equipment (fire extinguishers, irrigating fluid, smoke evacuators, and exhaust systems) must always be available and inspected periodically for proper function. Medical assistants or nursing staff in the office must have already received laser credentials and hands-on training in laser safety or they must attend courses for certification prior to assisting physicians performing laser procedures. All personnel should have in-service training from the manufacturer of the specific laser(s) being used in the office.

SPECIFIC SAFETY CONTROL MEASURES

Laser hazards can be classified into two major categories: (1) hazards directly caused by the unintended biologic effects of the laser beam itself (eg, corneal or retinal eye damage, skin or mucosal burns, and airway fires) and (2) injury related to nonbeam phenomena (eg, ignition of drapes or gowns or explosion of oxygen-containing tubing, laser plume biohazards, electrical shock, and exposure to unshielded electromagnetic fields or ultraviolet irradiation (11,12).

Safety Considerations in the Treatment Room

The treatment room must be of sufficient size to allow adequate dissipation of heat from the laser unit and enough space around the patient for unencumbered movement of the laser articulating arm or laser fiber. All basic life support and emergency equipment must also be available as in any ambulatory surgery environment. In the event of laser malfunction, traditional surgical instruments and hemostatic capabilities must be readily available. An electrocautery unit should always be present as well as silver nitrate to control minor bleeding. To avoid any potential fire hazard, all flammable liquids (eg, ethyl chloride, alcohol, acetone) should be removed from the treatment room when using the laser.

Paper drapes should be avoided whenever possible and the patient should be protected with wet towels, when appropriate. Pure oxygen should never be flowing during laser use because this could support combustion. Smoke detectors and fire extinguishers should be present at all times and regularly tested for proper function.

Specific electrical and plumbing requirements must meet local building codes and be in place prior to laser installation in the office. This may require consultation with an engineer or electrician to ensure adequate circuit breakers and fire protection.

Laser Quality Control and Lockout Features

The development and introduction of medical devices for use in the health care environment are heavily regulated by the United States Food and Drug Administration. All lasers manufactured or imported into the United States are regulated to conform to all safety regulations established by The Center for Devices and Radiological Health, a division of the U.S. Food and Drug Administration. These regulations classify each laser by power and wavelength and specify its mechanical and electrical requirements. Laser manufacturers are required to classify their laser into one of four major hazard categories (ANSI Z136.1 standard)—the laser hazard classifications depending on the type and power output. Each classification has specific operational safety guidelines (Table 2). All lasers must have an identifying decal stating its specific class and the need for eye protection (Fig. 1). Most medical lasers, with the exception of low-power diode lasers and lasers used specifically for alignment purposes (eg, the helium-neon [HeNe] laser) fall into class IV. Class IV lasers are hazardous to view either directly or indirectly; they will cause skin burns and are a fire hazard. Appropriate, ANSI-approved, laser-safety glasses must be worn at all times when the laser is turned on and in the treatment mode (see later).

TABLE 2. *American National Standard for the Safe Use of Lasers (ANSI Z136.1) Laser Classification*

Class I	Emission intensity below known hazard levels in range of 0.4 µW. Class I lasers are generally exempt from radiation hazard controls and are not considered to be hazardous.
Class IIA	Lasers not intended for viewing (eg, supermarket scanner), but may be a chronic hazard if the emission is viewed for a duration >1000 seconds and at a maximum power output of 4.0 µW.
Class II	Low-power visible lasers that emit above class I levels but at <1 mW. Only limited controls are specified since the aversion reflex to bright light will usually prevent injury. Considered to be a chronic viewing hazard.
Class IIIA	Intermediate-power lasers (1–5 mW). Considered to be an acute hazard for direct beam viewing or viewing through optical instruments. Some limited controls are recommended. This is the class for most solid-state laser pointers.
Class IIIB	Moderate-power lasers (5–500 mW). In general, not a fire hazard but acute eye and skin damage is possible. Specific controls are recommended.
Class IV	High-power lasers (≥500 mW). These lasers are considered acutely hazardous for viewing under any circumstances (direct or reflected), will cause a significant skin burn, and are potential fire hazards as well. Significant controls are required of class IV laser facilities.

Reprinted with permission from Public Health Service Food and Drug Administration: *Regulations for the administration and enforcement of the radiation control for health and safety act of 1968.* U.S. Department of Health and Human Services, Washington, DC, 1994: 514–515.

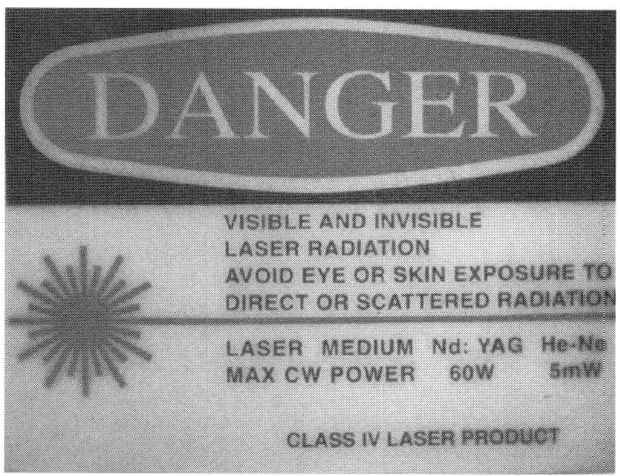

FIG. 1. Actual ANSI-approved identifying decal stating specific laser class and the need for eye protection.

used until it can be professionally serviced. Office-based lasers should be serviced by the manufacturer on at least a biannual basis to ensure proper output and alignment.

Eye Protection

Eye injury to either the cornea (focal cataract) or the retina (blind spot or permanent blindness) can occur from a direct hit from the laser beam, or from a side hit or a reflected beam hit. The specific injury will depend entirely on the wavelength of the laser energy and the energy density of the beam.

All lasers must have a key switch interlock or lock-out feature to ensure that only qualified individuals operate them. Most lasers have a key-actuated master control switch. The removable key ensures that the laser cannot be operated when it is not present. The laser should always be tested for proper functioning and, in the case of the CO_2 laser, the aiming and treatment beams should be in reasonable alignment and able to be tested on a wet tongue depressor (Fig. 2). If there is any doubt about the proper functioning of the laser, either the procedure should be rescheduled or more traditional surgical techniques

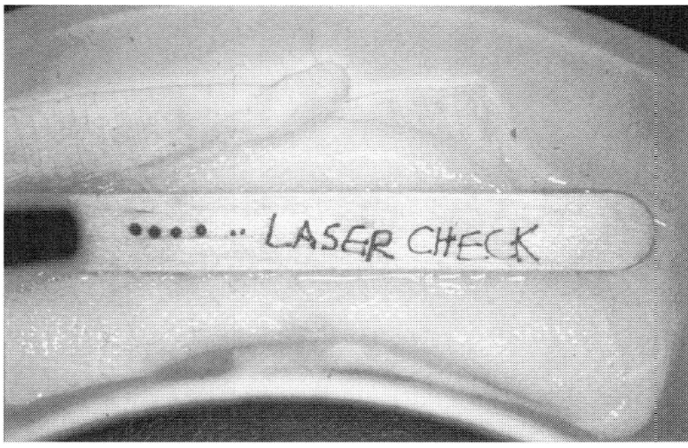

FIG. 2. Laser is checked for alignment (CO_2 and HeNe) and power output using a wet wood tongue blade on a bed of saline-soaked sponges.

TABLE 3. *Optical Densities for Protective Eye Wear for Various Lasers*

Laser Type and Power	Wavelength (m)	Optical Density for Exposure Durations			
		0.25 Second	10 Seconds	600 Seconds	30,000 Seconds
Argon (1 W)	0.514	3.0	3.4	5.2	6.4
HeNe (0.005 W)	0.633	0.7	1.1	1.7	2.9
Nd:YAG (100 W)	1.064[a]		4.7	5.2	5.2
Nd:YAG[b] (Q-Switch)	1.064[a]		4.5	5.0	5.4
Nd:YAG[c] (50 W)	1.33[a]		4.4	4.9	4.9
CO_2 (1000 W)	10.6[a]		6.2	8.0	9.7

[a] Repetitively pulsed at 11 Hz, 12-nanosecond pulses, 20 mJ/pulse.

[b] Optical density for ultraviolet and far infrared beams computed using a 1-mm limiting aperture, which presents a "worse-case" scenario. All visible and near infrared computations assume a 7-mm limiting aperture.

[c] Nd:YAG operating at a less-common 1.33 µm wavelength.

Reprinted with permission from Occupational Safety and Health Administration: *Laser hazards.* Office of Science and Technology Assessment, Section II, pp. 1–40. U.S. Department of Labor, Washington, DC, 1995.

Laser energy in the visible (argon, KTP/532, HeNe) and near infrared regions (Nd:YAG) of the electromagnetic spectrum (400–1400 nm) tends to pass through the cornea and cause a retinal burn, whereas the CO_2 laser in the far, infrared spectrum will be absorbed by the water content of the cornea and cause a thermal injury (cataract or scar).

Protective eye wear dedicated to the specific wavelength of the energy being used must be available for the patient, the surgeon, and any other personnel present in the operating or treatment room. The safety glasses should have side shields to prevent a side hit and be ANSI-approved with their optical density (Table 3) and wavelength stamped on the frame (Figs. 3 and 4). Al-though most plastic lenses are acceptable for the CO_2 laser, glass lenses tend to resist scratching and will better withstand a laser hit. Although laser-safety glasses are essential for eye protection, deeply colored lenses for the visible and near infrared lasers can obscure the operative field either by inadequate light or by color distortion. The operating surgeon must correct for these visual impairments and resist the temptation to operate the laser without safety glasses. Any currently available visible or near-infrared lasers are capable of emitting a laser beam of sufficient power and within a time frame of such short duration that an aversion reflex or blink will not be sufficient to prevent an irreversible retinal injury.

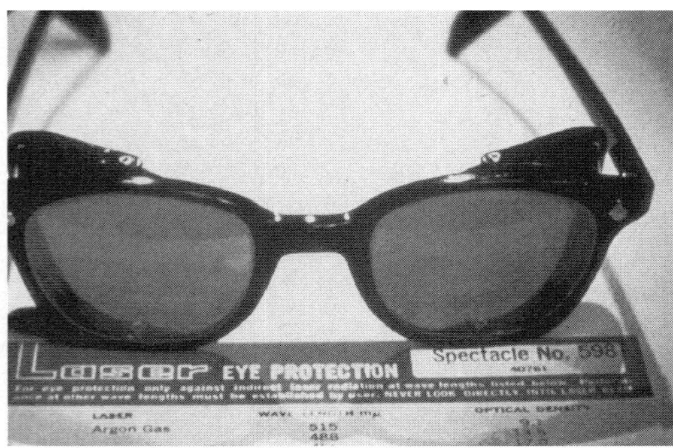

FIG. 3. Example of argon protective eye wear. Note specific wavelength and optical density imprinted on box or frame of glasses.

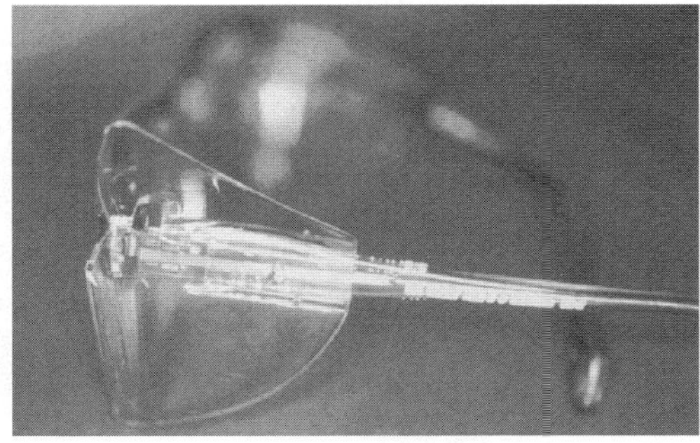

FIG. 4. Side guards help prevent stray laser hits to avoid ocular injury and prevent fluid or smoke plume exposure.

Protecting the patient's eyes from the laser is also mandatory. In addition to wearing appropriate laser-safety glasses, the patient's eyes should remain closed during laser use and be additionally protected with moist saline-saturated eye pads whenever possible.

Laser Warning Signs

A focused laser beam can traverse a room with very little attenuation and cause significant eye injury. It is essential that windows have black-out shades and that entrance and exit doors are closed at all times to protect personnel outside the treatment/operating room. The ANSI-approved laser warning sign indicating the laser's specific class, power, and wavelength (Fig. 5) should be hung in clear view outside the room. Ideally, a "laser in use" status should be indicated by either a lighted sign or flashing red light to ensure that the appropriate safety glasses will be selected. The laser warning sign, ideally, is affixed to the room door using Velcro strips, which permit repeated attachment and removal without damage to painted surfaces. Alternatively, if the door is metallic, a magnetic pad may be glued to the back of the sign to allow repeated removal. Safety glasses should be available in a box outside the door for visitors not present at the beginning of the procedure.

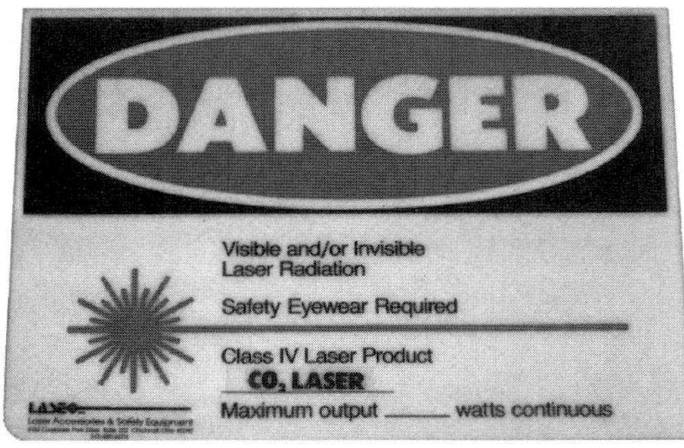

FIG. 5. Approved ANSI laser-safety sign. The specific type, power, and class of the laser must be specified as well as the need for eye protection.

Laser-safety glasses use must also be mandatory when operating waveguides, optical fibers, optical telescopes, and the microscope. Eye injuries from cracked fibers and malfunctioning mechanical shutter filters have been reported. Only when using CO_2 energy are the lenses within the optical telescopes and the microscope sufficient to prevent corneal injury.

The best protection against inadvertent laser hits away from the target area is coordination of laser actuation and standby modes. Any pause in laser activity should be immediately followed by depressing the standby switch. The surgeon must always have an assistant to operate the laser mode and have the standby mode actuated as soon as active lasering is suspended. For example, when working in the oral or nasal cavity, the laser should be in the standby mode as soon as the foot pedal is no longer depressed and prior to removal of the laser handpiece or fiber from the treatment area. Furthermore, when the laser is in the standby mode, confusing the laser foot switch with the foot pedal for the electrocautery or bipolar cautery will not cause any harm.

Skin Protection

Facial skin burns represented the second most frequently reported complication in a survey of otolaryngologists performing laser surgery of the larynx (13). This complication occurs both with inadequately protected skin and when the laser beam is misdirected either by user error or due to specular reflection from a metallic instrument in the surgical field. Use of a double layer of saline-soaked gauze sponges, lap pads, or towels is generally effective for the patient under general anesthesia. However, for office-based laser surgery on an awake patient, these items are seldom used. Therefore, it is crucial that the patient hold perfectly still during the procedure. For example, a rapid head turn during intraoral laser-assisted surgery could result in a facial or lip burn. Careful patient education with a videotaped demonstration of the procedure is quite helpful and reinforces the importance of a team approach.

Laser Plume Biohazard and Need For Universal Precautions

Although stringent regulations concerning eye protection have been established by the various regulatory agencies, little has been written about protection from smoke inhalation during laser use. Increasing concern exists within the medical community that the noxious smoke plume generated by laser surgery may represent a significant health hazard, both to the patient and to operating room personnel. The composition of plume generated during use of the CO_2 laser has been shown to contain particles ranging in size from $0.10\ \mu$ to $0.80\ \mu$. These particles are too small to be effectively filtered by currently available surgical masks. Although there are some commercially available laser masks that claim higher efficiency in filtering 0.1-μ particles, independent studies have shown that some of these masks are no better than standard surgical masks (14).

Several studies have also shown the laser plume to contain numerous gases and hydrocarbons that are toxic, potentially mutagenic, and carcinogenic. Bacteria and viral particles, which have also been isolated, may remain viable for up to 72 hours (15,16). In addition to obscuring the operative field and causing reflection of laser energy, laser smoke can be irritating to the eyes. Inhaled particles from laser plume fall into the size range of "lung-damaging dust" or particles that can travel to the most peripheral parts of the lung parenchyma. Inhalation of laser-generated smoke may cause transient nausea and hypoxia, pulmonary defense mechanism depression, and delayed airway inflammation (17). Repeated long exposures to unfiltered laser plumes could possibly cause or exacerbate existing lung disease or cause the so-called "black lung disease" (18,19). Live viral DNA, including papilloma viruses, hepatitis viruses,

and the human immunodeficiency virus, have been isolated from the airborne contents of the laser plume, and may be infectious (20,21). Therefore, laser plume must be treated as is any body fluid that may contain blood-borne pathogens, and universal precautions should be instituted, which should also be considered when handling and disposing used smoke evacuator filters.

Smoke Evacuation

To minimize the risk of smoke inhalation during laser surgery, adequate smoke evacuation is required at the site of generation, which will prevent the generation of airborne particulate matter and eliminate direct inhalation by either the surgeon, patient, or assistant. Specially designed laser handpieces, nasal specula, laser fiber holders, and metal tongue depressors must all incorporate smoke evacuation channels (Figs. 6 and 7). When one of these instruments is not in use, the smoke evacuator tubing should be connected to a pool tip suction to prevent suction of skin or sponges and held as close to the operative site as possible without interfering with the laser beam. The instruments are connected via tubing to efficient laser smoke evacuators capable of eliminating 99% of all particles in the range of $0.1\ \mu$ (Fig. 8). To maintain high efficiency and prevent malfunction, filters

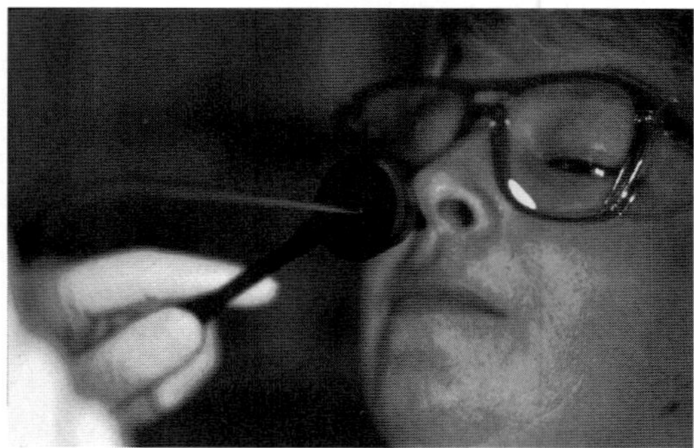

FIG. 6. Use of modified ebonized ear speculum allows both protection of the alar rim and efficient smoke evacuation.

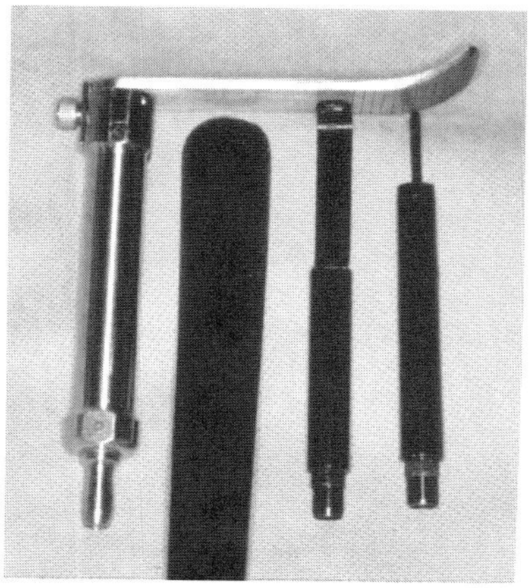

FIG. 7. Ebonized metallic tongue depressor and laser handpieces have separate suction ports to allow instantaneous smoke evacuation.

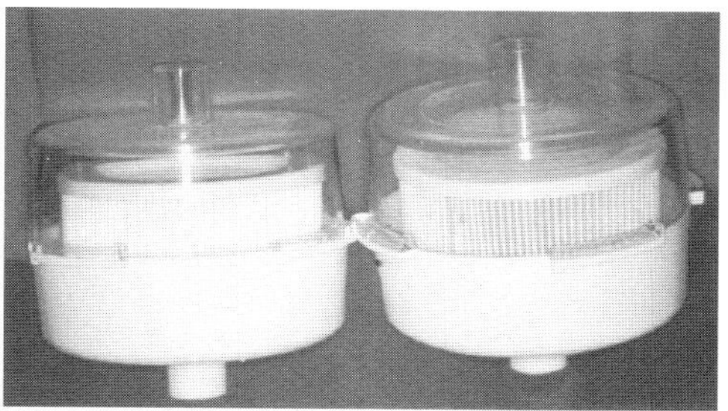

FIG. 9. Example of new and used smoke evacuator replacement filters. Discoloration of the initially white filter will eventually decrease filtration efficiency and must be replaced on a regular basis.

(Fig. 9) must be changed according to each manufacturer's recommendations and blood or secretions must never be suctioned into the smoke evacuator tubing. When operating in the upper airway on an awake patient, the physician should coordinate laser treatment with the patient's breathing so that tissue vaporization takes place while the patient exhales. Such coordination will divert the smoke plume toward the evacuation aperture of the laser instrument and minimize smoke inhalation.

Adequate room ventilation is also essential; room air must be exchanged and filtered according to local standards. Because the laser generates heat, fans and free-standing high-efficiency particulate air (HEPA) cleaners may also be needed in a small treatment room (Fig. 10). Ventilation ducts and vents should be strategically positioned relative to the treatment chair or table to maximize smoke evacuation.

Laser Instrumentation

Laser hits from a reflected beam can cause both skin burns and eye damage. Metallic instruments that appear dull in visible light may act like a mirror when exposed to the far infrared wavelength of the CO_2 laser. Reflected, misdirected laser hits can be avoided by using instrumentation that has a low specular or di-

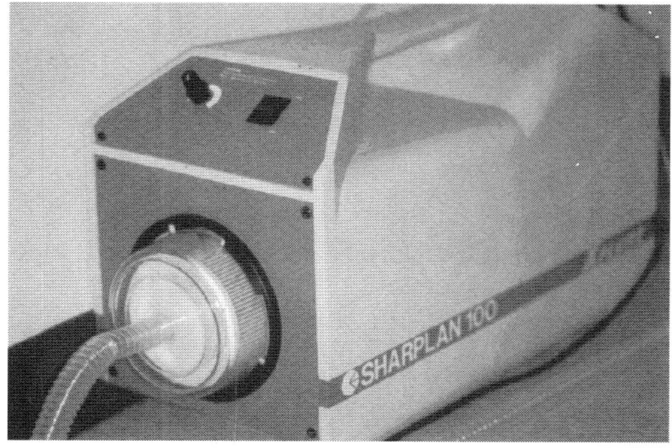

FIG. 8. High-efficiency smoke evacuator.

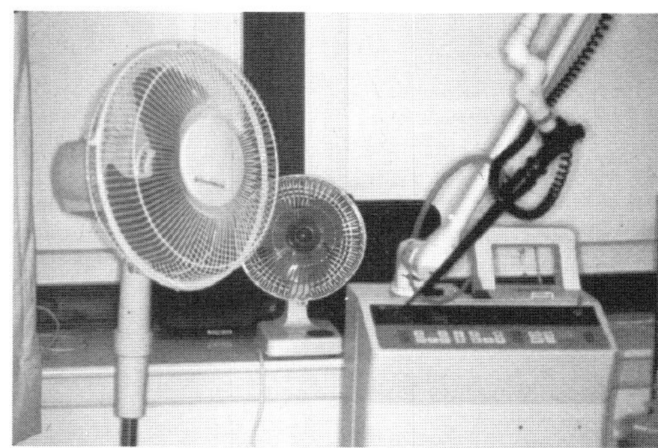

FIG. 10. Strategic placement of fans and/or HEPA cleaners will help direct nonevacuated smoke toward air return vents.

rect reflectance. Laser energy striking this type of instrument will produce a large diffuse or scattered and misdirected laser beam with little risk of tissue injury. Attempts to blacken or ebonize and roughen the surfaces of metallic instruments afford some, but incomplete, protection (22). Ebonized instruments often lose their black coating after several cycles of sterilization and may have no protective benefit over nonebonized instruments (23).

Instruments that are used in the upper airway must have a separate smoke evacuation channel, as discussed, to allow connection to the smoke evacuator. Some laser handpieces have a backstop to prevent laser hits beyond the target once vaporization is complete (Fig. 11). It is essential that continued, prolonged laser exposure of the backstop be avoided as this may cause excessive heating and potentially burn the anesthetized patient. Instruments should be lightweight to facilitate unencumbered movement especially when attached to smoke evacuator tubing (Fig. 12).

The laser has become a well-established surgical tool and little doubt exists of its role in "minimally invasive endoscopic surgery." Future novel applications, such as tissue welding and skin resurfacing, will further solidify its niche in our surgical armamentarium. Ambulatory and, more specifically, office-based laser surgery will continue to increase as pressure from managed care forces physicians and patients to accept their role in lowering the cost of health care in the United States. It is our responsibility as physicians to ensure the safety of both our patients

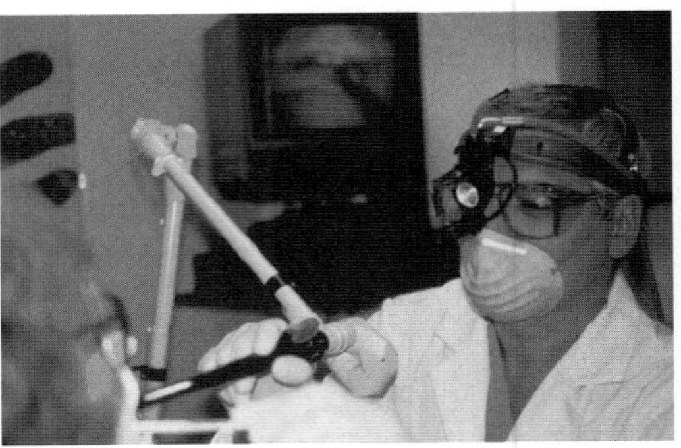

FIG. 12. Example of properly attired surgeon performing laser-assisted uvulopalatoplasty. Note protective eye wear, mask, gloves, and head light. Instrumentation must be lightweight and well balanced as shown here.

and co-workers. Without the protective surveillance formerly provided by the hospital laser-safety committee, it is now more critical than ever that laser-safety guidelines be implemented and monitored in our offices (24). Furthermore, because laser-assisted surgery exposes the patient to a small but added risk of injury compared with traditional techniques, its use must have clear advantages and always be in the best interest of the patient.

The appendix for this chapter provides an up-to-date list of organizations providing further information regarding laser safety in the office environment.

APPENDIX

Sources for Information Concerning Laser Surgery and Safety Issues

1. Laser Institute of America, 12424 Research Parkway, Suite 125, Orlando, FL 32826; Phone: (407) 380–1553; Fax: (407) 380–5588; Courses on Laser Safety, Phone: 1–800–34LASER

2. FDA Center for Devices and Radiological Health, 2098 Gaither Road, Rockville, MD 20850; Phone: (301) 594–4591.

3. Occupational Safety and Health Administration (OSHA) Office of Science and Tech-

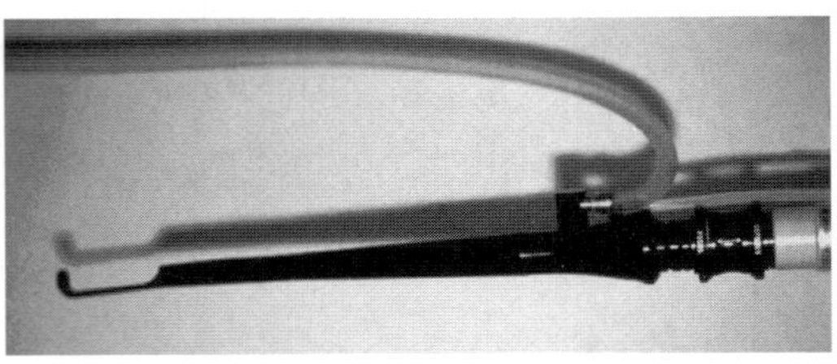

FIG. 11. Laser handpiece used for laser-assisted uvulopalatoplasty. Note presence of backstop and suction channel.

nology Assessment, U.S. Department of Labor, 200 Constitution Avenue, NW, Washington, DC 20210

4. American National Standards Institute (ANSI), 11 West 42nd Street, New York, NY 10036.

5. American College of Surgeons, 55 East Erie Street, Chicago, IL 60611–2797

REFERENCES

1. Schwalow AL, Townes CH: Infrared and optical masers. *Physiol Rev* 112:1940–,1958.
2. Maiman TH: Stimulated optical radiation in ruby. *Nature* 187:493–494, 1960.
3. Steven JL: Laser-tissue interaction. *Surg Clin North Am* 72:531–558, 1992.
4. American College of Surgeons: Guidelines for optimal office-based surgery. ACS, Washington, DC. November 1994.
5. American National Standards Institute: For the safe use of lasers. ANSI Z 136.1, New York, 1980.
6. American National Standards Institute: *Laser safety in the health care environment.* ANSI Z 136.3, New York, 1985.
7. Ossoff RH: Implementing the ANSI Z 136.3 laser safety standard in the medical environment. *Otolaryngol Head Neck Surg* 94:525–528, 1986.
8. Sliney D, Wolbarsht M, eds: *Safety with lasers and other optical sources: A comprehensive handbook.* New York: Plenum Press, 1980.
9. Healy GB, Strong MS, Shapshay S et al: Complications of CO_2 laser surgery of the aerodigestive tract: Experience of 4,416 cases. *Otolaryngol Head Neck Surg* 92:13–18, 1984.
10. Brodmahn M, Port M, Friedman F et al: Operating room personnel morbidity from carbon dioxide laser use during preceptored surgery. *Obstet Gynecol* 81:607–609, 1993.
11. Occupational Safety and Health Administration: Laser hazards. Office of Science and Technology Assessment, Section II, pp. 1–40. U.S. Department of Labor, Washington, DC, 1995.
12. Mohr RM, McDonnell BC, Unger M, Mauer TP: Safety considerations and safety protocol for laser surgery. *Surg Clin North Am* 64:851–859, 1984.
13. Fried MP: A survey of the complications of laser laryngoscopy. *Arch Otolaryngol* 110:31–34, 1984.
14. Kneedler JA, Purcell SK: Face masks as protection from laser plume. *AORN J* 50:520–521, 1989.
15. Winstin C: The effects of smoke plume generated during laser and electrosurgical procedures. *Minim Invasive Surg Nurs* 8:99–102, 1994.
16. McKinley IB, Ludlow MO: Hazards of laser smoke during endodontic therapy. *J Endod* 20:558–559, 1994.
17. Freitag L, Chapman GA, Sielczak M et al: Laser smoke effect on the bronchial system. *Lasers Surg Med* 7:283–288, 1987.
18. Wenig BL, Stenson KM, Wenig BM, Tracey D: Effects of plume produced by the Nd:YAG laser and electrocautery on the respiratory system. *Lasers Surg Med* 13:242–245, 1993.
19. Nezhat C, Winer WK, Nezhat F et al: Smoke from laser surgery: Is there a health hazard? *Lasers Surg Med* 7:376–382, 1987.
20. Garden JM, O'Banion MK, Shelnitz LS et al: Papillomavirus in the vapor of carbon dioxide laser-treated verrucae. *JAMA* 259:1199–1202, 1988.
21. Baggish MS, Poiesz BJ, Joret D: Presence of human immunodeficiency virus DNA in laser smoke. *Lasers Surg Med* 11:197–203, 1991.
22. Wood RL Jr, Sliney DH, Basye RA: Laser reflections from surgical instruments. *Lasers Surg Med* 12:675–678, 1992.
23. Friedman NR, Saleeby ER, Rubin MG et al: Safety parameters for avoiding acute ocular damage from the reflected CO_2 (10.6 µm laser beam). *J Am Acad Dermatol* 17:815–818, 1987.
24. Public Health Service Food and Drug Administration: *Regulations for the administration and enforcement of the radiation control for health and safety act of 1968.* Centers for Devices and Radiological Health (CDRH), Division of the Food and Drug Administration of the U.S. Department of Health, Education, and Welfare, Washington, DC, 1994:514–515.

Office-Based Surgery of the Head and Neck
Edited by Yosef P. Krespi, MD
Lippincott–Raven Publishers, Philadelphia © 1998

2

Sedation and Safety in Office-Based Surgery

Eric M. Kitain and Kurian Thomas

Surgery performed outside the hospital setting has increased significantly over the past several years. Although the driving force behind most of this increase is economic, much of it is patient driven. Patients today are seeking physicians who can perform procedures in their offices, to avoid the hassles, anxiety, and cost of going through a hospital's outpatient facility. Today, with the use of newer anesthetic agents and contemporary monitoring, physicians can safely provide sedation and even general anesthesia to most patients coming for office-based surgery.

This chapter provides the otolaryngologist with the necessary information to safely sedate patients undergoing office procedures.

WHO PROVIDES SEDATION AND MONITORING

Surgeon

Surgeons can safely sedate patients as long as they closely adhere to dosage and administration guidelines and properly monitor use.

Nurse or Physician's Assistant

A nurse or physician's assistant can be an excellent individual to monitor the patient during an office-based procedure. In addition, they play the dual role of surgical assistant, which is extremely important during any office-based surgical procedure. Generally, sedation must still be provided by the surgeon, as Food and Drug Administration regulations may not permit a nurse or physician's assistant to give intravenous sedatives or narcotics.

Anesthesiologist or Nurse Anesthetist

In an ideal setting, an anesthesiologist or nurse anesthetist should provide and monitor sedation. This allows the surgeon to concentrate solely on the surgical procedure and it provides the patient with a trained specialist in the field of sedation and monitoring. The increase in cost of an anesthesiologist can be offset by earlier discharge, fewer complications, and, most importantly, peace of mind for the otolaryngologist. Most insurance carriers allow for anesthesia costs and, in the case of cosmetic surgery, predetermined payment schedules let the patient know about these costs prior to surgery.

PATIENT SELECTION

The selection of appropriate patients will limit unanticipated complications and avoid emergency hospital admissions.

Age

The acceptability of very old and very young patients for outpatient surgical procedures is well documented (1,2). The factors that determine the acceptability of a geriatric patient for outpatient surgery are physiologic age, physical status, surgical procedure, level of anesthesia required, and quality of care available at home. Although infants can be safely operated on in an office-based practice, it is conservatively advisable to avoid procedures on premature infants who are younger than 60 weeks postconceptual age because postoperative apnea for 12–24 hours has been reported in this group of patients.

Medical Contraindications to Outpatient Surgical Procedures

The list below is a brief overview and guide to patients in which outpatient surgery is contraindicated; it does not replace a physician's medical judgment (1,2).

1. Any infant with a history of respiratory distress syndrome, who was intubated on ventilatory support, should have this surgery postponed until at least 6 months of age.
2. Any infant whose sibling has died of sudden infant death syndrome should not be operated on until 1 year of age.
3. Patients who have a history of malignant hyperthermia or who are susceptible to malignant hyperthermia.
4. Patients with a history of uncontrolled seizure activity.
5. Morbidly obese patients with other systemic diseases.
6. Any patient considered medically unstable.
7. Patients being treated with monoamine oxidase inhibitors.
8. Any patient giving a history of acute substance abuse.

EQUIPMENT

Oxygen and Nitrous Oxide Tanks

Oxygen tanks are generally supplied in two different cylinder sizes (2). The standard E cylinder, found on the back of most anesthesia machines, has an internal volume of 5 L and when full has an internal pressure of 1900 pounds per square inch gauge. A full E cylinder can deliver 660 L of gaseous oxygen at standard temperature and pressure (STP). The pressure in the tank directly reflects the

amount of gaseous oxygen remaining so that when the pressure gauge reads 1000 psig (pounds per square inch guage), the tank is (1000/1900) or 52% full and will provide only (660 × 52%) 340 L of oxygen. If space is available we recommend using the larger H cylinder. A full H cylinder (2200 psig) will deliver 6900 L of oxygen at STP.

Nitrous oxide also comes in both E and H cylinder sizes (2). An E cylinder will deliver 1590 L of nitrous oxide, whereas an H cylinder can provide 15,800 L. It is important to understand that nitrous oxide resides as a liquid within the cylinder at a pressure of 745 psig. As long as there is liquid nitrous oxide in the tank, the pressure will not change. Only when all of the liquid nitrous oxide in the tank has been used up and the tank contains only gaseous nitrous oxide will the pressure begin to fall.

Monitoring Equipment

Appropriate monitoring is the most important aspect of providing safe sedation for office-based surgery. Following is a list of monitors; some are routine for all procedures (denoted by *) and others are optional depending on the type of surgery performed.

*Pulse Oximetry**

Pulse oximetry has become the mainstay of patient monitoring because it provides continuous, real-time estimates of pulse rate and arterial hemoglobin saturation. The pulse oximeter will alert to hypoxemia from various causes, including apnea, loss of airway patency, or loss of oxygen supply. It is important to understand that pulse oximeters, placed on a finger, take measurements from the blood flowing to the extremity. Therefore, if there is inadequate circulation, either centrally or locally, to the extremity, pulse oximetry measurements may be erroneous. Anesthesiologists usually set the low alarm limits of oxygen saturation at 90% because the steep drop on the oxyhemoglobin dissociation curve begins at this point. It is advisable to set this limit somewhat higher, at 92% to 94%, when working alone.

ECG Monitoring

Electrocardiographic (ECG) monitoring is used to recognize arrhythmias and diagnose myocardial ischemia. For office-based surgery, this discussion is confined to cardiac arrhythmias. While pulse oximeters alert to significant changes in the heart rate, they do not aid in the interpretation of these changes. Both sinus bradycardia and heart block bradycardia appear similar on the pulse oximeter and can only be distinguished using electrocardiography. A three-lead system is all that is necessary for most ECG office monitoring, whereas a five-lead system is more appropriate for ischemia monitoring. We highly recommend the use of ECG monitoring for all procedures; however, pulse oximetry may suffice for many minor procedures.

Blood Pressure: Automatic versus Manual

For other than minor procedures, we recommend monitoring blood pressure. Vasocontrictors placed in the nasal passages can have profound effects on blood pressure. Automatic blood pressure cuffs are convenient, accurate, and reproducible when properly applied. Time intervals can be manually adjusted. We recommend setting the maximal time interval for taking blood pressure readings at 5 minutes. Manual blood pressure cuffs are inexpensive, but they require additional personnel and have been shown to be less accurate than the automated cuffs.

Capnography

Capnography, which measures end-tidal carbon dioxide ($etCO_2$) in exhaled gases, is especially useful during general endotracheal anesthesia; it is also desirable for patients who have been given significant sedation with hyp-

notics and narcotics. Capnography will alert the physician earlier than pulse oximetry to airway obstructions or apnea because it measures $etCO_2$ from each breath, whereas blood oxygen saturation will fall only after lung reserves are depleted.

Oxygen Analyzer

Oxygen analyzers should be used for cases wherein nitrous oxide is involved. Using nitrous oxide and oxygen mixtures can lead to low oxygen concentrations—below that of room air (21% oxygen).

Safety Equipment

The following equipment should be immediately available for all procedures no matter how minor. Medical emergencies occur even in the most controlled situations and not being prepared is tantamount to medical malpractice.

Ambu-Bag

An ambu-bag is essential for airway management. Most disposable ambu-bags come with their own mask and oxygen tubing.

Intubating Equipment: Basics

Among the basic intubating equipment is a laryngoscope with either Macintosh or Miller 3 and 4 blades. Add Miller 2 blade for pediatric patients. Also required are endotracheal tubes: sizes 6, 6.5, 7, and 7.5 should be available. For pediatric patients, add 4, 4.5, 5, and 5.5 cuffed or uncuffed tubes. The general rule of thumb for tube size in children is (4+age/4).

Laryngeal Mask Airway

The laryngeal mask airway (LMA) is ideal for securing the airway without intubating patients who have upper airway obstruction. The

LMA has not been shown to prevent aspiration of gastric contents. Skill in using this device can be acquired during advanced cardiac life support certification.

Emergency Cricothyroidotomy Set

Working around the head and neck can lead to airway obstruction where ventilation by ambu-bag is inadequate and intubation nearly impossible. A cricothyroidotomy set is inexpensive insurance and highly recommended.

Cardiac Resuscitation

A defibrillator is recommended. Working around the head and neck can lead to significant cardiac dysrhythmias. Drugs such as epinephrine, atropine, and lidocaine should be readily available. Certification in advanced cardiac life support is recommended for the appropriate use of cardiac resuscitative drugs.

DRUGS

The ideal agent for outpatient surgery should be capable of producing a rapid and smooth onset of action, adequate analgesia and amnesia, good surgical conditions, and a short recovery period with minimal or no side effects (3). In addition, the agent should be flexible enough for use in surgical procedures of varying duration. No single agent is available today that meets these demands; therefore, a combination of drugs is required to produce the desired effect. The drugs that can provide conscious sedation and optimal operating conditions in an office-based surgical practice are discussed below.

Sedatives and Amnestics

Benzodiazepines

Benzodiazepines, because of their rapid onset and short duration of action, have virtually replaced barbiturates as the drugs of choice for sedation. The favorable pharmacologic characteristics of benzodiazepines include:

1. Production of anterograde amnesia
2. Anxiolysis
3. Sedation
4. Minimal depression of respiratory and cardiovascular function
5. Elevation of seizure threshold
6. Centrally mediated muscle relaxation
7. Relative safety if taken in overdose

Benzodiazepine receptors occur almost exclusively on postsynaptic nerve endings in the central nervous system. Benzodiazepines enhance the chloride channel gating function of gamma-aminobutyric acid by facilitating the binding of this inhibitory neurotransmitter to its receptors (4). The resulting enhanced opening of chloride channels leads to hyperpolarization of cell membranes, which makes them more resistant to neuronal excitation.

Adverse Effects

Adverse effects include ventilatory depression, particularly after rapid intravenous administration or when combined with narcotics; residual drowsiness; impairment of mental function; dysarthria; ataxia; muscle weakness; and nausea and vomiting.

Diazepam (Valium)

Until recently, the parenteral form of diazepam was available in a solution of organic solvents, which caused severe pain from both intramuscular (IM) or intravenous (IV) injections. The recent introduction, in the United States, of diazepam in aqueous solution has helped to overcome this problem. Diazepam is a highly lipid soluble with a large volume of distribution. The drug is primarily metabolized by hepatic microsomal enzymes. The two principal metabolites of diazepam are desmethyldiazepam and oxazepam; they are active metabolites that may be responsible for the prolonged sedative effects of diazepam. It is likely that desmethyldiazepam contributes to the return of drowsiness that manifests 6–8 hours after the administration of diazepam. The elimination half-life of diazepam is variable and increases progressively with increasing age. Cirrhosis of the liver can increase the elimination half-life by as much as five times. Diazepam, rapidly absorbed from the gastrointestinal tract after oral administration, reaches peak concentration in about 1 hour in adults and as quickly as 15–30 minutes in children.

Dosage and Administration

Most patients may be given an oral dose of diazepam (0.1–0.2 mg/kg) (10 mg in most adults) on the morning of surgery. However, this may prolong the postprocedure recovery time. The aqueous injectable form can be used prior to the procedure in a dose range of 0.1–0.2 mg/kg. Titrating small doses until the patient has slurred speech is another method that produces desirable sedation and amnesia. The dose should be reduced by 50% in elderly patients. Due to its long half-life, diazepam may not be the ideal injectable agent for a busy office-based practice.

Recommendations

Diazepam usage should be limited to oral premedication because of its long-acting effects. Occasionally, however, it is desirable to have sedation well into the postoperative period, in which case diazepam may be appropriate.

Midazolam

Midazolam, available in water-soluble form, is two to three times more potent than diazepam. Compared with diazepam, midazolam produces a more rapid onset with greater amnesia and less postoperative sedation. The metabolites have pharmacologic activity, although prolonged sedative effects are uncommon.

Dosage and Administration

For sedation and anterograde amnesia, a dose range of 0.035–0.1 mg/kg IM or IV, should be given. As with diazepam, titrating small doses until the patient has slurred speech should provide ideal sedation and amnesia. Dosages in elderly patients should be reduced to a maximum of 2.5 mg.

Recommendations

Midazolam is an excellent sedative/amnestic. It is highly recommended for both IM and IV use. Intravenously, it should be administered slowly (1–2 mg at a time), as the onset of its clinical effects may be delayed. There is a danger of oversedation if midazolam is given rapidly, not allowing enough time to assess its effects.

Lorazepam (Ativan)

Lorazepam is a more potent amnestic than diazepam. Although formulated in organic solvents, there is minimal pain on injection. It is reliably absorbed after oral or IM injection and can be given intravenously. The drug has a very slow onset and prolonged duration of action.

Dosage and Administration

The recommended oral or IM dose of lorazepam for preoperative medication is 50 µg/kg, not to exceed 4 mg. Intravenously, 1–2 mg is all that is required for good sedation and amnesia.

Recommendations

Lorazepam may be difficult to titrate IV because of its slow onset and prolonged duration of amnesia and sedation. We discourage the use of lorazepam in office-based procedures where rapid awakening at the end of surgery is desirable.

Hypnotics

Propofol (Diprivan)

Propofol is a phenol derivative that has been commercially available for IV use since 1986. Propofol is one of the most versatile infusion agents in practice today. It is used for mild sedation as well as general anesthesia (3). Its popularity stems from its versatility, rapid onset, prompt recovery, minimal nausea and vomiting, and excellent patient satisfaction. Propofol is currently available as a 1% solution in an aqueous solution of 10% soybean oil, 2.25% glycerol, and 1.2% purified egg phosphatide (4). The medium for propofol now contains antibacterial preservatives; however, we still emphasize the importance of maintaining aseptic technique and discarding unused drug at the conclusion of each case.

Propofol is rapidly distributed after IV injection, and blood concentrations decline rapidly. Clearance of propofol from the plasma exceeds hepatic blood flow. The efficient clearance of propofol from the plasma, as well as the elimination half-time of 0.5–1.5 hours, minimizes the likelihood of cumulative drug effects.

Dosage and Administration

In healthy adults, a continuous infusion of 30–100 µg/kg/min provides excellent sedation. Higher infusion rates will cause loss of airway reflexes and should be avoided. The infusion rate should be reduced with the concomitant administration of an opioid. Maintaining verbal contact with the patient is essential to avoid oversedation and apnea. If an infusion pump is not available, incremental bolus doses of 10–30 mg can be administered as required.

Adverse Effects

Hypotension may occur in hypovolemic or elderly patients or in patients with impaired left ventricular function. Slow incremental titration of propofol infusion should minimize this complication. Respiratory depression can occur with rapid bolus injections or with the concomitant use of opioids. In our experience, if bolus injections are kept <30 mg apnea is unlikely to occur. Pain on IV injection occurs in about 40% of patients. Patient discomfort can be reduced by using a large vein, high flow rate, or administration of a small dose (20–30 mg) of lidocaine shortly before the administration of propofol. Lidocaine can also be mixed with propofol in the same syringe. Excitatory phenomena, such as hypertonus, tremor, or hiccoughs, can occur, although the incidence is very low. Allergic reactions, although extremely rare, may occur in those patients who are allergic to egg protein.

Recommendations

We highly recommend the use of propofol whenever there is someone designated to monitor the patient. Apnea and hypotension are minimized when propofol is administered by an infusion pump with slow incremental increases in the infusion rate. Propofol can be used as the sole anesthetic agent, but we recommend combining it with a benzodiazepine and an opioid. Remember, start with lower infusion rates when concomitantly administering other agents.

Ketamine

Ketamine is a phencyclidine derivative introduced in 1965. It is available as a solution containing 10 mg/mL for IV use or 50 mg/mL for IM injection. Ketamine produces a dissociative state in which the eyes remain open with a slow nystagmic gaze. The patient is often noncommunicative, although appearing awake. Ketamine provides excellent amnesia and analgesia while not depressing respiratory function or blood pressure (3,5).

Ketamine has a rapid onset of action and a relatively short duration. It is a highly lipid soluble and not significantly bound to plasma proteins. Peak plasma levels occur within 1 minute following IV injection and within 5 minutes following IM injection. Ketamine is metabolized extensively by the liver. The elimination half-life of ketamine is 1–2 hours. The metabolite norketamine is pharmacologically active and may contribute to prolonged effects.

Dosage and Administration

A single dose of 0.25–0.5 mg/kg IV or an infusion of 50 µg/kg/min may be used to produce intense analgesia without loss of consciousness while maintaining spontaneous ventilation and airway reflexes. If an IM injection is preferred, we recommend using 3–5 mg/kg, which should also produce profound analgesia. Ketamine causes significant salivation, which, besides being problematic for intraoral procedures, can stimulate coughing and laryngospasm. For this reason it is highly recommended to administer an antisialogue, such as glycopyrrolate, in conjunction with ketamine.

Adverse Effects

Emergence delirium, nightmares, and hallucinations have all been associated with ketamine. Factors associated with these emergence phenomena are female gender, age >16, dosage >2 mg/kg IV, and history of personality problems or frequent dreaming. The incidence of emergence phenomena can be minimized by pretreating with a benzodiazepine. Because ketamine stimulates the sympathetic nervous system, hypertension and tachycardia are very common. This may be harmful in patients with existing hypertension, pulmonary hypertension, or ischemic heart disease.

Recommendations

The occasional prolonged recovery period, profound salivation, and emergence phenomena make ketamine a second choice for many office ear, nose, and throat (ENT) procedures.

However, smaller doses of ketamine in conjunction with benzodiazepines and opioids have been used with excellent results in busy outpatient practices.

Opioids

Opioid is an inclusive term that describes all drugs (natural or synthetic) that bind to opioid receptors. Many different classes of opioid receptors are available, and the actions and side effects of various opioids differ depending on the class of receptor on which they act. The drugs that are useful for outpatient surgical procedures include morphine, meperidine (Demerol), fentanyl, and alfentanil. The initial distribution of opioids is related to the degree of drug ionization in the blood and to the lipid solubility of the un-ionized portion. The more lipid soluble the drug, the faster its onset and the shorter its duration of action (3,6). For instance, alfentanil has effects within 2–3 minutes and they last only 30 minutes.

Narcotics are most effective when given prior to a painful stimulus. To blunt existing pain, the patient must be given either larger doses of narcotics or the narcotics must be supplemented with other medications, such as nonsteroidal anti-inflammatory drugs (NSAIDs) or sedatives. We recommend NSAIDs as adjunctive medications because they provide superior pain relief and are devoid of sedative or ventilatory depressive effects.

The following must be taken into consideration when selecting an opioid and its proper dosage to minimize the risk of postoperative ventilatory depression.

1. Anticipated duration of action of the opioid should match the duration of the surgical procedure.
2. Increased sensitivity to opioids in the elderly and in patients with chronic obstructive pulmonary disease, hypothyroidism, and obesity should be considered.
3. Increased sensitivity to opioids in patients with chronic infection, cirrhosis, malignancy, and debility should be considered.

Adverse Effects

Dose-dependent respiratory depression may occur. With fentanyl, there can be a biphasic depression of ventilation, but it is uncommon if doses <150 μg are given. Most of the narcotics have minimal effect on blood pressure and heart rate; however, orthostatic hypotension does occur, most commonly with meperidine or morphine. Dysphoria, rather than euphoria, may occur when opioids are given to patients not experiencing pain. Some patients experience nausea and vomiting. Miosis is commonly seen except with meperidine, which can cause mydriasis. Some have decreased peristalsis and increased contraction of the smooth muscles of the sphincters of Oddi, the ureter, and the bladder. Histamine release may occur with morphine and meperidine. Skeletal muscle rigidity may occur with high doses, especially with fentanyl. Convulsions have been reported with high doses, particularly with meperidine. Hypertensive crisis may occur in patients on monoamine oxidase inhibitors with meperidine.

Morphine

Although morphine has a number of undesirable side effects, such as histamine release and nausea, it is an excellent analgesic and remains the mainstay for postoperative intravenous analgesia. Although it is effective against pain of any origin, it is more effective against dull continuous pain than sharp intermittent pain. The pain threshold is elevated and the physiologic and emotional components of pain are diminished.

Pharmacokinetics

Morphine is well absorbed following IM administration, with peak effects in 45–90 minutes and a duration of action of about 4 hours. After an IV dose, the onset is within 5 minutes and the peak effect is within 20 minutes. Metabolism occurs predominantly in the liver. One of the metabolites, morphine-6-glucuronide, is pharmacologically active. Consequently, clinical effects of morphine may exceed that expected, particularly in patients with impaired renal function.

Dosage and Administration

In a healthy adult, we recommend giving 2–5 mg IV bolus doses at 20-minute intervals while monitoring the patient's respiratory rate. If the respiratory rate falls below 10 breaths per minute additional boluses could cause the patient to become apneic.

Recommendations

Although morphine can be used for any surgical procedure, it should be used judiciously intraoperatively because side effects are common within the analgesic dose range. It is an excellent drug for postoperative pain management because of its euphoric and sedative effects.

Meperidine (Demerol)

Meperidine is a synthetic opioid with analgesic potency one tenth that of morphine. It produces sedation but little euphoria. The drug has mild atropinelike qualities and is commonly associated with orthostatic hypotension.

Pharmacokinetics

Meperidine is more lipid soluble than morphine; consequently it has a faster onset and shorter duration of action. The drug is extensively metabolized by the liver. One of the metabolites, normeperidine, is pharmacologically active and possesses twice the convulsive properties of meperidine with half the analgesic effect.

Dosage and Administration

Meperidine can be used in dosages of 25–50 mg IV or 100–150 mg IM.

Recommendations

We do not recommend meperidine for intraoperative use, but find it very useful for postoperative analgesia. Orthostatic hypotension is more of a concern with meperidine than with the other opioids.

Fentanyl

Fentanyl is a synthetic opioid with analgesic potency approximately 100 times that of morphine. Fentanyl is one of the two most commonly used opioids in outpatient surgical procedures because of its greater potency, more rapid onset, shorter duration of action, and minimal side effects compared with morphine. It can produce skeletal muscle rigidity, but only rarely in the dose range used for outpatient procedures.

Pharmacokinetics

Fentanyl is extremely lipid soluble and has a rapid onset and short duration of action. After a single IV dose, onset is within 1–2 minutes and the duration of action is only 20–30 minutes.

Dosage and Administration

Fentanyl comes as 50 μg/mL and is supplied in ampules of 2 or 5 mL. For most procedures analgesia can be achieved with bolus doses of 1–2 μg/kg or 50–100 μg IV that can be repeated as necessary.

Recommendations

Fentanyl is an excellent choice for intraoperative analgesia. As with all the opioids, it is best to administer it prior to a noxious stimulus, titrating the dose to respiratory rate. Supplementing narcotics with a sedative, such as midazolam, is common, but it increases the potential for respiratory and circulatory depression. We do not recommend using fentanyl for postoperative pain management because of its shorter duration of action and higher incidence of respiratory depression.

Alfentanil

Alfentanil is a synthetic derivative of fentanyl and is the most commonly used opioid for short surgical procedures. Its analgesic potency is approximately one tenth that of fentanyl, but it comes as 500 μg/mL, which is 10 times the concentration of fentanyl. It, too, is supplied in ampules of 2 or 5 mL. In this respect, equivalent volumes of both alfentanil and fentanyl would be used for analgesia.

Pharmacokinetics

Although alfentanil is less lipid soluble than fentanyl, it has a faster onset because of its low pKa. After a single IV dose, the onset is within 1 minute and the duration of action is <15 minutes. Unlike other opioids, repeated doses or a continuous infusion of alfentanil does not result in significant cumulative effects, which eases any concerns of possible postoperative ventilatory depression, even after prolonged infusions of the drug.

Dosage and Administration

Alfentanil can be given as intermittent boluses or as a continuous infusion. An initial bolus of 5–10 μg/kg, or 250–500 μg, can be followed by boluses of 3–5 μg/kg every 10–15 minutes as needed. Infusions are generally begun at a rate of 0.5 μg/kg/min and incrementally increased by 0.25 μg/kg/min.

Recommendations

We strongly recommend the use of alfentanil for intraoperative pain control as its rapid onset and metabolism make it ideally suited for outpatient surgical procedures. Although it is most suitable as a continuous infusion, it is also quite amenable to intermittent boluses. This, however, may require a dedicated individual because of the frequent dosing regimen.

Local Anesthetics

Local anesthetics produce reversible conduction blockade of impulses along the nerves. Adequate infiltration of local anesthesia at the operative site is essential to prevent patient discomfort. Many agents have been developed since the introduction of cocaine as the first local anesthetic in 1884.

Local anesthetics are classified as aminoesters or aminoamides based on their structure (3,4). The aminoester used in ENT procedures is cocaine; the aminoamides are mainly lidocaine and bupivacaine.

The amount of local anesthetic that reaches a nerve depends to a large extent on the proximity of injection, the intervening connective and adipose tissue, the pKa, and the concentration of the local anesthetic and its lipid solubility. Absorption of local anesthetic from the injection site into the central circulation is influenced by the injection site (areas of high blood flow have more rapid absorption), dosage, vasoconstrictor use, and drug pharmacologic characteristics. The local anesthetic's systemic absorption rate thus influences both its neural blockade duration and its toxicity. The aminoesters are rapidly cleared from the plasma by plasma cholinesterases. The aminoamides are metabolized by the liver.

Local Anesthetic Toxicity

Allergic Reactions

The ester class of local anesthetics is more allergenic than are the amides because of its relationship to p-aminobenzoic acid. Prior exposure to paraben, which is present in many foods and cosmetics, may sensitize patients. The subsequent administration of local anesthetic solutions containing these materials may lead to an allergic reaction unrelated to the local anesthetic.

Systemic Toxicity

Toxic reactions, which most frequently occur from accidental intravascular injection, can be secondary to systemic absorption. Both mechanisms produce a concentration-dependent effect on the brain and heart; the difference is the time onset of symptoms. Central nervous system toxicity manifests as numbness of the tongue, circumoral paresthesia, and lightheadedness. It progresses to visual disturbances, muscular twitching, unconsciousness, convulsions, and coma if not recognized and treated immediately with benzodiazepines or barbiturates. The cardiovascular system is more resistant to the toxic effects of local anesthetics. Cardiac toxicity results from blockade of the cardiac sodium channels by the local anesthetic, which may manifest as bradycardia, hypotension, or cardiac arrest. Bupivacaine is much more cardiotoxic than the other local anesthetics; an accidental intravascular injection may result in precipitous hypotension, cardiac dysrhythmias, or atrioventricular block. Cardiovascular toxicity is often resistant to treatment despite administration of large doses of epinephrine, atropine, and bretylium.

Cocaine

Cocaine has enjoyed immense popularity among ENT surgeons because it combines local anesthesia with intense vasoconstriction. Its use has declined in recent years because of its side effects, abuse potential, and availability of better alternatives. Substantial absorption of cocaine occurs from the upper respiratory tract within minutes of application with peak plasma concentrations occurring within 30–60 minutes. Cocaine has a biologic half-life of 0.5–1.5 hours (7). In addition to metabolism by plasma cholinesterases, cocaine undergoes oxidative metabolism by the liver.

Cocaine is available as 4% or 10% solutions for topical application or as a nasal spray.

Complications and Toxicity

Cocaine produces intense sympathetic nervous system stimulation. Cardiac arrhythmias are common; myocardial work and oxygen consumption are increased, which may lead to ischemia or infarction. Cocaine toxicity may lead to sudden death. Severe reactions are characterized by unpredictability and rapidity of onset, which may manifest as seizures, cardiac arrhythmias, or cardiorespiratory collapse. Cardiovascular toxicity may be treated with esmolol, and seizures may respond to benzodiazepines.

Recommendations

We recommend giving a benzodiazepine prior to using cocaine because it will blunt the sympathetic response and raise the seizure threshold. The use of cocaine in hypertensive patients and in patients with known cardiovascular disease should be avoided.

Lidocaine

Lidocaine, one of the most commonly used agents in practice today, is an amide local anesthetic. The addition of epinephrine prolongs its duration, allows increased dosage, decreases systemic absorption, and provides the necessary vasoconstriction often needed for ENT surgery. Epinephrine, because it in-

TABLE 1. *Comparative Pharmacology of Local Anesthetics for Infiltration Anesthesia*

Drug	Onset	Duration of Action (min)	Maximum Single Dose (mg/kg)
Cocaine	Fast	20–30	2 (topical)
Lidocaine	Fast	60–90	4–5
Lidocaine with epinephrine	Fast	120–360	7–8
Bupivacaine	Slow	120–240	3

creases blood pressure and heart rate, should be used cautiously in patients with hypertension or coronary artery disease. To prevent central nervous system toxicity, it is advisable to stay within the dosing guidelines as outlined in Table 1.

Bupivacaine

Bupivacaine is an amide local anesthetic with a long duration of action. The addition of epinephrine does not significantly prolong the duration of bupivacaine. Keeping within the dosing guidelines, as listed in Table 1, should prevent the cardiotoxicity associated with this drug.

Reversal Agents

Even the most cautious physician can overestimate a patient's need for narcotics or sedatives. Fortunately, there are new agents available today that can readily reverse the effects of sedatives as well as narcotics. We highly recommend having these drugs immediately available whenever sedatives or narcotics are utilized.

Naloxone

Naloxone is the classic narcotic reversal agent. It is provided in 1-mL ampules containing 0.4 mg. Naloxone, 1–4 µg/kg IV, will promptly reverse the opioid-induced depression of ventilation and analgesia. The lower dose range may preserve some analgesia while reversing ventilatory depression. We recommend diluting an ampule into a 10-mL syringe with normal saline and giving it in 2-mL aliquots until the desired effect is achieved, which may prevent the undesirable sympathetic response that often accompanies opioid reversal. It is also noteworthy that reversal of opioids is associated with nausea and vomiting in approximately 20% of patients. Naloxone, given as an IV bolus, only lasts 30–45 minutes, and may require supplemental doses for sustained antagonism. A naloxone infusion at a rate of 5 μg/kg/h can be used to prevent renarcotization.

Nalmefene

Nalmefene is the first long-lasting injectable opioid antagonist. Its approximate 8-hour duration of action should outlast any residual narcotic effect and, therefore, allow earlier patient discharge. Nalmefene is supplied in ampules containing 1 mL at a concentration of 100 μg/mL. It should be titrated in 0.25-μg/kg doses IV and given every 2–5 minutes until the desired degree of reversal is achieved to a maximal dose of 1.0 μg/kg. Using it in this manner may effectively reverse ventilatory depression while maintaining reasonable analgesia. As with naloxone, sympathetic stimulation and nausea and vomiting are common side effects. In patients with significant cardiovascular disease, the recommended titration dose should be decreased to 0.1 μg/kg.

Flumazenil

Flumazenil, an imidazobenzodiazepine, is a specific and exclusive benzodiazepine antagonist. It will reverse, in a dose-related manner, all the agonist effects of benzodiazepines. This antagonism is not followed by acute anxiety, hypertension, tachycardia, or increased pain. It is supplied in vials of 5 mL at a concentration of 0.5 mg/mL. The IV administration of incremental dosages of 0.2 mg to a maximum of 1 mg is usually sufficient to abolish the effects of therapeutic doses of benzodiazepines within 1–2 minutes. The duration of antagonism may last only 1–2 hours and, therefore, may need to be repeated if prolonged sedation is expected.

REFERENCES

1. Barash PG, Cullen BF, Stoelting RK: *Clinical anesthesia*, 2nd ed. Philadelphia: JB Lippincott, 1992.
2. Miller RD, ed: *Anesthesia*, 3rd ed. New York: Churchill Livingstone, 1990.
3. Stoelting RK: *Pharmacology and physiology in anesthetic practice*, 2nd ed. Philadelphia: JB Lippincott, 1991.
4. Gilman AG, Rall RW, Nies AS, Taylor P: *The pharmacological basis of therapeutics*, 8th ed. New York: McGraw-Hill, 1993.
5. Aitkenhead AR, Smith G, eds: *Textbook of anesthesia*, 2nd ed. New York: Churchill Livingstone, 1990.
6. Estafanous FG: *Opioids in anesthesia* II. Butterworth-Heinemann, 1991.
7. Barash PG, Fleming JM: *Cocaine: Therapeutic uses and problems anesthetizing the abuser*. ASA Annual Refresher Course Lectures, 1991.

Office-Based Surgery of the Head and Neck
Edited by Yosef P. Krespi, MD
Lippincott–Raven Publishers, Philadelphia © 1998

3

Instrumentation for Office Laser Surgery

Michael Slaktine

With more than 2000 lasers currently being used in an office environment in North America to treat snoring, transportable carbon dioxide (CO_2) lasers have already fostered significant surgical advances in ear, nose, and throat (ENT) ambulatory health care (1–4). The ability to treat a multitude of nasal, pharyngeal, laryngeal, and oral disorders within minutes with the same equipment keeps the laser almost constantly busy in ENT clinics. Moreover, the same equipment is now widely used in hundreds of clinics to perform important aesthetic and plastic surgical procedures with only local anesthesia. The most popular applications are skin resurfacing (5–7) and hair transplantation (8). Two novel and unique features previously unavailable with CO_2 lasers have revolutionized the position of these lasers in the office:

1. The ability to instantly switch the laser from a high-precision 100-µm incision mode to a mode that can achieve layer-by-layer char-free vaporization of large surface areas without damaging subjacent tissue even at low-power levels. This ability was achieved by computerized flashscan technology, which has added an unprecedented degree of control and simplicity of laser surgical procedures.
2. The ability to transmit the superpulse mode through thin optical waveguides to induce char-free ablation in deep and narrow nasal subcutaneous and other cavities.

We review the operating principles and tissue effects generated by surgical accessories optimally designed to perform ENT and aesthetic procedures in an office setting with a CO_2 laser. We also list the peripheral accessories necessary for each procedure (Table 1).

Both neodymium:yttrium aluminum garnet (Nd:YAG and diode) lasers have important clinical benefits in performing nasal procedures in an ambulatory setting. They provide a simple and excellent way to shrink hypertrophic turbinates using only local anesthesia and to control endoscopically control epistaxis. We devote a brief section of this chapter to describe Nd:YAG and diode laser instrumentation used in nasal procedures.

INSTRUMENTATION FOR ENT OFFICE SURGERY WITH A CO$_2$ LASER

Laser-Assisted Uvulopalatoplasty

Laser-assisted uvulopalatoplasty (LAUP) is performed in three to five stages in the office with a CO_2 laser, using two different laser modalities (1–4): incision or vaporization to create inverted U-shaped trenches in the soft palate, and char-free vaporization of the uvula from the bottom (fish-mouth technique). The uvula is reshaped to produce a new uvula in each stage without noticeable bleeding and with minimal thermal damage (Fig. 1). These operating modalities are available with a 220-mm focal length oral-pharyngeal handpiece and a SwiftLase flashscanner (Fig. 2) integrally attached to the handpiece. The focusing lens can be slid with the thumb to a defocus position necessary for coagulation. The autoclavable oral-pharyngeal handpiece incorporates a detachable protective

TABLE 1. *Equipment Necessary for the Performance of Multiple Ear, Nose, and Throat Procedures in an Office Setting With a CO_2 Laser*

Procedure	Surgical Accessories	Laser Power Setting
LAUP	22-mm oral-pharyngeal handpiece with SwiftLase attachment and smoke evacuation channel Laser tongue depressor with smoke evacuation channel	18 W for soft palate fine incision, focused beam 18 W for char-free ablation of the uvula bottom and inverted U shape trenching of soft palate with the SwiftLase mode
Tonsil cryptolysis Lingual tonsils	Oral-pharyngeal handpiece with extended 90° and 120° folding mirrors	15 W char-free ablation SwiftLase mode
Reduction of hypertrophic turbinates Postoperative adhesions	1-mm-diameter optical hollow waveguides, curved and straight shapes with suction channel Laser coupler Sinoscope or headlight illuminator	8 W superpulse
Laryngeal lesions	FlexiLase fiber—endoscope protection Flexible endoscope Endoscopic anesthetic delivery unit	15 W superpulse

Oral
  Periodontal diseases
  Gingivectomy
  Salivary gland pathologies
  Leukoplakia
  Hairy tongue
  Mucous cysts
	125-mm focusing handpiece
	Straight and curved 1-mm hollow waveguides
	SwiftLase, F = 125 mm
	Laser tongue depressor
		5 to 15 W
		5 to 15 W

Basic equipment: transportable CO_2 laser, TEM_{oo} 1 to 30 W with superpulse mode capability; smoke evacuator, 54 L/min; protective eyeglasses.

Additional applications of office laser in operating room setting: stapedectomy with 300-mm micromanipulator and microscope; laryngology (vocal cords) with 400-mm micromanipulator and microscope.

LAUP, laser-assisted uvulopalatoplasty.

backstop and a smoke evacuation port. Incision is performed with the laser power level set to 18 W. The TEM_{oo} mode assures precise incisions (200–300 μ width). Char-free vaporization of the uvula (or inverted U soft palate trenching) is performed by turning the SwiftLase flashscanner to its ablating mode (ON) at the same power level. Char-free ablation prevents bleeding and provides excellent depth control of the ablated crater. It also reduces deep burn caused by heat retention of carbonized tissue. As a result, the procedure is less painful and healing is improved.

SwiftLase Flashscan Technology

The SwiftLase (Sharplan model 755, Allendale, NJ) is a miniature optomechanical flashscanner compatible with any CO_2 laser. The SwiftLase consists of two nearly parallel

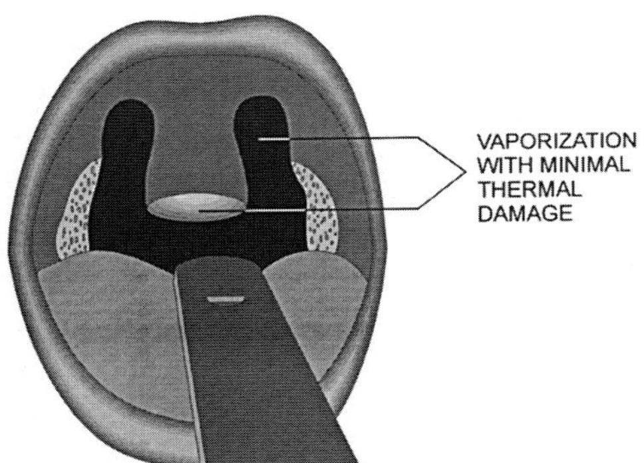

FIG. 1. Inverted U-shape trenching of the soft palate and ablation of the uvula bottom for the treatment of snoring. Both are best performed with the SwiftLase scanner in ON position for char-free vaporization.

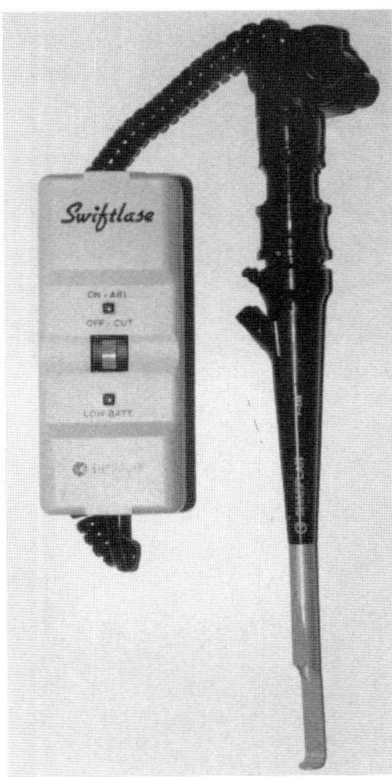

FIG. 2. Oral-pharyngeal handpiece with the integrated SwiftLase attachment.

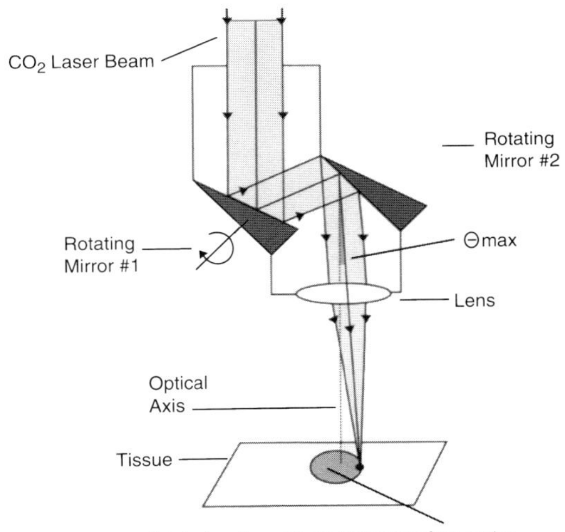

FIG. 3. The operating principles of the SwiftLase technology for single-layer char-free ablation.

theta-folding mirrors. Optical reflections of the CO$_2$ laser optical beam from the mirrors cause the beam to deviate from its original direction by an angle θ (Fig. 3). The mirrors constantly rotate at slightly different angular velocities, thereby rapidly varying the off-axis angle θ with time, between zero and a maximal value θ ($θ_{max}$). By attaching a focusing delivery system of focal length F to the SwiftLase, the CO$_2$ laser generates a small focal spot that rapidly and homogeneously scans and covers a round area of diameter 2F Tan $θ_{max}$ on tissue at the focal plane. For the Sharplan oral-pharyngeal handpiece delivery system F = 225 mm. The maximal off-axis angular deviation $θ_{max}$ was selected to provide a round treated area 3 mm in diameter. The rapid movement of the beam over the tissue ensures a short duration (about 1 millisecond) or exposure on individual sites within the area, and very shallow vaporization.

Because the oral-pharyngeal handpiece used for the treatment of snoring generates a focused beam <0.3 mm in diameter on tissue, using the SwiftLase with a typical laser power level of 18 W will generate an optical power density of about 225 W/mm^2 on tissue. This is considerably higher than the threshold for vaporization of tissue without residual carbon char (the threshold for char-free tissue ablation is about 50 W/mm^2). The time required for the SwiftLase to homogeneously cover a 3-mm round area is about 100 milliseconds. During this time, the 18-W operating laser will deliver 1800 mJ to the tissue. Because the typical energy required to ablate the tissue completely is approximately 3000 mJ/mm^3 (9), keeping the oral-pharyngeal delivery system precisely on a single site for 0.1 second will generate a clean char-free crater <0.15 mm deep.

However, the handpiece can be smoothly and evenly moved across an extended lesion intended for treatment, consequently vaporizing tissue layers as thin as 50 μm. Histologies of New Zealand white rabbit skins irradiated with the SwiftLase showed residual thermal necrosis to a depth <160 μ (Fig. 4) (10).

In addition to the laser oral-pharyngeal surgical handpiece described, some peripheral equipment is necessary: an ebonized laser tongue depressor that incorporates a cleanable

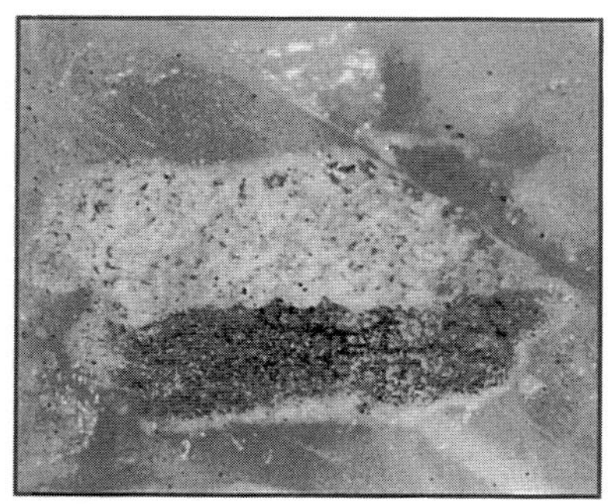

A

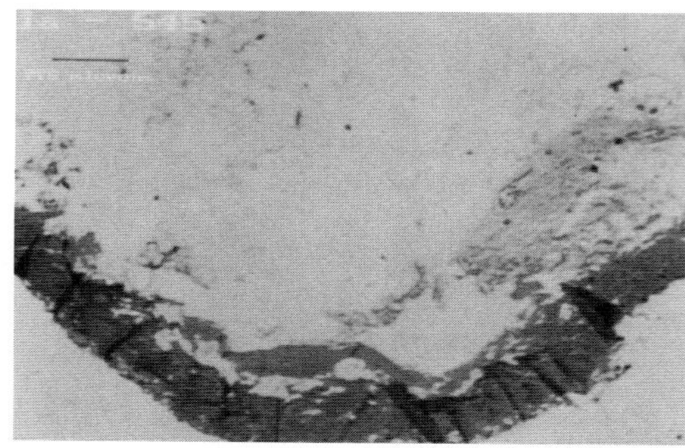

B

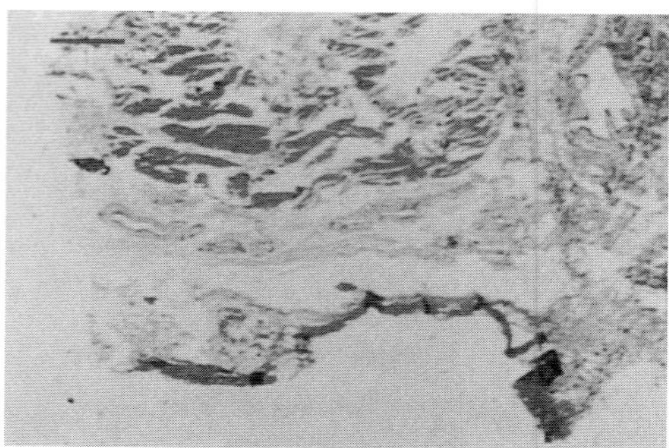

C

FIG. 4. SwiftLase tissue interaction. **(A)** Top section shows the char-free effect of SwiftLase; at bottom is conventional ablation of tissue without the SwiftLase. Histologies of a laser-irradiated skin of a New Zealand white rabbit. **(B)** Without SwiftLase, 10 W, 3-mm laser beam spot, thermal necrosis, 512 µm. **(C)** With Swift-Lase, thermal necrosis, 186 µm.

smoke evacuation channel such as the Krespi tongue depressor (Sharplan model 15205), smoke evacuation tubing, and a smoke evacuator (Fig. 5).

So far, we estimate approximately 50,000 snorers have been treated with SwiftLase technology by >800 ENT offices and ambulatory surgery centers in the United States with success rates of >85%.

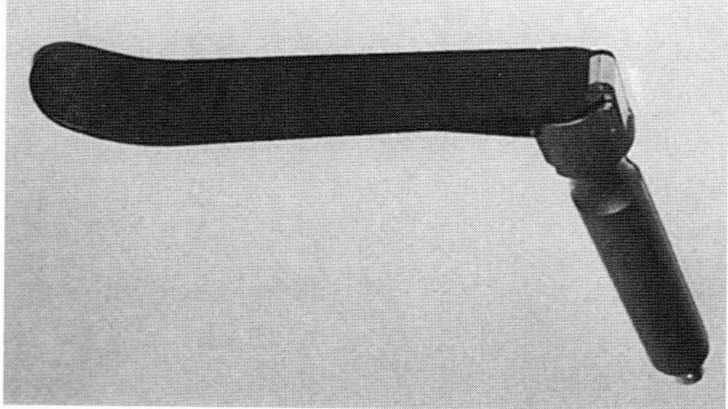

FIG. 5. Laser tongue depressor incorporating a cleanable smoke evacuation channel.

Tonsil Ablation and the Treatment of Bad Breath

Tonsil ablation (cryptolysis) is an office procedure that has been done with great success in the last 4 to 5 years (11). The procedure involves vaporization of the tonsil crypts without any char using the SwiftLase at a 15-W power level. This procedure uses a regular straight tip or a large-diameter (1″) 90° silvered folding mirror tip attached to the oralpharyngeal handpiece. The mirror is large enough to enable the SwiftLaser beam to bounce toward the tonsil surface and, simultaneously, the surgeon to see the target tissue clearly (Fig. 6). An important application of tonsil cryptolysis is the treatment of bad breath, which is often caused by inflamed crypts.

The tonsil mirror tip can also be used to ablate lingual tonsils without gag reflex in a cooperative patient. While treating lingual tonsils the surgeon should slightly pull the patient's tongue to better expose the tonsils.

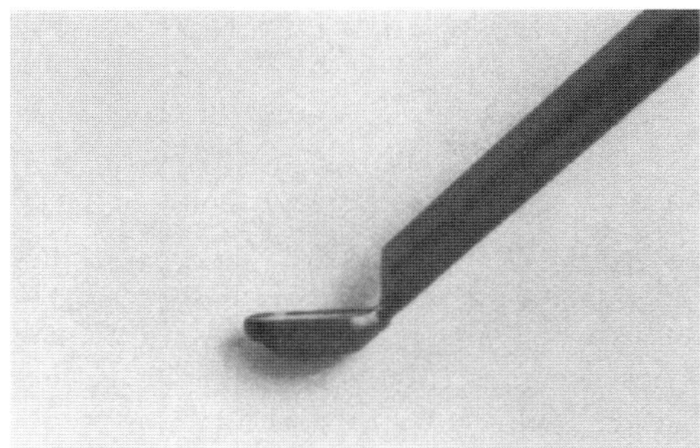

FIG. 6. Ninety-degree oral-pharyngeal hand-piece attachment for the treatment of tonsils.

Nasal Applications of the Office CO_2 Laser

Nasal obstructions caused by turbinate hypertrophy can be treated in the office with the same compact CO_2 laser used for LAUP. The laser is operated in the superpulse mode at an average power level of 7 W. The peak power of each superpulse is 350 W, and the pulse duration is 100 µs. The laser beam is coupled to a thin optical waveguide (1-mm diameter, 10 cm long) that delivers the laser energy to the turbinate surface deep inside the nose (Fig. 7A). The straight or curved tip waveguide also transmits the helium neon pilot beam. The nasal tip incorporates a thin smoke evacuation channel.

Activation of the laser causes evaporation of the tissue hit by the 1-mm beam at the end of the fiber. The superpulse mode is crucial because it assures that tissue is evaporated layer by layer (about 0.1 mm per pulse) without any char and with good control of depth and tissue effect. Most importantly, there is no bleeding.

Air cooling is necessary both to cool the tissue and to keep the waveguide channel clean and cool. A tiny rotary pump incorporated in the laser provides the necessary air flow.

The procedure lasts for a few minutes, using only topical anesthesia. No packing is required. Complete healing occurs within 7–8 days (12).

Endoscopic CO_2 Laser Surgery for the Treatment of Laryngeal Lesions

In addition to nasal applications, flexible CO_2 waveguides are used for endoscopic treatment of laryngeal lesions in an ambula-

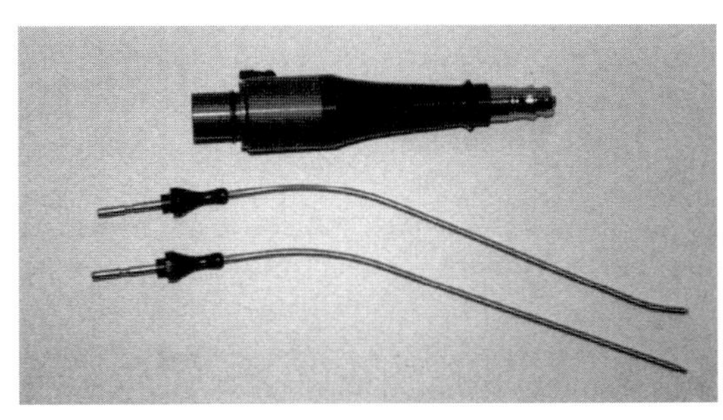

A

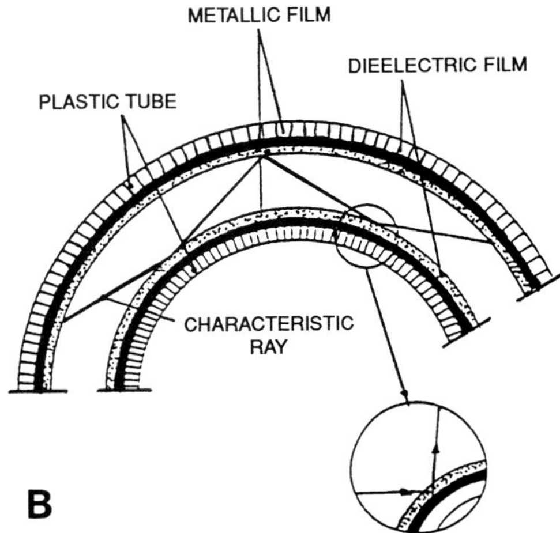

FIG. 7. (A) Flexible FlexiLase CO_2 fibers for the treatment of nasal and narrow cavity lesions. **(B)** Operating principles of a flexible hollow waveguide. View of a section of plastic hollow fiber showing the internal metal and dielectric coating and a path of characteristic ray.

tory environment with only local anesthesia. One meter long, up to 1-mm-diameter flexible CO_2 waveguides (Sharplan model 2222, specifically designed to protect the endoscope) are introduced into the working channel of a flexible endoscope. The flexible video endoscope is introduced through the nasal cavity and pushed down the pharynx up to the laryngeal lesion. The CO_2 laser is operated at 10–15-W power level, preferably in the superpulse mode. Breathing is through the mouth. Prior to the surgical procedure, local anesthesia is administered through the endoscope operating channel (Krespi Endoscopic Anesthetizer, Sharplan model 1111).

Optical Waveguide Technology

The operating principles of optical hollow fibers (13) are depicted in Figure 7B. The operating laser beam is coupled via a focusing lens into the center of a thin plastic tubing. The flexible tube is coated with a dielectric silver-iodine film covered by a second metallic silver film. The optical coating is highly reflective from the multilayer at a 10.6-μm wavelength. Multiple reflections from the waveguide walls enable the trapped optical radiation to propagate along the fiber and produce a 1-mm spot at a distance of 1 mm from the fiber distal end. The optical beam divergence is 80°, thus enabling considerable defocusing by slightly pulling back the fiber. The airflow through the fiber is synchronized with laser activation, the fiber walls do not warm up, and the optical channel is kept clean of debris. FlexiLase (Sharplan) fibers used for nasal surgery (straight and curved) (Fig. 7A) can efficiently transmit laser radiation generated in the superpulse mode (transmissivity, 80%–90%). Consequently, when the 12-cm fibers are used in the near contact mode (spot size, 1 mm), peak power densities of 200 W/mm^2 are attained on tissue, when used with a CO_2 laser that generates pulses of 350 W peak power, and 100-μs pulse duration in the superpulse mode. This is high enough to produce char-free ablation. Longer fibers used in flexible endoscopy have a lower transmissivity, closer to 60%.

Oral and Dental Surgery

The CO_2 laser has been shown to have many advantages over a scalpel in surgery of soft tissue of the oral cavity. The major reason for this is the laser's ability to seal blood vessels during surgery with minimal thermal damage to surrounding tissue. Three accessories are used in the ambulatory environment: FlexiLase 1-mm, short-stem (125 mm) CO_2 waveguides for gingivectomy (power levels 15 to 20 W), and 50-mm and 125-mm focal length handpieces to excise sublingual glands (14,15), locate sialoliths, and excise fibromas, granulomas, and other oral lesions (power levels 8 to 10 W). The 50-mm focused handpiece in conjunction with the laser superpulse mode is extremely useful for tissue excision in dental implant procedures because of the minimal thermal damage and heat conductivity properties of titanium implants. The char-free ablation SwiftLase, mostly used in oral surgery, is a 125-mm focal length version for vaporization of leukoplakia and hairy tongue. The laser power level is set to 10 W.

INSTRUMENTATION FOR AESTHETIC OFFICE SURGERY WITH A CO_2 LASER

Skin Resurfacing in Aesthetic Surgery

Cosmetic facial skin resurfacing, particularly for the removal of perioral, lip, periorbital, and nasolabial wrinkles, is performed in the office under local anesthesia with a focused microprocessor-controlled spiral flashscanner (SilkTouch, Sharplan) that vaporizes variable size (2–9 mm diameter) craters in the epidermis down to the papillary layer, with no thermal injury to the underlying dermis. The SilkTouch flashscanner provides the aesthetic surgeon with an unprecedented control of peeling depth by enabling collagen denaturation just in the papillary layer for long-term permanent results. Wrinkles are removed by ablating their shoulders with the CO_2 laser, typically operated at 18 W in the pulsed or re-

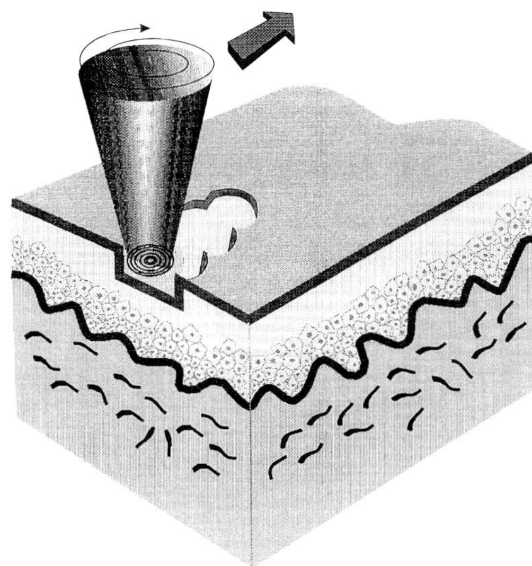

FIG. 8. Wrinkle removal with a SilkTouch microprocessor-controlled flashscanner at low CO_2 laser power level.

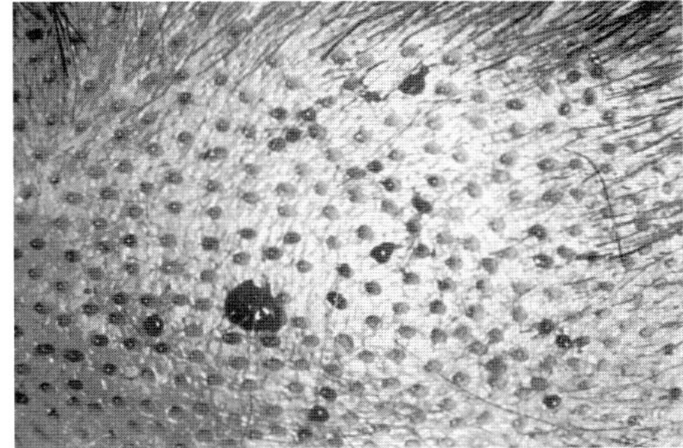

FIG. 9. Recipient holes created by a SilkTouch scanner in a Megasession hair transplantation.

peat mode, with ON time set to 0.2 second and tissue vaporization diameter set to 6 mm; 0.2 second is the necessary duration for the SilkTouch to complete one spiral revolution period (Fig. 8). Residual necrotized tissue above the papillary dermis is wiped off with a saline-moisturized gauze. So far, >1000 facial peels have been performed with the Silk-Touch laser without complications. In addition, the flashscanner has found extensive use in the treatment of scars, including punch grafting of ice pick scars.

Postoperative follow-up consistently shows excellent cosmetic results (5–7). A comprehensive, thorough understanding of the surgical technique, skin types, laser parameters, and postoperative treatment is mandatory for consistent success.

Laser-Assisted Hair Transplantation

The CO_2 flashscanner is an extremely useful tool that replaces the mechanical driller in preparing recipient holes for hair transplantation. The SilkTouch flashscanner, when operated in its hair transplantation mode, vaporizes recipient holes of standard 0.9 mm and 1.2 mm diameters for micrograft transplantation and 1.5 mm for minigrafts. The laser used for hair transplantation should deliver higher power levels than are normally used for ENT or skin

TABLE 2. *Equipment Necessary for the Performance of Multiple Aesthetic Procedures in an Office Setting With a CO_2 Laser*

Procedure	Surgical Accessory	Laser Settings
Skin resurfacing	SilkTouch flashscanner	
Wrinkle removal	f = 200 mm, 6-mm diameter	0.2 sec, 18 W
Full facial peel	f = 125 mm, 3-mm diameter	0.2 sec, 7 W
Rhinophyma	SilkTouch flashscanner painting mode	Continuous, 10 W
Viral warts	f = 125 mm, 3-mm diameter	
Hair transplantation	SilkTouch flashscanner	0.05–0.1 sec, 40–80 W*
	Hair transplant mode	
	f = 80 mm with smoke evacuation channel	
	Diameter = 0.6, 0.9, 1.2 mm	
	Slit	

*Minigraft (d >1.2 mm) holes and slits are still experimental.

resurfacing. Typical operating power level is 80 W (Sharplan 150XJ) with time duration of 0.1 second for the generation of 5-mm-deep holes. The advantage of using a laser in hair transplantation is lack of bleeding and complete removal of tissue in the recipient site, which considerably speed up the procedure and improve Megasession's capability (8) (Fig. 9).

Table 2 summarizes the equipment used in aesthetic laser surgery.

NASAL APPLICATIONS OF ND:YAG AND DIODE LASERS IN AN OFFICE SETTING

The Nd:YAG lasers operated at a 1.06-μm wavelength are not often found in an office setting because of their relatively high prices and lower versatility. The reduced versatility stems from the fact that, in contrast to the superficial tissue effects generated by CO_2

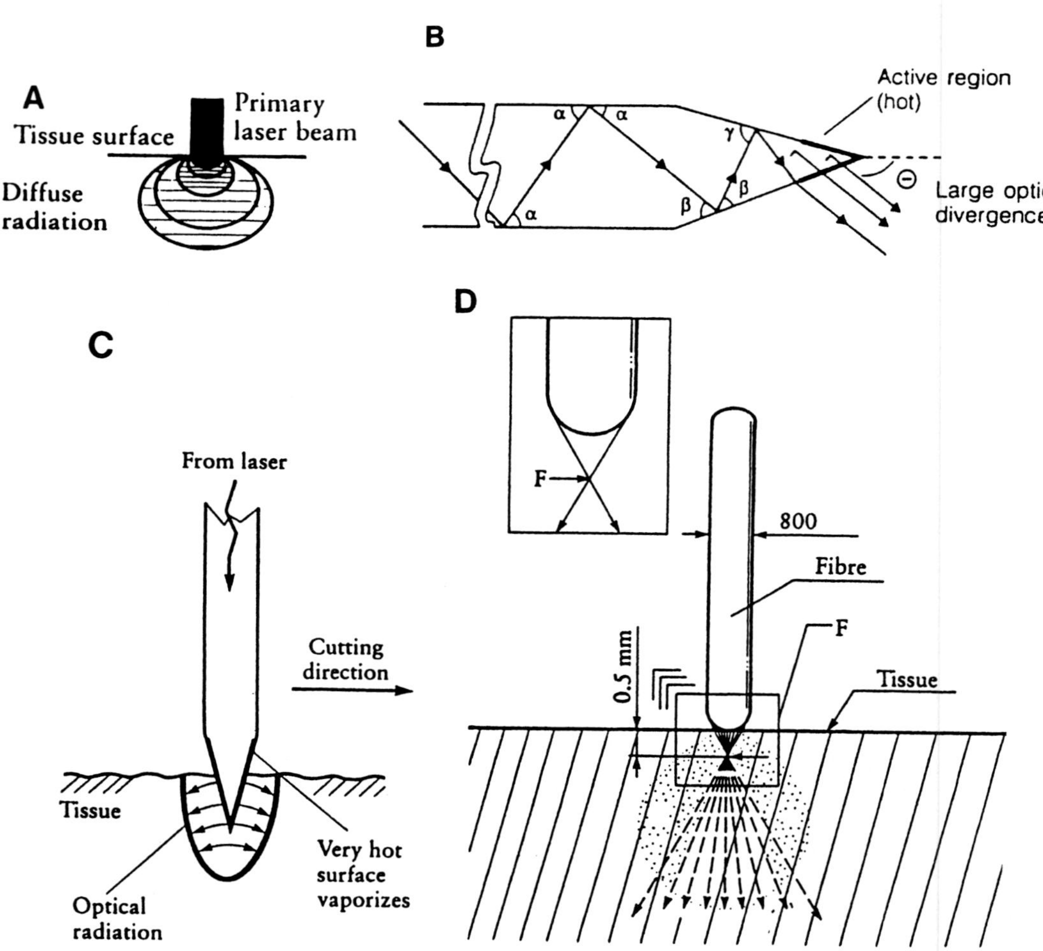

FIG. 10. Operating principles of Nd:YAG laser fibers. **(A)** Coagulation of tissue with Nd:YAG laser radiation emitted by noncontact fibers. **(B)** Optics of a conical sculpted fiber. The angle of incidence of internally reflected rays gradually increases along tapered tip until it exceeds the total internal reflection-critical angle. A light-emitting zone is thus defined. Contact with tissue causes this zone to be hot and therefore active. **(C)** Origin of high incision efficiency of a conical sculpted fiber. **(D)** Optics and operating principle of a hemispherical sculpted fiber. F is the point where the power density is maximal and around which there is divergence of the radiation.

lasers, they produce deeper and less controllable tissue reaction. Nevertheless, they are useful in three nasal applications performed in ambulatory conditions, namely: shrinking of hypertrophic turbinates (16), endoscopic control of nasal epistaxis (17), and ablation of benign nasopharyngeal lesions (18). The recent development of less expensive diode lasers with tissue effects almost identical to Nd:YAG has made this laser an excellent tool for office nasal procedures. The diode laser is well suited for the office setting owing to its small size and low current consumption.

The Nd:YAG laser radiation can induce deep (4 mm) thermal coagulation in the non-contact fiber mode, or it can incise tissue with a 0.5-mm residual thermal necrosis along the incision line in the contact fiber mode. The optical fibers used in the contact mode are specially sculpted at their distal tip to optimize incision control. (See Fig. 10 for the operating principle of Nd:YAG surgical fibers.)

Interstitial Coagulation of Nasal Hypertrophic Turbinates

Interstitial coagulation of hypertrophic turbinates with the consequential production of submucosal scar and turbinate shrinking without damaging the mucosa is accomplished with a flat bare fiber at 8-W Nd:YAG power level.

The 0.4 numerical aperture, 600-μm diameter, silica-silicon fiber is pushed along the turbinate at the rate of 1–2 cm per second for 2 seconds with laser activation. The fiber is then pulled out at the same rate with the laser once again being activated (Fig. 11). The total lasing time is about 3 seconds. Figure 12 depicts the physical effect attained during this procedure.

A thin (2.5 mm) diameter cylindrical tissue volume is directly coagulated by the Nd:YAG laser forward emitted (20° divergence) laser radiation. This cylinder is surrounded by a 6-mm-diameter coaxial zone coagulated by heat escaping the inner zone, directly coagulated by laser radiation. Figure 12B shows the submucosal temperature distribution around the fiber track, indicating very high safety. The power level should not be higher than 8 W. So far, more than 50 patients have been treated with an interstitial fiber in the office with excellent results (16).

Control of Nasal Epistaxis

Laser surgery for the control of nasal epistaxis is performed with a 600-μm flat optical

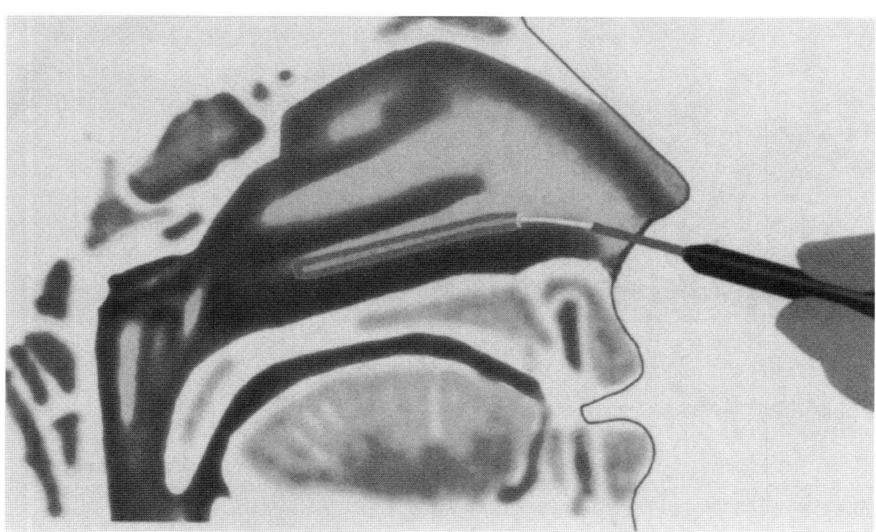

FIG. 11. Interstitial thermal therapy with a flat-end Nd:YAG optical fiber.

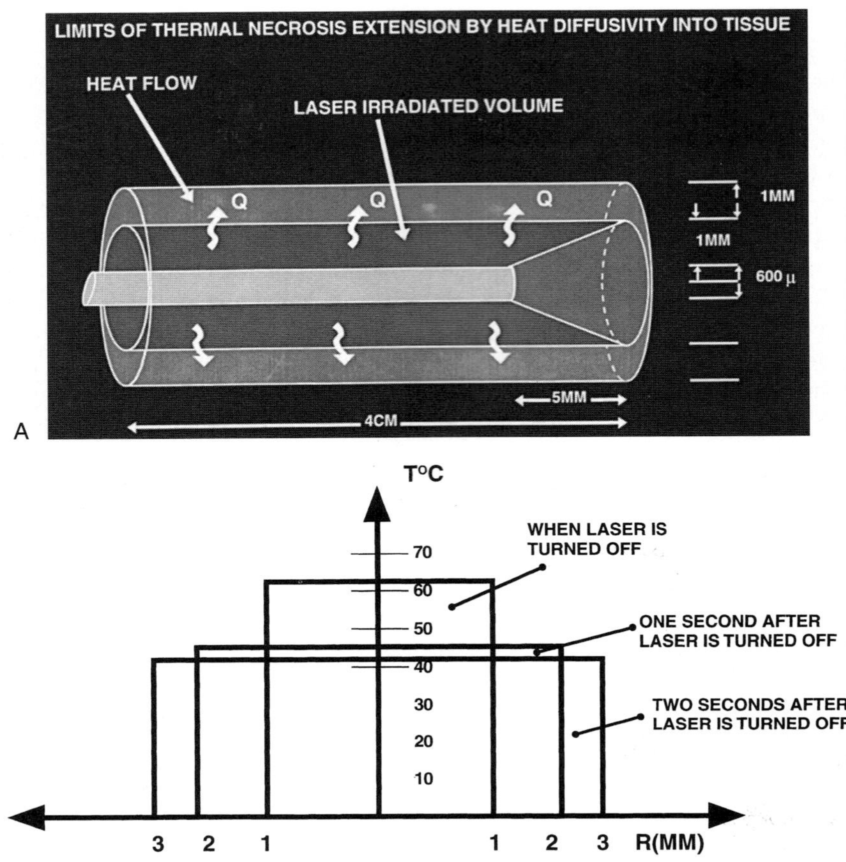

FIG. 12. Tissue coagulation with an interstitial thermal therapy fiber. **(A)** Schematic presentation of the tissue effect. **(B)** Temperature distribution during and after interstitial laser radiation.

fiber in the noncontact mode. The fiber, incorporated in a malleable handpiece, is inserted into the nose and aimed at a blood vessel with the aid of a sinoscope. In the case of recurrent anterior epistaxis for the septum, the laser ablation is performed through the septal flaps directly over the blood vessel. The laser is operated at 10 W for 1–2 seconds until coagulation is observed. The microendoscopic procedure enables extremely accurate coagulation of blood vessels without damaging surrounding tissue (17).

Table 3 summarizes the equipment required for an Nd:YAG laser or a diode laser in an ambulatory setting.

TABLE 3. *Equipment Required for the Ambulatory Use of an Nd:YAG Laser/Diode Laser*

Nd:YAG laser, 1 to 40 W; diode laser 1 to 20 W
600-μm flat optical fiber for coagulation (interstitial and noncontact)
800-μm hemispherical fibers for incision
Fiber holders
Protective eyeglasses for 1.06-μm wavelength
Sinoscope

REFERENCES

1. Kamami YV: Laser CO_2 for snoring, preliminary results. *Acta Otorhinolaryngol Belg* 44:451–456, 1990.

2. Krespi YP, Pearlman SJ, Keidar A et al: Laser assisted uvulopalatoplasty for snoring. *Insights of Otolaryngology* 9:2–7, 1994.
3. Krespi YP, Coleman JA, Pearlman SJ et al: Laser assisted uvulopalatoplasty for snoring. *Lasers Surg Med* 179(suppl 6, abstract), 1994.
4. Krespi YP, Pearlman SJ: L.A.U.P.: Results and complications in 1000 patients. Presented at annual meeting of AAO-HNS, New Orleans, September 1995.
5. Chernoff WG, Slatkine M, Zair E, Mead D: SilkTouch: A new technology for skin resurfacing in aesthetic surgery. *J Clin Laser Med Surg* 15:170–173, 1995.
6. Ross EV, Grossman MC, Anderson RR, Grevelink JM: Treatment of facial rhytides: Comparing a pulsed CO_2 laser with a collimated beam to a CO_2 laser enhanced by a flashscanner. *Lasers Surg Med* 6(suppl 6, abstract 235), 1995.
7. Kauvar ANB, Geronemus R, Waldorf HA: Char free tissue ablation: A comparative histopathological analysis of new CO_2 laser systems. *Lasers Surg Med* (suppl 7, abstract 236), 1995.
8. Villnow M, Slatkine M, Mead D: Laser assisted hair transplantation with flashscanner technology. *J Clin Laser Med Surg* 15:330–333, 1995.
9. Carruth JAS, McKenzie AL: Medical lasers: Science and clinical practice. Bristol, Great Britain: Adam Hilger, 1986.
10. Raif J, Zair E: SwiftLase: A new CO_2 laser scanner for reduced tissue carbonization. *Lasers Surg Med* (suppl 5, abstract 126), 1993.
11. Krespi YP: Tonsil cryptolysis utilizing CO_2 SwiftLase. *Lasers Surg Med* (suppl 5, abstract 197), 1993.
12. Krespi YP, Mayer M, Slatkine M: Laser photocoagulation of the inferior turbinates. *Op Tech Otolaryngol Head Neck Surg* 5:287–291, 1994.
13. Kaplan I, Glen S, Dror J et al: Experimental surgery on dog's stomach and liver using CO_2 laser plastic hollow fibers: Technical methods. *J Clin Laser Med Surg* 12:115–118, 1992.
14. Mints S, Barak S, Horowitz I: Carbon dioxide laser excision and vaporization of nonplunging ranulas: A comparison of two treatment protocols. *J Oral Maxillofac Surg* 52:370–372, 1994.
15. Krespi YP, Slatkine M: Nd:YAG fiber delivery system for submucosal interstitial photocoagulation of nasal turbinates. *Lasers Surg Med* (suppl 6, abstract 183), 1994.
16. Krespi YP, Ling E: Control of anterior epistaxis utilizing YAG laser. *Op Tech Otolaryngol Head Neck Surg* 5:209–210, 1994.
17. Krespi YP, Khosh M, Blitzer A: Transnasal endoscopic laser surgery for the treatment of benign nasopharyngeal lesions. *Op Tech Otolaryngol Head Neck Surg* 5:225–226, 1994.

PART 2

The Oral Cavity

Office-Based Surgery of the Head and Neck
Edited by Yosef P. Krespi, MD
Lippincott–Raven Publishers, Philadelphia © 1998

4

Office-Based Laser Surgery of the Oral Cavity

Philip T. Ho and Andrew Blitzer

Since the introduction of the first red ruby laser by Maiman in 1960 (1), lasers have continually gained interest, acceptance, and use in surgical procedures. Nearly all surgical and surgically related fields have incorporated lasers into their operative practices—from coagulation of bleeding gastric ulcers to radial keratotomy to urethral anastomoses (2,3). In head and neck surgery, lasers have been used for procedures as diverse as microlaryngeal surgery to nasal turbinectomy to stapes surgery (4–6).

The oral cavity has been an anatomic area of great interest for laser surgical applications because of the easy accessibility and relatively high vascularity. Traditional "cold steel" methods have been fraught with problems such as bleeding, difficult access, and unsatisfactory cosmetic results. Although electrocautery improved hemostasis, it increased pain, scarring, and cosmetic deformity. Lasers can deliver precise cutting, wide ablation, and dependable coagulation in a single instrument (7,8).

The laser wound differs from those of the scalpel and electrocautery in that the zone of cell damage peripheral to the excision is much narrower. The depth and radius of the tissue ablation and damage depends on the laser's spot size, power density, and tissue exposure time. As the light wavelength of the laser is decreased, the tissue disruption is increased. Low wavelength-high frequency energy, such as gamma and x-rays, can cause damage at the nucleic acid level, whereas excimer lasers at the ultraviolet range (100–380 nm) break chemical bonds with minimal heat damage. Higher wavelength energy causes more heat, more gross tissue effect, and, thus, more thermal damage. Therefore, very short, intermittent pulses of high power density (high power with small spot size) maximizes tissue cutting with minimal tissue thermal effects (9–11).

After a laser excision in the oral cavity, a layer of fibrin or collagen coagulum forms in the wound. This layer, which is seen within 24 hours after the procedure, acts to protect the wound. It seems to reduce the pain of exposed subcutaneous tissue and muscle and acts as a scaffold for epithelial migration. The laser wounds of the oral cavity also produce less edema because the energy coagulates and "seals" blood vessels and lymphatics. This sealing of lymphatics is thought to help reduce metastatic seeding of tumor and infection. The lasers are also reported to be directly bacteriocidal (11–13).

Epithelial healing has been reported to be slower with a laser than with cold steel surgery. Within the first 4 days after laser surgery, there is less closure of a surgical wound and decreased tensile strength. After 2 weeks, however, the wound healing is identical. The initial delay of wound closure appears to be secondary to less collagen formation and a decreased wound contracture from a decreased myofibroblast stimulation and infiltration. The decrease in myofibroblasts is also responsible for the decreased scar formation and wound contracture. Reduction in scarring allows for improved functional and cosmetic results (10,11).

Laser wounds also have been found to be less painful. Aside from the decrease in both tissue edema and thermal tissue damage, the fibrin coagulum and the nonchromatic, low water characteristics of nerves contribute to the decreased nerve damage found in the laser wound (10,11).

CARBON DIOXIDE LASERS

The carbon dioxide (CO_2) laser, which was developed by Patel et al. in 1964 at Bell Laboratories, is currently the most frequently used laser in surgery. CO_2, helium, and nitrogen are the active elements used to produce an energy wavelength of 10,600 nm. Because this energy is in the infrared spectrum, it is invisible; therefore, a helium-neon (HeNe) beam is added for visual aiming of the laser energy. The CO_2 lasers are highly efficient, requiring only a 110-V energy source and no special cooling mechanisms. Most of the systems available have articulated arms with mirrors and prisms to reflect the energy. Because of the wavelength, the energy cannot be delivered via fiberoptic cables efficiently. Some systems offer hollow waveguides with polished internal surfaces that allow transmission of the energy, but even in this system, there is an energy loss proportional to the length of the waveguide (14,15).

The CO_2 laser energy is primarily absorbed by the intracellular water, causing a vaporization of surface cells. Most of the incident energy is absorbed no greater than 0.2 mm into the surrounding tissues, which makes the CO_2 laser ideal for vaporizing many oral cavity lesions. The small spot size and high-power density of the laser enable precise tissue ablation with coagulation of vessels (5,14,16).

NEODYMIUM:YTTRIUM-ALUMINUM-GARNET (ND:YAG) LASER

The Nd:YAG laser was first introduced by Johnson in 1961. The active medium of 1% to 3% neodymium on a yttrium-aluminum-garnet crystal, pumped by a xenon or krypton arc lamp, produces a light of 1060 nm wavelength. This near-infrared light requires an HeNe aiming beam. The light energy can be delivered purely by fiberoptics to hand-held probes or through endoscopes. The cutting energy can be used in a contact or noncontact mode. The Nd:YAG laser beam is poorly absorbed by body tissues; consequently, there is a deeper penetration of the energy (3–5 mm in depth) with considerable tissue scatter and reflection with significant thermal tissue damage. The transmission through clear fluids makes the Nd:YAG laser well suited for urologic and ophthalmologic procedures. In the head and neck, the Nd:YAG laser is better for deep coagulation than for precise cutting (4,6,14,17).

ARGON (AR) LASER

The AR laser was first introduced by Bennett in 1962. This laser passes high electrical current through AR gas, producing a blue-green light of 488 nm and 515 nm. Because it is visible light, no special aiming beam is needed. The light energy is delivered via flexible fiberoptics through hand-held probes or endoscopes. The energy is primarily absorbed by pigmented tissues, such as melanin or hemoglobin. Therefore, these lasers are used more frequently for coagulation than for vaporization. The depth of penetration is about 1 mm. The AR laser is used most often for superficial vascular lesions, such as port wine hemangiomas and telangiectasias (9,18,19).

LASER APPLICATIONS IN THE ORAL CAVITY

When evaluating the oral cavity for surgery in the office setting, the airway must be monitored and protected. Bleeding and postoperative edema may be critical problems, particularly in posterior and tongue base lesions.

Benign Oral Cavity Lesions

Many benign lesions occur on the lips because of chronic exposure to sunlight, irritation, and trauma. Classic examples are actinic or solar keratoses from prolonged sun exposure. These are small superficial lesions present as erythematous areas with varying degrees of hyperkeratosis, atrophy, or lichenoid areas. There may be a precancerous nature to many of these lesions, making biopsy imperative. The CO_2 laser is an ideal instrument for complete excision, hemostasis, and ablation, with minimal thermal damage and scarring. The decreased contracture and scar formation associated with lasers may be beneficial for multiple and recurrent excisions (4–6,20).

Fibromas and papillomas may occur anywhere in the oral cavity, such as the buccal mucosa, tongue, and palate (Fig. 1). These are readily amenable to laser excision or ablation under local anesthesia. The fibromas are fibroepithelial inflammatory lesions usually resulting from repeated local trauma and irritation (Fig. 2) (21). The treatment is simple excision or total laser ablation in conjuction with removal of the source of trauma. Papillomas are exophytic, cauliflower-shaped growths that are linked to the human papilloma virus. They can be singular or multiple, and are often recurrent. Preoperatively, a thorough examination of the upper aerodigestive tract should be done, including a fiberoptic examination, to rule out other papillomatous lesions. Removal can be achieved with laser ablation, with ablation of a margin of "healthy" tissue deep and adjacent to the papilloma(s). Extra precautions must be taken to minimize the vapor plumes to minimize the potential possibility of seeding

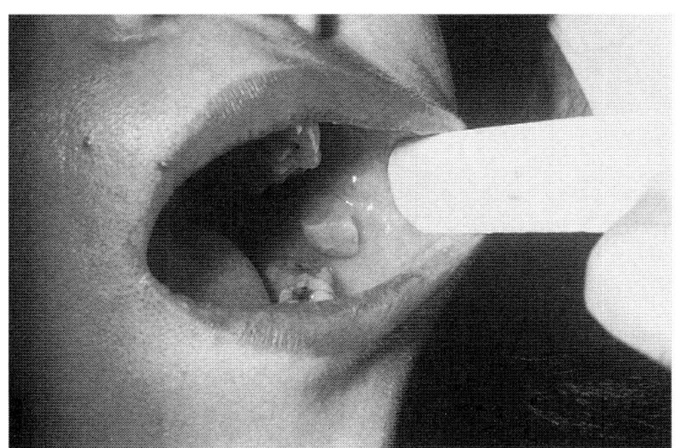

FIG. 1. Pyogenic granuloma of left buccal mucosa.

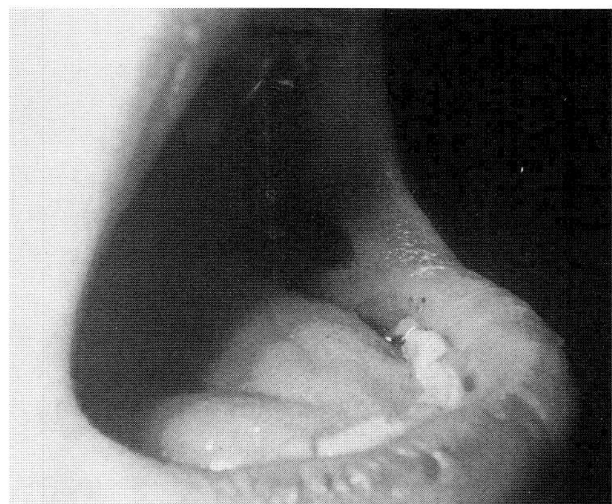

FIG. 2. Status after excision with CO_2 laser.

other areas of the patient's aerodigestive tract, or of infecting the operator via live virus in the laser plume (13,22).

On the buccal mucosa, mass lesions such as irritation granulomas or epuli, which result from chronic irritation such as that caused by ill-fitting dentures or cheek biting, can also be excised or ablated by laser. The wound site is allowed to close by secondary intention and granulation to minimize scarring. Highly vascular epuli or granulomas may also be ablated by prochromophoric AR or Nd:YAG lasers if bleeding is an issue. Chronically infected oral ulcers can be safely treated with lasers because of the laser's bacteriocidal properties and strong vascular and lymphatic coagulating abilities (19,23).

Chronic use of dilantin often causes hyperplasia of the gingiva that frequently leads to severe gingivitis and bleeding. The gingiva can easily be vaporized under local anesthesia with minimal bleeding using a CO_2 laser. The teeth, however, have to be protected, because they will act as a heat sink, and the laser energy can injure the pulp. Festooned aluminum foil can be used to cover the enamel surface while exposing the gingiva. Then using a handpiece, the surgeon can remove the gingiva layer by layer until a more normal contour is established. There is minimal bleeding and scarring, and the procedure can be repeated when necessary (19,20).

Many other types of gingival hyperplasia can be surgically treated with lasers. The most common cause of hyperplasia is trauma and irritation from ill-fitting dentures, producing a diffuse erythema, swelling, and polypoid changes of the gingiva and hard palate. Epulis fissurata are elongated growths of hyperplastic fibrous and epithelial tissue in the gingivolabial fold. The treatment involves laser excision with ablation of hyperplastic tissue and proper fitting of dentures. Gingival hyperplasia can also result from chronic use of certain types of medications (phenytoin, cyclosporin, cardizem, nifedipine), pregnancy, and poor oral hygiene. For pregnancy-related hyperplasia, it is recommended to wait several months after completion of the pregnancy to evaluate whether or not surgical therapy is needed. CO_2 laser gingivectomy has also been shown to be effective in the treatment of gingival and mucosal disease found in Sturge-Weber disease (24–26).

Granulomas and operculi, other types of hyperplastic gingival lesions, can be treated easily with laser surgery. These lesions often present with intraoperative bleeding and access problems, which make complete excision difficult. The use of a CO_2 laser for soft tissue removal and ablation often solves these problems. A unique use of lasers is the removal of soft tissue for second stage osseous titanium implant recovery. This procedure is done with CO_2 lasers, because Nd:YAG lasers have been shown to damage titanium (27).

Gingivoplasty and gingivectomy can be performed for irregular crown margins and for general crown lengthening. Some of these procedures have been done without local anesthesia. Good cosmetic results have been shown. Gingival troughing can be done in preparation for mold impressions or crown placements (25–27).

Lichen planus is a white lacy lesion, possibly stress-induced, that can be symptomatically erosive and painful. It is most often found along the buccal mucosa, but can occur anywhere in the oral cavity. Atrophic and ulcerative forms have been linked to increased malignancy rates. Topical pain medications

have been the mainstay therapy, with biopsy of uncertain or suspicious lesions. If necessary, CO_2 laser ablation can provide ablation of the lesions if they are symptomatic or dysplastic.

Leukoplakia is ubiquitously defined as "a raised white patch which can neither be scraped off, nor attributed to any other diagnosable disease" (28). Clinically, it can appear in several different forms, ranging from homogeneous white keratinized mucosa to a mixed white and red lesion (speckled) to an erosive lesion with ulcerations. Although not actually cancer itself, leukoplakia is considered a precancerous lesion with a reported three times higher incidence of malignant transformation. Erythroplakia, with a red velvety appearance, has a 3–17 times increased incidence of cancer versus simple white leukoplakia. In one study, nearly 10% of leukoplakia lesions with negative preoperative biopsies later showed carcinoma *in situ* or microinvasive carcinoma on final pathology following total excision. Carcinoma seemed to be more frequent with mixed white and red lesions, which also often have associated chronic fungal infection. In addition, although leukoplakia seems to be found more frequently on the buccal mucosa, carcinoma frequency seemed to be greater with lesions in other locations such as the tongue and floor of mouth (Fig. 3) (29–33).

The premalignant potential of these lesions suggests that leukoplakia and erythroplakia should be removed with oncologic surgical

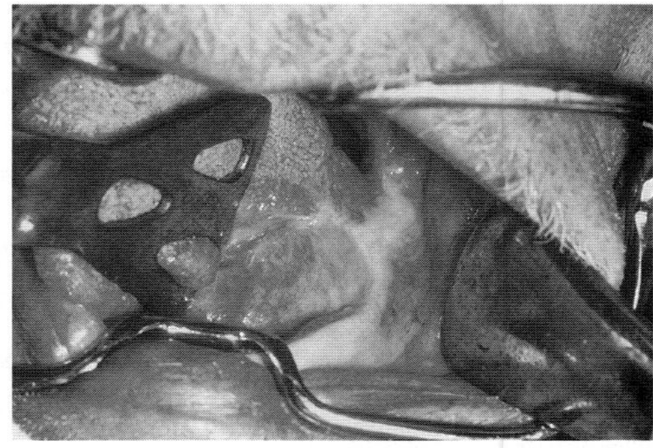

FIG. 3. Adhesive band from previous reconstruction of tongue and buccal mucosa.

principles. This ensures complete excision and reduces the chance of recurrence. Many still advocate the use of toluidine (tolonium) blue dye (2%) to help identify and better delineate suspicious lesions prior to excision. A supravital stain, tolonium stains nucleic acids, which are increased in dysplastic and malignant cells. Stained atypical cells appear deep violet. Benign leukoplakia, however, remains white, whereas trapped oral debris stains dark black-purple. The sensitivity and specificity have both been reported to be 90%. Unfortunately, the dye has a limited penetration of only four to five cell layers, which makes it effective for only shallow or superficial lesions (33–35).

Once the lesion's (or lesions') margins are well established, the laser can be used to precisely remove the lesions with adequate normal tissue around the lesion. The edges or margins can be further laser ablated to further clear the margins while coagulating blood vessels and lymphatics. Wounds are left open to heal by secondary intention. Reported postoperative complications have included wound infection, sloughing, granulation tissue, bleeding, and recurrences, both at the primary site and at new sites in the mouth (33,34).

Lasers have also been used to treat a number of salivary tissue lesions of the oral cavity. Ranuli and mucoceles can be incised and marsupialized easily using a CO_2 laser, with care not to damage the surrounding structures such as Warthin's ducts. Interestingly, there is a lower incidence of Warthin's and Stenson's duct stricture or obstruction with laser surgery. With ranuli, good results have been shown using the laser to vaporize the cyst wall while removing the associated minor salivary gland. The laser can also be used to incise the salivary ducts to expose and remove intraoral sialoliths, with little or no bleeding and minimal stimulation of fibroblasts to form scar (33).

On the hard and soft palates, many of the lesions involve the minor salivary glands. Benign mixed tumors (pleomorphic adenomas) require wide excision. A thorough preoperative evaluation is required to assess the histology and the tumor extent. Sometimes fine needle aspiration can define the tissue type

with minimal manipulation of the tumor. For small tumors, the laser may allow resection with minimal bleeding and scarring. In larger tumors, the laser may be used in the office for biopsy of the lesion. Warthin's tumors (papillary cystadenoma lymphomatosum) may also occur in the hard palate minor salivary glands and may require biopsy or excision.

Lasers are also useful for incising adhesions and releasing strictures that may occur on the floor of mouth in patients with previous oral cavity surgery or trauma. Laser wounds themselves cause minimal scarring. Frenulectomies including "tongue-tie" are quickly, easily, and bloodlessly performed by CO_2 lasers. The laser needs to cut through the anterior band of the hypertrophic genioglossus muscle. Because the laser causes minimal tissue damage, scarring and recurrences are rare and pain and discomfort are minimal. The CO_2 laser has also been very useful in releasing scar bands and contractures after reconstructive surgery of the oral cavity. These bands can easily be lysed with the laser. The laser has also been used to perform a sulcoplasty to increase the

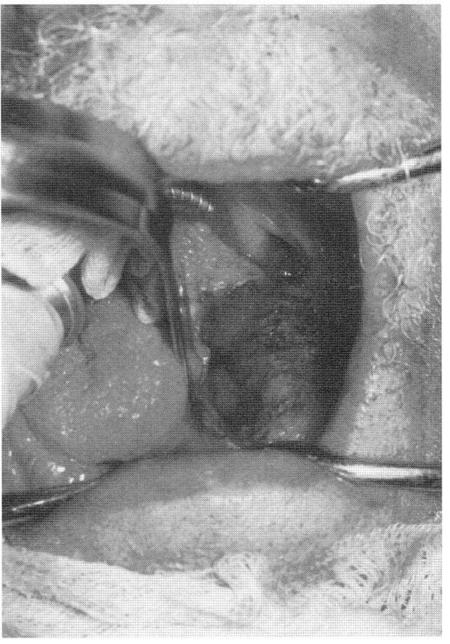

FIG. 4. Laser lysis of band.

available retentive tissue for prosthetic rehabilitation. Then the sulcus can be maintained with a denture or a stent inserted at the time of the surgery.

Aphthous ulcers (recurrent aphthous stomatitis, "canker sores") occur nearly anywhere in the predominantly nonkeratinized oral cavity (tongue, buccal mucosa, oropharynx). These ulcers present as transitory (7–40 days), recurrent, painful ulcers of unclear origin, and have been treated medically with pain medicines (oral and topical), tetracycline rinses, high-dose vitamin therapy, and topical prostaglandin E (PGE)-2 and recombinant interferon alpha-2a. Low- power CO_2 lasers have been used successfully to ablate ulcers under local anesthesia with no pain medications required postoperatively, no primary site recurrences, and good patient satisfaction (33,35).

Granular cell tumors (myoblastomas) are firm, small, nontender tumors sometimes found on the tongue of middle-aged adults. Their unclear origin and sometimes hyperplastic histology can be confused with carcinoma, and complete surgical excision is required to avoid recurrence (Fig. 5). The tongue is better viewed as two parts: the mobile anterior two thirds and the posterior one third to the base of tongue. Anteriorly, lesions can be easily visualized, manipulated, and removed. Small excision sites can be left open, while some larger defects may be partially closed with sutures. Partial closure has been advocated in certain subset populations, such

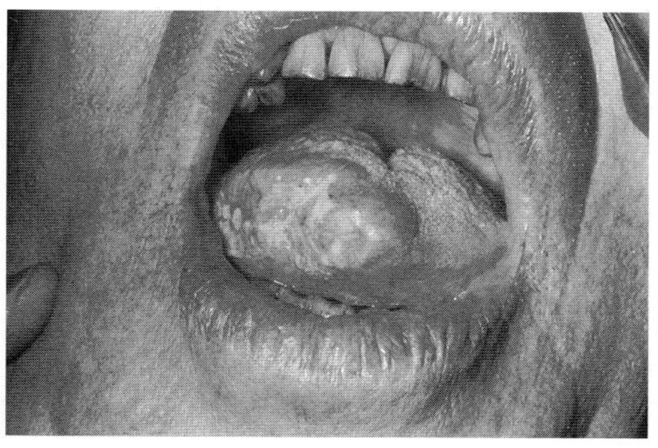

FIG. 5. Carcinoma *in situ* of tongue.

as diabetics and the elderly. If possible, preservation of taste function involving the circumvallate papillae and the tip of the tongue should be attempted during resection (21,25).

The posterior oropharynx and base of tongue must be approached with extreme caution, owing to exposure and visualization difficulties and to potential airway complications. Thus, major procedures on the base of tongue or posterior oropharynx are better done in the operating room under general anesthesia and with good airway management. Laser procedures involving the uvula and soft palate (laser-assisted uvulopalatoplasty [LAUP]), the palantine tonsils (laser-assisted serial tonsillectomy [LAST]), and the lingual tonsils are discussed in Chapters 12, 11, and 13, respectively.

Some vascular lesions are ideal for laser excision and management. It has been estimated that 50% of all hemangiomas and 70% of all lymphangiomas occur in the head and neck region (36,37). They may occur as singular or multiple lesions, or as part of systemic or congenital syndromes. The most common site is the tongue, although areas such as the buccal mucosa and the lips may also be affected. Traditional therapies have included observation, medications (steroids, 5-fluorouracil), radiation, embolization, sclerotherapy, cryotherapy, cauterization, and excision. Small superficial lesions, such as capillary hemangiomas and lymphangiomas, are easily amenable to CO_2 laser excision or ablation or the use of the AR laser, which is preferentially red absorbed. Vascular granulomas and epulis can be precisely excised or ablated with minimal blood loss and pain. For more diffuse vascular lesions, such as telangiectasias (Osler-Weber-Rendu disease), varicosities, and venous lakes, use of clear microslides to compress the lesions allows diffuse laser coagulation to work more effectively and quickly. The AR or YAG lasers are also useful in treating such lesions because they cause endothelial damage with occlusion of the lesions and shrinkage (Fig. 6) (36,37).

For deeper and larger vascular lesions, such as diffuse angiomatosis of the tongue, cav-

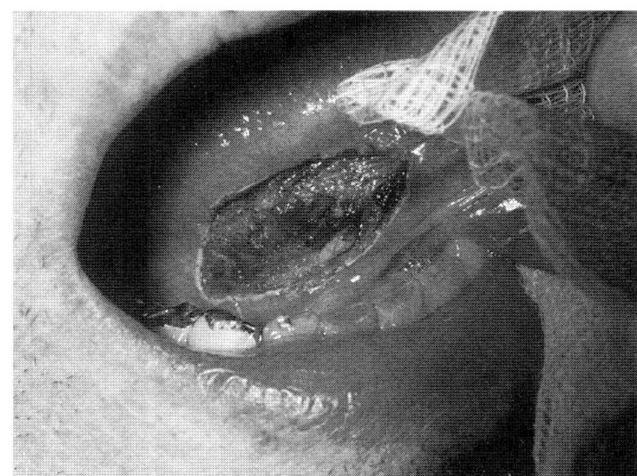

FIG. 6. Postoperative YAG laser partial glossectomy.

ernous hemangiomas, and larger capillary hemangiomas and lymphangioma lesions, the AR or Nd:YAG lasers should be employed (Fig. 7). Good to excellent results have been reported using either the AR (2–3 W, continuous, 2-mm spot, 75 W/cm^2, total 1000–4000 J delivered) or the Nd:YAG (30–50 W, pulsed, 2-mm spot size, 0.2–0.5 second pulse duration, 1000–3000 W/cm^2, total 400–6000 J delivered) for several different vascular tongue lesions (36,37). The laser can be used in conjunction with vascular embolization to correct highly vascular lesions. Complications have included sloughing, mild infection, and some airway obstruction. The Nd:YAG laser should be used with a "punctate nonoverlapping technique" (maintaining 2–4 mm separation

between the 2-mm laser spots) to prevent overlap due to scattering that can produce necrosis. This punctate nonoverlapping technique has been combined with clear slide compression with larger and thicker vascular malformations (36,37).

Malignant Oral Cavity Lesions

Basic oncologic principles allow for the adequate removal of malignant lesions (margins of at least 0.5–1.0 cm) by laser. Well-labeled biopsies and frozen sections should be sent from the remaining margins. The tissue bed and edges can be coagulated or ablated with the laser in the defocused mode. The wound should be left open for direct observation and palpation during follow-up visits.

As discussed, leukoplakia and erythroplakia are both amenable to laser excision and ablation. Carcinoma *in situ*, small verrucous carcinomas, and early invasive T1 lesions can be easily managed with a CO_2 laser or an Nd:YAG laser in a contact mode. In addition, laser surgery can be used for palliation of some malignant lesions that may be unresectable, or in patients with advanced metastatic disease who have symptomatic oral lesions. Partial debulking and control of hemorrhage may be provided with few complications. Painful lesions or functionally impaired lesions can be treated with the laser. Patients with oral or pharyngeal Kaposi's sarcomas can be managed with Nd:YAG laser energy, which makes excision bloodless and allows for both a diminution in the lesion size and decreased bleeding (38–40).

Postoperative Care

Postoperative care is minimal after laser surgery of the oral cavity. Pain, described as soreness to mild burning, can be controlled with Tylenol (McNeil Pharmaceuticals, St. Paul, MN), Tylenol with codeine, or nonsteroidial anti-inflammatory drugs. Most pain subsides within 3–14 days. A course of penicillin is sometime prescribed depending on

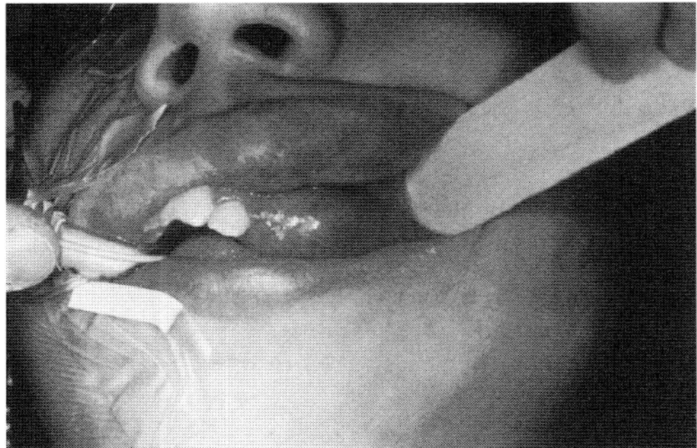

FIG. 7. Cavernous hemangioma of maxillary alveolar ridge.

the type and extent of the surgical lesions. Perioperative intravenous, intraoperative injected, and postoperative oral steroids have been used by some physicians. Normal saline rinses or half strength peroxide rinses have also been used at times. For lesions involving the adjacent buccal-gingival surfaces, postoperative stenting with dressings or packing (dental roll with bacitracin) may reduce adhesion formation, stenoses, or granulation tissue. Postoperative oral exercises may also be beneficial for certain tongue lesions. Again, most lesions heal well with minimal suturing, dressings, and medicines.

The laser affords the surgeon the ability to operate on the oral cavity as an outpatient for many lesions, with decreased pain, bleeding, scarring, and functional loss. It allows for precise excision and delivery of energy that ablates surface or other lesions, leaves the surface unharmed, and coagulates a deep vascular lesion.

REFERENCES

1. Maiman TH: Stimulated optical radiation in ruby. *Nature* 187: 493–494, 1960.
2. Council on Scientific Affairs: Lasers in medicine and surgery. *JAMA* 256(7):900–907, 1986.
3. Ball K: *Lasers: The perioperative challenge.* St. Louis: C.V. Mosby, 1990.
4. Fried MP: Lasers in clinical otolaryngology: Current uses and future applications. *Ear Nose Throat J* 70(12): 843–847, 1994.
5. Ossoff RH, Coleman JA, Courey MS et al: Clinical applications of lasers in otolaryngology-head and neck surgery. *Lasers Surg Med* 15:217–248, 1994.
6. Parkin JL, Davis RK: Laser use in otolaryngology and head and neck surgery. In: Dixon JA, ed. *Surgical application of lasers.* Chicago: Year Book Medical Publishers, 1987:144–159.
7. Schuller DE: Use of the laser in the oral cavity. *Otolaryngol Clin North Am* 23(1):31–42, 1990.
8. Stevens MH: Laser surgery of tonsils, adenoids, and pharynx. *Otolaryngol Clin North Am* 23(1):43–47, 1990.
9. Fuller TA: Fundamentals of laser surgery. In: Fuller TA, ed. *Surgical lasers: A clinical guide.* New York: Macmillan Publishing, 1987:1–17.
10. Fisher SE, Frame JW, Browne RM et al: A comparative histological study of wound healing following CO2 laser and conventional surgical excision of canine buccal mucosa. *Arch Oral Biol* 28(4):287–291, 1983.
11. Parrish JA: Laser photomedicine: Selective laser-tissue interaction. In: Dixon JA, ed. *Surgical application of lasers.* Chicago: Year Book Medical Publishers, 1987: 34–51.
12. White JV, Milner R: Laser-tissue interaction. In: Weisberger EC, ed. *Lasers in head and neck surgery.* New York: Igaku-Shoin, 1991: 17–34.
13. Matchette LS, Faaland RW, Royston DD et al: In vitro production of viable bacteriophage in carbon dioxide and argon laser plumes. *Lasers Surg Med* 11:380–384, 1991.
14. Unthank JL: Fundamental principles of surgical lasers. In: Weisberger EC, ed. *Lasers in head and neck surgery.* New York: Igaku-Shoin, 1991:1–15.
15. DeRowe A, Ophir D, Katzir A: Experimental study of CO2 laser myringotomy with a hand-held otoscope and fiberoptic delivery system. *Lasers Surg Med* 15: 249–253, 1994.
16. Wilder-Smith P, Arrastia AMA, Liaw LH et al: Incision properties and thermal effects of three CO_2 lasers in soft tissue. *Oral Surg Oral Med Oral Pathol* 79(6):685–691, 1995.
17. Barroso EG, Haklin MF, Staren ED: Characteristics of Nd:YAG sculptured contact probes after prolonged laser application. *Lasers Surg Med* 16:76–80, 1995.
18. Bennett WR Jr, Faust WL, McFarlane R, et al. Dissociative excitation transfer and optical maser oscillation in NeO_2 and ArO_2 rf discharges [letter]. *Physiol Rev* 8: 470–473, 1962.
19. White JM, Goodis HE, Rose CL: Use of the pulsed Nd:YAG laser for intraoral soft tissue surgery. *Lasers Surg Med* 11:455–461, 1991.
20. Crawford BE, Callihan MD, Corio RL et al: Oral pathology. *Otolaryngol Clin North Am* 12(1):29–42, 1979.
21. Nash, HS Jr: Benign lesions of the oral cavity. *Otolaryngol Clin North Am* 5(2):207–229, 1972.
22. Baggish MS, Poiesz BJ, Joret D et al: Presence of human immunodeficiency virus DNA in laser smoke. *Lasers Surg Med* 11:197–203, 1991.
23. Wilson M: Photolysis of oral bacteria and its potential use in the treatment of caries and periodontal disease. *J Appl Bacteriol* 75:299–306, 1993.
24. Frame JW: Removal of oral soft tissue pathology with the CO_2 laser. *J Oral Maxillofac Surg* 43:850–855, 1985.
25. Abt E, Wigdor H, Lobraico R et al: Removal of benign intraoral masses using the CO_2 laser. *JADA* 115:729–731, 1987.
26. Hylton RP: Use of CO_2 laser for gingivectomy in a patient with Sturge-Weber disease complicated by dilantin hyperplasia. *J Oral Maxillofac Surg* 44:626–648, 1986.
27. Nanami T, Shiba H, Ikeuchi S et al: Clinical applications and basic studies of laser in dentistry and oral surgery. *Keio J Med* 42(4):199–201, 1993.
28. WHO Collaborating Centre for Oral Precancerous Lesions: Definition of leukoplakia and related lesions: An aid to studies in oral precancer. *Oral Surg* 46:518–539, 1978.
29. Banoczy J: Followup studies in oral leukplakia. *J Oral Maxillofac Surg* 5:69–75, 1977.
30. Silverman S Jr, Gorsby M, Lozada F: Oral leukoplakia and malignant transformation: A follow-up study of 257 patients. *Cancer* 53:563–568, 1984.
31. Chiesa F, Tradati N, Sala L et al: Follow-up of oral leukoplakia after carbon dioxide laser surgery. *Arch Otolaryngol Head Neck Surg* 116:177–180, 1990.
32. Chu FW, Silverman S, Dedo HH: CO_2 laser treatment of oral leukoplakia. *Laryngoscope* 98:125–130, 1988.
33. Frame JW, Gupta RD, Dalton GA et al: Use of the carbon dioxide laser in the management of premalignant lesions of the oral mucosa. *J Laryngol Otol* 98:1251–1260, 1984.
34. Vaughan CW: Supravital staining for early diagnosis

of carcinoma. *Otolaryngol Clin North Am* 5(2): 301–302, 1972.
35. Colvard M, Kuo P: Managing aphthous ulcers: Laser treatment applied. *JADA* 122:51–53, 1991.
36. Dixon JA, Davis RK, Gilbertson JJ: Laser photocoagulation of vascular malformations of the tongue. *Laryngoscope* 96:537–541, 1986.
37. Rebeiz E, April MM, Bohigian RK et al: ND-YAG laser treatment of venous malformations of the head and neck: An update. *Otolaryngol Head Neck Surg* 105: 655–661, 1991.
38. Nagorsky MJ, Sessions DG: Laser resection for early oral cavity cancer: Results and complications. *Ann Otol Rhinol Laryngol* 96:556–560, 1987.
39. Guerry TL, Silverman S, Dedo HH: Carbon dioxide laser resection of superficial oral carcinoma: Indications, technique, and results. *Ann Otol Rhinol Laryngol* 95:547–555, 1986.
40. Strong MS, Vaughan CW, Jako GJ et al: Transoral resection of cancer of the oral cavity: The role of the laser in cancer of the oral cavity. *Otolaryngol Clin North Am* 12(1):207–225, 1979.

Office-Based Surgery of the Head and Neck
Edited by Yosef P. Krespi, MD
Lippincott–Raven Publishers, Philadelphia © 1998

5

Management of Malignant and Premalignant Lesions of the Oral Cavity in the Office

C. Gaelyn Garrett, Brian B. Burkey, and Robert H. Ossoff

Oral cavity cancers account for slightly less than one third of new head and neck cancers each year. The average age at diagnosis is 60 years. Overall, oral cavity cancers represent 4% of cancers in men and 2% in women. Squamous cell carcinomas (SCCA) account for approximately 95% of these cases (1). As in other head and neck regions, tobacco and alcohol exposure have been directly implicated as causative agents in oral cavity squamous cell carcinomas. In addition, the use of snuff has resulted in a higher incidence of oral cavity cancers secondary to prolonged direct mucosal contact with the carcinogens.

ANATOMY, PATHOLOGY, AND STAGING

The anatomic boundaries of the oral cavity include the vermilion border of the upper and lower lips anteriorly; the junction of the hard and soft palate posterosuperiorly; and the circumvallate papillae of the tongue posteroinferiorly. Therefore, the regions of the oral cavity are the lips, the alveolar ridges, the buccal mucosa, the retromolar trigone, the oral tongue, the hard palate, and the floor of mouth.

Premalignant lesions of the head and neck are often picked up on routine examination by the primary-care physician or dentist. Leukoplakic lesions appear clinically as whitish plaques that on histologic examination show hyperkeratosis with or without dysplasia. Erythroplastic lesions are reddish areas that microscopically show a higher rate of dyspla-

sia. These latter lesions have a greater potential for malignant change.

Epidemiologic reviews have shown that most squamous cell carcinomas arise in an area of the oral cavity from the anterior floor of the mouth extending to the retromolar trigone along the gingivobuccal sulcus (1). This is most likely related to the chronic contact of carcinogens found in chewing tobacco and snuff. Less common neoplasms occurring in the oral cavity include those of minor salivary gland origin, such as adenoid cystic carcinoma, adenocarcinoma, and mucoepidermoid carci-

TABLE 1. *TNM Staging for Oral Cavity Squamous Cell Carcinoma*

Primary Tumor (T)	
Tx	Carcinoma *in situ*
T1	≤2 cm in greatest dimension
T2	2–4 cm in greatest dimension
T3	>4 cm in greatest dimension
T4	Invasion of adjacent structures including bone, deep tongue musculature, maxillary sinus, skin
Regional Lymph Nodes (N)	
Nx	Data unavailabe
N0	No nodal metastases
N1	Single ipsilateral node, ≤3 cm
N2	N2a single ipsilateral node, 3–6 cm
	N2b multiple ipsilateral nodes, none >6 cm
	N2c bilateral or contralateral nodes, none >6 cm
N3	Node >6 cm
Distant Metastases (M)	
Mx	Data unavailable
M0	No distant metastases
M1	Distant metastases

Reprinted with permission from American Joint Committee on Cancer: *Manual for staging of cancer*, 4th ed. Philadelphia: JB Lippincott, 1992:29.

noma. Other malignant neoplasms that may be found in the oral cavity include sarcoma, malignant fibrous histiocytoma, lymphoma, and malignant melanoma. Human immune deficiency virus (HIV)-positive patients are at increased risk for SCCA, Kaposi's sarcoma, and non-Hodgkin's lymphoma. Only SCCA are discussed in this chapter.

Staging of oral cavity SCCA is according to the 1992 American Joint Committee on Cancer (Table 1).

CRITERIA FOR OUTPATIENT SURGERY

Select lesions of the oral cavity can be safely resected via outpatient surgery. A 1992 study by Helmus et al. reported on 30 patients with oral cavity lesions who were managed with outpatient surgery (2). Most lesions were T1 cancers of the tongue, palate, floor of mouth, and buccal mucosa. Only one of the patients was eventually admitted postoperatively. No mention was made concerning the type of anesthesia used. However, based on other procedures mentioned, general anesthesia was most likely available.

By definition, the patient arrives for outpatient surgery, and is discharged to home the same day as the procedure. Determining eligibility for outpatient surgical management of select oral cavity carcinomas requires intensive presurgical planning. Factors that need to be considered include both patient and lesion characteristics:

1. Depending on the resources available in the office setting, anesthesia may be limited to local with monitored intravenous sedation, but more extensive excisions may be performed if general anesthesia is available.
2. Pain management and hydration must be achieved with oral intake; therefore, the patient must be able to take fluids by mouth when discharged.
3. Perioperative swelling is expected to be minimal.
4. Closure of the resulting surgical defect should be via primary or secondary closure without the need for extensive reconstruction.
5. There should be no plan for surgical management of the neck at the time of primary excision.

Each of these criteria requires a significant investment in surgical and medical evaluation and planning. Any center wishing to perform ambulatory surgery must be committed to this degree of planning.

All preoperative evaluations must be completed prior to the patient arriving for the day of surgery. Routine laboratory data and other information appropriate to the individual patient are collected and reviewed. Chest radiographs and electrocardiograms are obtained as appropriate. All information necessary for correct TNM staging should be available. This may include imaging studies to evaluate the neck and the extent of the primary tumor in addition to a complete examination of the head and neck. Computed tomography may be necessary to determine bony involvement, especially in the floor of mouth and alveolar ridges.

The overall general health of the patient is important in determining eligibility for ambulatory surgery. Appropriate preoperative medical consultations should be obtained as indicated. Certain patients, regardless of factors related to the oral cavity lesion itself, may not be appropriate candidates for ambulatory surgery. Risk factors, especially tobacco use, associated with the development of head and neck SCCA are also associated with other medical problems, such as heart disease and pulmonary disorders. A significant percentage of head and neck cancer patients will have problems such as coronary artery disease, hypertension, or chronic bronchitis. Perioperative care in these patients may be beyond the scope of an ambulatory surgery center. Patients with cardiac disorders may need perioperative monitoring. Hypertensive patients may require indwelling arterial monitoring. These issues need to be addressed in conjunction with the surgical planning.

Anesthesia support also determines eligibility for ambulatory surgery. Certain sites within the oral cavity are more amenable to excision via local anesthesia (eg, lips, anterior tongue, and floor of mouth). Other sites, although easily accessible clinically, are more difficult to manage in an awake patient without a secure airway or adequate control of secretions. In general, these include the more posterior sites, such as the palate and retromolar trigone. If general anesthesia is an option, these areas may be more easily managed in an outpatient situation.

Adequate hydration and pain management in the immediate postoperative period are mandatory. Therefore, the inability to take fluids by mouth the day of surgery is a relative contraindication for ambulatory surgery. Excision of even small lesions within the oral cavity can be disabling enough in some patients to prevent oral intake soon after the operation. An option would be the temporary insertion of a nasogastric tube for liquid enteral feeding. Pain medication in liquid form would then be prescribed. Another consideration is management of the nausea and vomiting that frequently accompanies surgery. Promethazine suppositories may be given every 4 hours as needed. Inability to control these factors may result in overnight hospital admission to maintain intravenous hydration and patient comfort.

Perioperative swelling is an important factor in determining whether a patient may be safely discharged home after excision of an oral cavity lesion. Unlike other locations in the body, even minimal swelling in the oral cavity can be life-threatening because of airway compromise. Swallowing may also be affected by sufficient swelling. Perioperative steroids may be given to decrease edema. Patients must be evaluated prior to discharge to ensure a safe airway.

Certain defects following oral cavity excision are more appropriately reconstructed using grafts or flaps to preserve function and cosmesis. Factors determining this include size and location of the surgical defect. In general, patients with oral cavity lesions whose resulting excision defect would require more than primary or secondary closure are not candidates for ambulatory surgery.

Discussion of the management of the neck in oral cavity SCCA is beyond the scope of this chapter. If, based on currently accepted criteria, some type of neck dissection is indicated for the specific oral cavity malignancy, then that patient is not eligible for outpatient management of the primary tumor.

LESIONS ELIGIBLE FOR OFFICE EXCISION

A great deal of judgment needs to be used in deciding which oral cavity lesions are eligible for office-based excision. Certainly, many early cancers of the oral cavity are amenable to outpatient management. However, even many early lesions have characteristics that may preclude management of this type. Some small-diameter lesions may have involved deeper structures earlier, necessitating more extensive resection. For example, a floor of mouth cancer <2 cm in size may involve the bone or periosteum of the mandible, necessitating at least a partial mandibulectomy. Further, the site and size of the resulting defect after adequate margins are taken need to be considered. Excision of certain T1 lesions approaching 2 cm may result in a defect approximately 4 cm in diameter to ensure adequate margins. A defect this large in the floor of mouth, for example, usually requires reconstruction with a graft to maximize function. Outpatient management would be precluded in this situation, whereas a similar superficial lesion of the palate will leave a defect that can be allowed to heal secondarily.

Based on the above criteria, only few select oral cavity lesions can be appropriately managed on an outpatient basis. Premalignant lesions, which by definition do not invade beyond the mucosa and do not require a large superficial excision, can be safely excised on an outpatient basis. Similarly, select malignancies can be managed in this manner provided that the surgeon ensures that all the previously mentioned criteria are fulfilled.

Unfortunately, despite their easy clinical access, many oral cavity malignancies tend to be of greater stage when the patient initially presents, necessitating extensive excision, which dictates inpatient perioperative care.

The following lesions by site within the oral cavity may be considered for outpatient management and are the subject of further elaboration:

1. Lips: premalignant lesions or malignant SCCA <2.0 cm that do not involve the commissure; primary closure usually suffices.
2. Alveolar ridges: premalignant lesions or malignant SCCA <2.0 cm not involving periosteum or bone of mandible; closure may occur by secondary intention.
3. Buccal mucosa: premalignant lesions or malignant SCCA ≤2.0 cm with superficial involvement and located more anteriorly; primary closure or closure by secondary intention usually suffices.
4. Retromolar trigone: premalignant lesions or malignant SCCA ≤2.0 cm without bone involvement; closure may occur by secondary intention.
5. Oral tongue: premalignant lesions or malignant SCCA ≤2.0 cm; primary closure usually suffices.
6. Hard palate: premalignant lesions or malignant SCCA ≤2.0 cm with superficial involvement only; closure may occur by secondary intention.
7. Floor of mouth: premalignant or malignant SCCA ≤1.5 cm; closure may be primary or secondary.

These criteria should serve as guidelines only and are not absolute. Each patient should be evaluated individually for management options.

Management of lip carcinomas, which account for most oral cavity carcinomas, is well described. In general, defects one half or less the length of the lip can be closed primarily after full-thickness wedge resection. Most surgeons accept 5–10-mm margins of normal-appearing mucosa around the lesion. As the average transverse length of the upper and lower lips is 7–8 cm, the resulting defect can

approach 3–4 cm. Therefore, the actual size of the lesion can be up to 2 cm to result in a surgical defect that can be closed primarily. These are potentially manageable by outpatient surgery. Superficial carcinomas and carcinoma *in situ* can be managed with vermilionectomy and advancement of mucosa.

Alveolar ridge carcinomas are relatively uncommon, with most occurring on the inferior alveolus. Only those lesions that are superficial and not involving bone or periosteum should be considered for outpatient management. In general, safe margins should be approximately 8–10 mm around the lesion. Reconstruction of the resulting defect depends on the size and the extension onto the floor of mouth or buccal mucosa. Defects with minimal or no involvement of these adjacent areas can be left to granulate in by secondary intention. Larger defects should be closed with split-thickness skin grafts to prevent contracture. As a general guideline, defects from lesions <2.0 cm in length along the alveolus can be left to granulate.

Buccal mucosa carcinomas are also uncommon, accounting for 5%–10% of all oral cavity neoplasms. Unfortunately, few cases of buccal carcinomas present early, with approximately 50% of patients presenting with evidence of cervical metastases. Verrucous carcinomas have a better prognosis than ulcerative lesions, as do more anteriorly located lesions. Involvement of Stensen's duct creates a greater complexity of the excision, and therefore may limit the appropriateness of outpatient surgery. Surgical management of superficial and exophytic lesions can be accomplished via transoral excision with local anesthesia. Acceptable margins are between 10 and 20 mm around the lesion. Well-differentiated and verrucous lesions may have the smaller margins. It is important to note that buccal defects tend to be larger than the size of the excised tissue owing to unopposed elastic forces. In general, superficial lesions ≤2.0 cm in diameter can be managed with local excision and primary closure of the defect (Fig. 1). Larger lesions will most likely require closure with a skin graft or flap to prevent contracture.

Isolated lesions of the retromolar trigone are uncommon as they frequently involve the soft palate or anterior tonsillar pillar. Carcinomas in this area often invade the periosteum or bone of the mandible earlier owing to the adherence of the mucosa over the ascending ramus. This involvement would obviously preclude outpatient management. However, select T1 carcinomas (ie, ≤2.0 cm) and small premalignant lesions may be amenable to excision with local anesthesia on an outpatient basis if the resulting surgical defect with adequate margins allows for closure via granulation and secondary healing. Grafting is not usually necessary for these lesions in the retromolar trigone because the support of surrounding structures prevents contracture.

The major concerns for outpatient management of oral tongue lesions are speech and swallowing functions following excision and closure. Consequently, larger defects, especially those involving the floor of mouth, usually require skin graft or flap closure to prevent tethering of the tongue. Certain lesions ≤2.0 cm can be managed with excision and primary closure and still maintain adequate speech and swallowing. Superficial T1 carcinomas and premalignant lesions, which require a smaller margin around the defect, are obviously more amenable to outpatient management (Fig. 2). The issue concerning prophylactic neck therapy in T1 lesions of the oral tongue is controversial, but must be considered prior to planning management of the primary lesion.

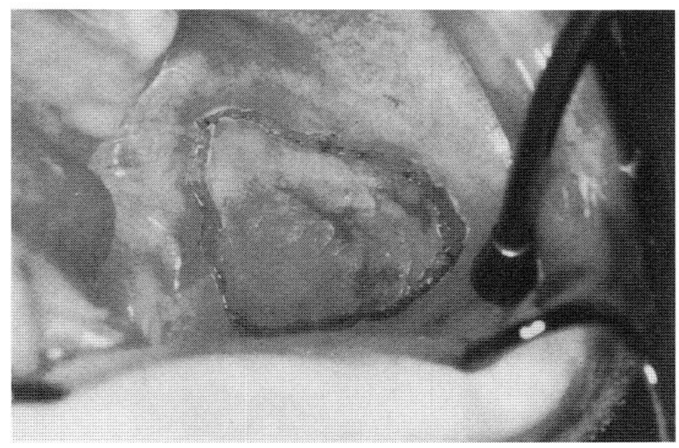

FIG. 2. Photograph of a T1 SCCA of the buccal mucosa. The margin of excision has been outlined prior to excision with the CO_2 laser. The defect was left to close secondarily.

Superficial T1 hard palate carcinomas and premalignant lesions ≤2.0 cm can be managed by local resection under local anesthesia in select patients. The resulting defect would be left to granulate and heal by secondary intention. A prosthodontics evaluation may be obtained for fitting of a temporary palate guard to improve patient comfort postoperatively. Deeper lesions may involve the bone of the maxilla, thus necessitating some type of maxillectomy. An apparently small hard palate lesion may also represent extension from a primary maxillary sinus cancer that has eroded bone. Therefore, computed tomography scanning may be indicated as part of the preoperative evaluation.

Small, superficial T1 floor of mouth cancers and premalignant lesions can be excised on an outpatient basis with the defect left to granulate. Because of the potential for contracture and resulting tethering of the tongue, only lesions ≤1.5 cm should be considered for closure without grafting. In addition, larger T1 lesions usually require prophylactic treatment of the neck with possible dissection.

SURGICAL TECHNIQUE

Once the decision is made to proceed with outpatient management of the oral cavity lesion, other factors need to be considered. These include the type of anesthesia available and the surgical technique to be used. Outpatient surgery in an office-based setting would

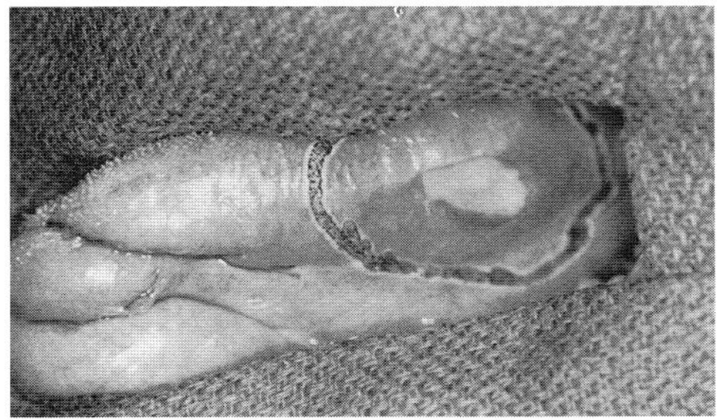

FIG. 1. Photograph of a small T1 SCCA of the lateral oral tongue. The margin of excision has been outlined with a hand-held CO_2 laser. The defect was closed primarily.

most likely be limited to local anesthesia with or without intravenous sedation. Appropriate cardiopulmonary monitoring should always be available along with personnel trained in its use. Emergency code or crash carts are also required if intravenous sedation is used.

Several methods are available for the resection of oral cavity carcinomas and premalignant lesions. These include cold steel instrumentation, electrocautery, and various lasers, which may be used alone or in combination. Oncologically, these modalities offer no advantage over one another (3). Also, studies have shown no difference in final wound strength between the laser and scalpel (4). Instrument selection is according to the surgeon's personal preference; however, certain advantages do exist for each modality.

The cold knife is the traditional instrument used for excision. It is the least expensive method providing precise cutting with sparing of surrounding tissue. Electrocautery is a useful adjunct to cold steel to control bleeding. Cautery may also be used to resect the lesion without the use of a cold scalpel. However, cautery artifact may hamper histologic analysis of tissue margins.

The carbon dioxide (CO_2) laser is a popular instrument for resection of oral cavity carcinomas and premalignant lesions (3,5–7). Its wavelength of 10.6 μm is in the infrared portion of the spectrum. When applied to tissue, the CO_2 laser results in the conversion of water to steam, causing cell membrane disruption, heating of cell contents, and cell death. The surrounding zone of thermal injury is less than with standard electrocautery, especially with the newer generation of microspot manipulators. Tissue margins, therefore, are preserved for histologic examination. Other cited advantages of the laser are its hemostatic effect on blood vessels <0.5 mm in diameter and decreased postoperative edema and pain. These features are important in treating lesions located in the richly vascular tissue of the oral cavity.

The CO_2 laser can be used with either an operating microscope and attached micromanipulator or with a hand-held adaptor. Supravital staining with toluidine blue may enhance areas of dysplasia in and around the lesion. Anterior lesions, especially those on the oral tongue, are amenable to resection with the hand-held adaptor, which has a focal length of 125 mm. Other lesions can be resected using the microscope adaptor. This is a hands-free method offering a magnified view of the lesion without the interference of a hand-held device. Unfortunately, frequent repositioning of either the patient or the microscope may be necessary as a result of the size of the lesion or the movement of an awake patient. Use of the CO_2 laser dictates strict adherence to laser safety protocols. These include protection of exposed areas on the patient with moist towels or drapes. Moist eye pads should be used. All personnel in the procedure room also need protective eyewear.

Some surgeons have described using the CO_2 laser to ablate leukoplakic lesions in the oral cavity rather than excising them (8). Equipment used for office-based laser-assisted uvulopalatoplasty can be used. This consists of a SwiftLase laser scanner (Sharplan, Allendale, NJ) that sweeps the focused laser beam over the affected area based on the principle of space modulation. The beam moves rapidly and homogeneously over the area ensuring an exposure time of <1 ms on individual sites within the area. The resulting shallow wound bed is free of char and is left to heal secondarily. Adequate tissue biopsies should be performed on all these lesions before proceeding with ablation rather than excision.

POSTOPERATIVE CARE

Regardless of technique used, patients undergoing outpatient transoral excision of an oral cavity lesion should be observed postoperatively for at least 4 hours for signs of bleeding and airway obstruction. Adequate pain management may consist of an intramuscular injection of narcotic immediately after the procedure and oral medication to take at home.

Broad spectrum oral antibiotics will decrease bacterial contamination within the mouth and decrease the duration of postoperative pain in those patients with open wounds. These should be continued until the wound has healed. Oral rinses after meals with a half-strength mixture of hydrogen peroxide and water will enhance oral hygiene. A bland soft diet, such as a post-tonsillectomy diet, is recommended. Follow-up should consist of a telephone call the next day by an office nurse or physician's assistant and an office visit within 7–10 days. The results of permanent histopathologic examination should be reviewed to determine whether adequate margins were taken. Routine cancer follow-up is then initiated.

CONCLUSION

Physicians and administrators of health care are dedicated to developing the most efficient system while maintaining excellent patient care. Outpatient or office-based management of disease is a cornerstone of the continuing evolution in health care. Such management of certain head and neck cancers, including oral cavity cancers, may be safely accomplished when the previously described criteria are satisfied.

REFERENCES

1. Baden E: Prevention of cancer of the oral cavity and pharynx. *Cancer J Clin* 37:49–62, 1987.
2. Helmus C, Grin M, Westfall R: Same-day-stay head and neck surgery. *Laryngoscope* 102:1331–1334, 1992.
3. Panje WR, Scher N, Karnell M: Transoral carbon dioxide laser ablation for cancer, tumors, and other diseases. *Arch Otolaryngol Head Neck Surg* 115:681–688, 1989.
4. Buell BR, Schuller DE: Comparative analysis of tensile strength in CO_2 laser and scalpel skin incisions. *Arch Otolaryngol Head Neck Surg* 109:465–467, 1983.
5. Duncavage JA, Ossoff RH: Use of the CO_2 laser for malignant disease of the oral cavity. *Lasers Surg Med* 6:442–444, 1986.
6. Guerry TL, Silverman S, Dedo HH: Carbon dioxide laser resection of superficial oral carcinoma: Indications, technique, and results. *Ann Otol Rhinol Laryngol* 95:547–555, 1986.
7. Roodenburg JLN, Panders AK, Vermey A: Carbon dioxide laser surgery of oral leukoplakia. *Oral Surg Oral Med Oral Pathol* 71:670–674, 1991.
8. Barak S, Mintz S, Katz J: The role of lasers in ambulatory oral maxillofacial surgery. *Op Tech Otolaryngol* 5(4):244–249, 1994.

PART 3

The Pharynx and Larynx

Office-Based Surgery of the Head and Neck
Edited by Yosef P. Krespi, MD
Lippincott–Raven Publishers, Philadelphia © 1998

6

The State of the Art in the Evaluation of Snoring and Sleep-Related Breathing Disorders

Gary K. Zammit and Lynn Weatherby

The advent of laser-assisted uvulopalatoplasty (LAUP) (1,2) has contributed to a recent increase in the number of patients who undergo sleep laboratory evaluation for snoring and sleep-related breathing disorders. This is owing to the need to document the complaint of snoring, as well as to determine the presence and extent of upper airway resistance or obstructive sleep apnea prior to surgery. Sleep laboratory studies are essential to the development of appropriate treatment plans, especially with respect to the identification of patients who require mechanical or other treatments for sleep-related breathing disorders. This chapter defines the features of snoring and sleep-related breathing disorders, offers clinical practice guidelines for use in the evaluation of these disorders, and reviews the state of the art in clinical polysomnography as an essential diagnostic tool for the evaluation of snoring and sleep-related breathing disorders.

SNORING

Epidemiologic studies indicate that snoring is common in the general population. One study of 5713 individuals has shown that approximately 19% of adults describe themselves as habitual snorers (3). This corresponds to 24.1% of the male and 13.8% of the female population. Up to the age of 30 years, approximately 10% of men and less than 5% of women are habitual snorers, whereas more than 60% of men and 40% of women between

the ages of 60 and 65 years describe themselves as such. Obesity is one factor that contributes to snoring (4,5). When survey samples are divided between normal-weight individuals and those >15% above ideal body weight, only 34% of the normal-weight group reported habitual snoring, whereas >50% of the overweight group reported habitual snoring.

Snoring may be defined as an audible and typically loud recurrent breath sound during sleep that occurs on inspiration and that varies in intensity with breath volume and frequency. It is produced by the vibration of soft tissue, including the tonsils, soft palate, uvula, and other structures of the oropharyngeal airway (6). Snoring is the result of several contributing factors, including conditions that compromise upper airway patency, such as a small or narrow airway, nasal polyps, deviated septum, or enlarged turbinates. Such conditions produce an increase in airway resistance (7) and negative intraluminal pressure during inspiration, resulting in traction and vibration of tissues in the upper airway. Other functional factors that contribute to snoring include the decrease in upper airway muscle tone that occurs during sleep. It has been shown that the function of the dilator muscles in snorers may be delayed or absent on inspiration, resulting in pharyngeal collapse at lower negative intraluminal pressures than normal (8).

Snoring never arises spontaneously during wakefulness, but may occur immediately at sleep onset. It is possible for snoring to begin during the transition from wakefulness to sleep, at the first signs of stage I sleep, or at subsequent points in the sleep period. Its occurrence may be continuous or intermittent throughout the night, and it appears to be found with equal intensity in all sleep stages. However, some reports have suggested that snoring is worse during non-rapid eye movement (non-REM) sleep (6). REM sleep, which is associated with a decline in respiratory efficiency, does not appear to be associated with an increase in snoring frequency or volume.

Body position during sleep is one important factor in the occurrence of snoring. Snoring is most likely to occur when the patient is in the supine position, and less likely when prone or lateral (9,10). The transient improvement in snoring when adopting the latter position is obvious to spouses who request that the offending sleeper "roll over," which has led to the development of devices that can be used in the treatment of snoring (eg, use of a body position monitor or alarm, sewing a tennis ball in the back of one's pajamas to discourage sleeping in the supine position) (10–12). Hypothyroidism (6) and tobacco use (4,5) have also been found to be associated with snoring, which contributes to greater long-term risk. Acute and prominent increases in snoring may result from nasal congestion due to common colds or allergies, sleep deprivation, and the use of alcohol or sedative or hypnotic agents (13–15).

For many years, snoring was considered an annoying but otherwise benign problem. The International Classification of Sleep Disorders includes a category of "primary snoring" that is characterized by loud upper airway breathing sounds in the absence of apnea, hypoventilation, or serious medical sequelae (16). However, recent data suggest that snoring may be associated with serious health risks (17). Habitual snoring is known to be associated with hypertension (3,14,18–20) and heart disease (21), and has also been found to be associated with myocardial (22) and brain infarct (23,24). It has been shown that habitual snorers are as much as 10.3 times more likely to suffer a stroke than those who never or only occasionally snore (21,25). Snoring

may also result in significant sleep disruption or fragmentation (19), which may lead to daytime fatigue, sleepiness, or occupational and safety risks due to performance impairment (19, 26,27).

Perhaps the most significant health risk of snoring is its association with serious sleep-related breathing disorders such as obstructive sleep apnea. Snoring may be the "alarm mechanism" that alerts the sleeper or bed partner to the occurrence of periods of hypopnea or upper airway resistance, or the termination of apneic events. In fact, it may be the only reported symptom of obstructive sleep apnea or upper airway resistance, and the only symptom that prompts the patient to seek treatment, even when severe obstructive sleep apnea is present.

OBSTRUCTIVE SLEEP APNEA

Sleep apnea is a sleep-related breathing disorder that is thought to affect between 1% and 10% of the general population (28–30). The most recent epidemiologic data indicate that 2% of women and 4% of men between the ages of 30 and 60 years meet the minimal diagnostic criteria for sleep apnea syndrome (31). This may be a lower estimate of prevalence than is suggested by studies of elderly samples, as it appears that respiratory events during sleep increase with advanced age (32). In studies of people over the age of 65 years, it has been reported that 24% of people living independently, 33% in acute care inpatient facilities, and 42% in nursing homes have more than five apneic events per hour of sleep, which is the minimal criterion typically used to diagnose sleep apnea in adults (33).

There are several factors that predispose patients to sleep apnea. The disorder is more common in men, with the male-to-female ratio estimated between 3:1 and 20:1 (31,34). Although sleep apnea may first appear at any age, most cases are identified when patients are between the ages of 40 and 60 years. In women, the disorder is more commonly diagnosed after menopause (33), possibly due to the increased risk associated with aging or hormonal changes. Obesity is a significant risk factor and is thought to contribute significantly to the development of sleep apnea (35). Recent surveys of patients presenting with the complaint of loud snoring found that obesity is the only clinical variable that has predictive value in identifying patients with sleep apnea, with body weight accounting for 41% of the variance in the sample (36).

Sleep apnea is characterized by multiple respiratory pauses during sleep. These pauses, or apneas, are defined as the complete cessation of airflow measured at the level of the nose and mouth lasting at least 10 seconds (35). The duration of most apneic events exceeds this minimal criterion. The average duration of apneic events in an individual with sleep apnea is between 30 and 40 seconds, and there have been documented events lasting as long as 3 minutes (37).

Partial reductions in airflow are known as hypopneas. Hypopneas are defined as the reduction of airflow measured at the level of the nose and mouth lasting at least 10 seconds. They are associated with oxygen desaturation and evidence of electroencephalographic (EEG) or electromyographic (EMG) arousal. The mean duration of hypopneic events in an individual with sleep apnea tends to be similar to the duration of apneic events.

Obstructive apneas and hypopneas result from similar mechanisms that impede airflow during sleep. Consequently, individuals with sleep apnea often have both apneic and hypopneic events during the sleep period. Another pattern of sleep-disordered breathing that has been recently described is known as the "upper airway resistance syndrome" (38,39). This disturbance is associated with modest reductions in airflow during sleep that often are not detected by conventional recording methods. Measures of intraesophageal pressure may be required to detect the subtle respiratory characteristic of upper airway resistance. These changes in respiration can result in EEG arousals during sleep that are similar to those seen in sleep apnea. Arousals as short as 3 seconds may be characteristic of upper airway resistance in some cases. Episodes of upper airway resistance may occur in patients with sleep apnea, although the upper airway resistance syndrome has been found to occur independently of sleep apnea.

Individuals with sleep apnea experience multiple respiratory events during sleep. These events recur throughout the sleep period, and may worsen during REM sleep (37). A minimum of five apneic or hypopneic events per hour of sleep is required to diagnose sleep apnea (16) and, therefore, at least 40 events should be detected during a normal 8-hour sleep recording. However, most people with sleep apnea have many more events. It has been found that the average number of apneic events per hour of non-REM sleep is 65 (range, 48–79), and the average number of apneic events per hour of REM sleep is 42 (range, 17–90) in patients with sleep apnea (40). The recurrence of respiratory events during the sleep period appears to have two main consequences: It results in sleep fragmentation and intermittent transient declines in oxygen saturation. Sleep fragmentation can be so severe that it interferes with sleep architecture and with the occurrence of delta and REM sleep (41). There appears to be a relationship between sleep fragmentation and the severity of daytime sleepiness associated with sleep apnea (42–44). Oxygen desaturation may possibly contribute to complaints of daytime sleepiness, but it is more likely a contributor to the cognitive deficits seen in some patients with sleep apnea (45).

The diagnosis of sleep apnea syndrome is not made exclusively on the basis of respiratory disturbance during sleep. Clinical signs and symptoms that define this disorder are listed in Table 1. Perhaps the two most common signs are snoring and excessive daytime sleepiness. Virtually all patients with obstructive sleep apnea snore, with 94% reporting the development of loud snoring before the age of 21 (40). Snoring is frequently loud, stridorous, and interrupted by snorts or other unusual sounds. It is commonly a source of annoyance or embarrassment, and can be quite disturbing to a bed partner. Many individuals with sleep

TABLE 1. *Symptoms of Obstructive Sleep Apnea*

Night-time Symptoms
  Loud, bothersome snoring
  Witnessed apneas
  Awakenings secondary to gasping for air/choking
  Awakenings associated with a sense of dread or
    anxiety
  Restless or fitful sleep
  Nocturnal or morning confusion ("sleep
    drunkenness")
  Polyuria
Daytime Symptoms
  Morning sluggishness, fatigue
  Excessive daytime sleepiness
  Dry mouth/sore throat upon awakening
  Early morning headaches
  Impaired memory
  Difficulty concentrating
  Personality changes such as irritability, anxiety, or
    depression
  Decreased motivation or "laziness"
  Diminished libido
Associated Physical Symptoms/Findings
  Cardiac arrhythmia
  Hypertension
  Stroke
  Angina
  Peripheral edema
  Polycythemia
  Hypothyroidism

---

apnea have been evicted from their bedrooms because of loud snoring, and some can relate memorable stories of disturbing others in adjoining rooms or apartments.

Excessive daytime sleepiness is considered the primary daytime manifestation of sleep apnea (46). Subjective complaints of daytime sleepiness are common among individuals with sleep apnea, who often report drowsiness, napping, or falling asleep at inappropriate times. When given the opportunity to sleep during the day on the multiple sleep latency test (MSLT), individuals with sleep apnea have been shown to have a mean latency to stage I sleep of 2.6 minutes across four naps, revealing that this group of patients is excessively sleepy during the day (47). It must be kept in mind that there is variability among individuals with respect to the severity of daytime sleepiness and to the likelihood that they will report these problems to a physician. Mild symptoms, such as fatigue or the ten-

dency to doze in sedentary situations, may be the only evidence of daytime sleepiness. These symptoms may not be immediately recognized as a problem (48), and can be easily dismissed if the patient is not questioned carefully. Fatigue-related cognitive impairment may reveal itself as occasional attention or memory lapses (45), which may be another indicator of daytime sleepiness. Severe symptoms of sleepiness are often characterized by reports of difficulty sustaining alertness in virtually any situation, with some patients reporting that they fall asleep at work, while socializing, at meal times, or when operating a motor vehicle. The latter has been documented by studies of actual and simulated driving showing that individuals with sleep apnea perform more poorly than normal control subjects (49,50). Severe daytime sleepiness can be debilitating owing to its impact on social and occupational functioning, and can result in the risk of accident or injury due to performance failure. Other common symptoms of sleep apnea are listed in Table 1.

Sleep apnea presents a serious health risk. Hypertension is common. Podszus (51) has reported that the prevalence of systemic hypertension averaged 58% among 461 sleep apnea patients evaluated in four studies (52–55). Hypertension correlates with the risk factors that are commonly associated with sleep apnea, especially age and weight. These findings are complemented by sleep laboratory studies of hypertensive patients with no sleep complaints showing that up to one half meet minimal criteria for the diagnosis of sleep apnea, and one third have apnea indices $\geq$20 (56). Cardiac arrhythmias are also common. Approximately 48% of patients with sleep apnea have cardiac arrhythmias (57). The most common types of cardiac events observed are premature ventricular contractions and sinus arrest between 2.5 and 13 seconds in duration (40). In some patients, transient periods of bradycardia occur during apneic or hypopneic events, followed by tachycardia when respiration resumes. Oxygen desaturation during the night can lead to hypoxemia, and there have been reports of seizures occurring in association with desaturation (40). The frequent desaturation associated with sleep apnea occasionally results in polycythemia. One evaluation of 1000 patients has found that 7% of those with unexplained polycythemia have sleep apnea (35). One of the most important health risks associated with sleep apnea is increased mortality (24,58). A 9-year longitudinal study of untreated patients with sleep apnea (59) found that those with ≥20 apneic events per hour of sleep had a high mortality rate, with a cumulative probability of survival of only 0.63, whereas those with <20 had a cumulative probability of survival of 0.96. These data underscore the need for the early detection and treatment of sleep apnea.

CLINICAL EVALUATION OF SNORING AND SLEEP-RELATED BREATHING DISORDERS

Consultation

The evaluation of snoring and sleep-related breathing disorders begins with a thorough diagnostic interview. The presence of loud snoring alone is not pathognomonic of sleep apnea or other respiratory disturbance during sleep. However, snoring that occurs in association with obesity or other associated features (see Table 1) may be indicative of a serious sleep-related breathing disorder. It is critically important that a careful inquiry be made during consultation, as many patients will deny the presence of clinically significant symptoms. Interview of the patient's spouse or bed partner often yields helpful information regarding night-time symptoms, daytime sleepiness, and social and occupational functioning. Current practice guidelines acknowledge the serious health and safety risks associated with sleep apnea syndrome, and dictate that practitioners exercise caution and thoroughness in the evaluation and follow-up of snoring and sleep-related breathing disorders. Snoring, the warning signal that often prompts the patient to seek medical care, may be eliminated by procedures such as LAUP or uvulopalatopharyngoplasty without significant impact on serious breathing disorders such as upper airway resistance or sleep apnea syndrome.

Polysomnography

The diagnosis of sleep-related breathing disorders is usually confirmed using standard all-night polysomnography (level I polysomnography) (Table 2). Polysomnography is usually performed in a sleep laboratory environment, although advances in technology have made it possible to perform this procedure at the patient's home or hospital bedside. The essential feature of polysomnography is the EEG. The EEG, usually obtained from parietal leads placed in the C_3 or C_4 positions, is used to determine the occurrence of wakefulness and the distinctive patterns of brain electrical activity that are characteristic of sleep. Relaxed wakefulness is characterized by low-voltage fast EEG activity in the 8–13 Hz range. This is usually observed just prior to sleep onset and during awakenings. There are five stages of sleep (60) (Fig. 1). Stage I sleep may be associated with the appearance of slow, rolling eye movements, and is characterized by low-voltage, slow-frequency EEG activity in the 3–7 Hz range. Stage I is a transitional stage of sleep that typically occurs at sleep onset, during sleep stage shifts, and following arousal. This is of importance, as patients with sleep-related breathing disorders often have an elevated percentage of stage I sleep due to respiratory events. Stage II sleep is characterized by low-voltage mixed EEG activity that is punctuated by phasic events known as k-complexes and sleep spindles. A k-complex is a sharp negative wave ≥75 μV that is immediately followed by a sharp positive wave. They are typically about 0.5 second in duration. A sleep spindle is a burst of fast EEG activity in the 12–15 Hz range that lasts at least 0.5 second. Stage II sleep comprises most of the night for most healthy adult sleepers. Stages III and IV sleep, otherwise known as slow-wave sleep or delta

TABLE 2. *Diagnostic Studies for Snoring and Sleep-Related Breathing Disorders*

	Level I Standard Polysomnography	Level IA Standard Portable Polysomnography	Level II Comprehensive Portable Polysomnography	Level III Modified Portable Sleep Apnea Testing
Parameters	Minimum of 7, including EEG (C_4–A_1 or C_3–A_2), EOG, chin EMG, ECG, airflow, respiratory effort, SaO_2	Minimum of 7, including EEG (C_4–A_1 or C_3–A_2), EOG, chin EMG, ECG, airflow, respiratory effort, SaO_2	Minimum of 7, including EEG (C_4–A_1 or C_3–A_2), EOG, chin EMG, ECG, airflow, respiratory effort, SaO_2	Minimum of 4, including ventilation (at least 2 channels of respiratory movement or respiratory movement and airflow), heart rate or ECG, SaO_2
Body Position	Documented or objectively measured	Documented or objectively measured	May be objectively measured	May be objectively measured
Leg Movement	EMG or motion sensor desirable but optional	EMG or motion sensor desirable but optional	EMG or motion sensor desirable but optional	May be recorded
Personnel	In constant attendance	In constant attendance	Not in attendance	Not in attendance
Interventions	Possible	Possible	Not possible	Not possible
Location	Laboratory	Laboratory/home/institution	Home/institution	Home/institution

EEG, electroencephalogram; EOG, electro-oculogram; EMG, electromyogram; ECG, electrocardiogram; SaO_2, oxygen saturation.

Adapted from Ferber R, Millman R, Coppola M et al: Portable recording in the assessment of obstructive sleep apnea. *Sleep* 17:378–392, 1994.

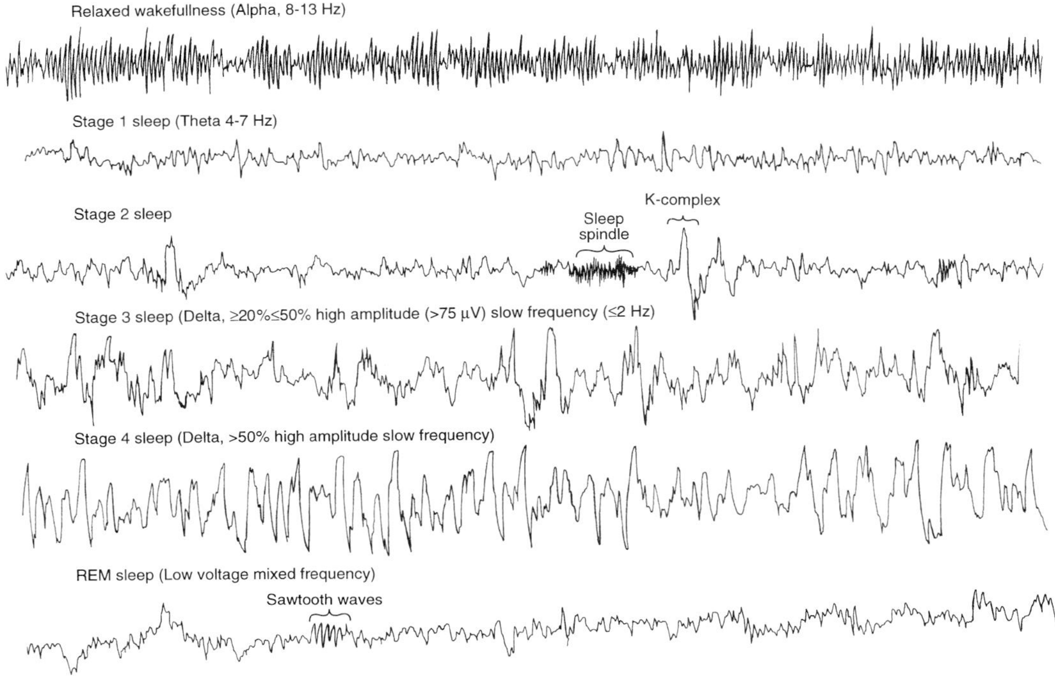

FIG. 1. Recording samples of electroencepalographic (EEG) activity obtained during relaxed wakefulness and the five stages of sleep. Stage I sleep is characterized by slowing of the electroencephalograph (EEG) into the 4–7 Hz range. Stage II sleep is distinguished by the appearance of phasic events known as sleep spindles and k-complexes. Stages III and IV sleep are characterized by slow-frequency, high-amplitude delta waves. The EEG during rapid eye movement (REM) sleep is a low-voltage, mixed-frequency pattern that is accompanied by electromyographic (EMG) hypotonia and rapid conjugate eye movements (not shown).

sleep, are characterized by high-amplitude (<75 µV), low-frequency (1–2 Hz) waves. Delta sleep usually comprises less than 20% of the sleep period in healthy young adults, but is thought to be associated with deep and restful sleep. REM sleep is characterized by a low-voltage, mixed-frequency EEG with occasional "sawtooth" waves and is accompanied by phasic rapid conjugate eye movements and a tonic decrease in muscle tone.

Night-time sleep is organized. Figure 2A depicts the sleep architecture of a healthy young adult sleeper. Note that the subject begins the night with a brief episode of stage I sleep, which cascades into stages II, III, and IV sleep. The first REM period, which is brief, occurs approximately 90 minutes following sleep onset. This pattern, known as a sleep cycle, repeats itself multiple times over the course of the night. As the sleep period continues, the percentages of stages III and IV (delta) sleep normally decline and the percentage of REM sleep increases. The organization of night-time sleep is critical to the evaluation of snoring and sleep-related breathing disorders because these disorders often disrupt or fragment the normal architecture of sleep. Figure 2B is a representation of sleep architecture in a patient with severe obstructive sleep apnea. Note the frequent shifts into stage I sleep, the low amounts of delta and REM sleep, and the fragmentation of REM sleep during the sleep period.

When polysomnography is used clinically to detect sleep-related breathing disorders, multiple variables are measured. Standard

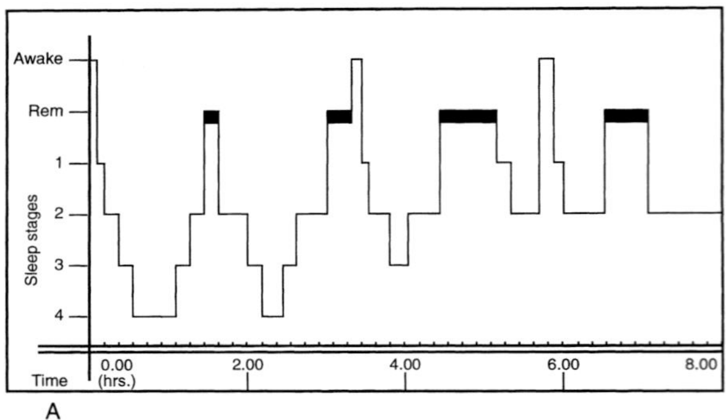

A

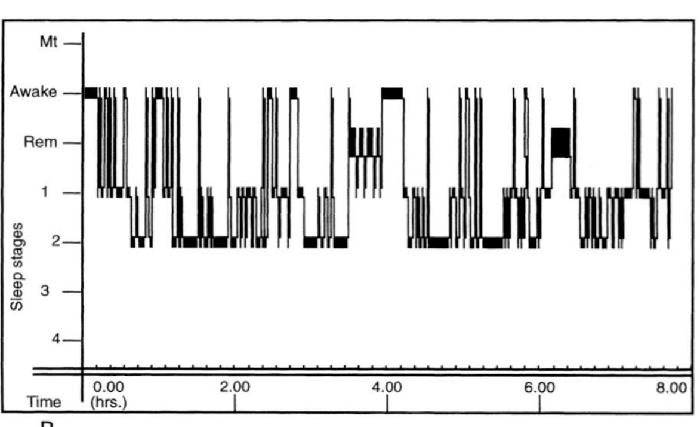

B

FIG. 2. A. Graphic representation of sleep architecture in a healthy young adult. The night is initiated with a brief period of stage I sleep, which is followed in orderly succession by stages II, III, IV, and rapid eye movement (REM). It is normal for the percentage of delta sleep to decline and the percentage of REM sleep to increase as the night progresses. **B.** Graphic representation of sleep architecture in a patient with severe obstructive sleep apnea. There are multiple arousals and brief awakenings secondary to apneas, hypopneas, and upper airway resistance. There is also a marked disruption of sleep architecture, characterized by the absence of delta sleep and the fragmentation and reduction of REM sleep.

measures are those performed in standard level I polysomnography (see Table 2). These recordings are sufficient to quantify and characterize sleep stages and architecture as well as the occurrence, nature, and severity of episodes of apnea, hypopnea, and possibly upper airway resistance. The key diagnostic indicators used to determine the presence and severity of a sleep-related breathing disorder include the number of awakenings, number of arousals, and sleep efficiency (the percentage of time in bed that is spent asleep). These measures indicate the degree of sleep fragmentation that may be due to respiratory disturbance. Sleep stage percentages provide a measure of the disruption of sleep architecture. As the severity of the disorder increases, the percentage of stage I sleep increases, and the percentages of delta and REM sleep tend to decrease. Measures of airflow and respiratory effort are used to detect respiratory events, which are often reported in the apnea/hypopnea index or respiratory disturbance in-

dex. These values indicate the average number of apneic and hypopneic events per hour of sleep. Baseline, average, and nadir SaO_2 values during desaturation provide a measure of apnea severity and hypoxemia during sleep. These values are often used to determine the number of times that SaO_2 falls below normal, which is considered to be an SaO_2 of 90%. Finally, the single-lead electrocardiogram (ECG) is a measure of heart rate and rhythm that provides an index of the cardiac arrhythmias that are commonly observed in patients with sleep apnea.

In addition to measures that are obtained at night, it is frequently useful to have data from the MSLT. The MSLT is a test of daytime sleepiness that provides the patient with multiple scheduled opportunities to nap during the day. The latency to sleep onset for each nap period is calculated and an average is obtained. This average is compared with normative data to determine if the patient is pathologically sleepy. Healthy normal subjects have a mean sleep latency between 10 and 20 minutes, and many subjects will not fall asleep at all. Mean latencies of <5 minutes are indicative of a pathologic degree of daytime sleepiness (61). This finding may be crucial in deciding whether or not to treat mild cases of sleep-related breathing disorders. The MSLT is also one critical measure of treatment effectiveness. For example, a patient with obstructive sleep apnea who is restricted from driving because of excessive daytime sleepiness may require documentation that treatment has resulted in normal levels of daytime alertness.

Postoperative Follow-Up

Postoperative follow-up with level I polysomnography is an important consideration for patients who have undergone upper airway surgery for snoring or sleep-related breathing disorders. If surgery was performed to treat primary snoring as documented by polysomnography, short-term postoperative follow-up in the sleep laboratory may not be necessary. However, long-term office follow-up is advised to ensure that sleep-related breathing disorders do not develop in the absence of snoring. It is critical to avoid the development of "silent" sleep apnea, which potentially increases morbidity and mortality without warning the patient. This is especially important to consider as the patient ages or increases body weight. When upper airway surgery is performed as a treatment for sleep apnea or another sleep-related breathing disorder, follow-up with polysomnography is crucial to determine treatment efficacy, as well as the need for adjunctive treatments (eg, nasal continuous positive airway pressure). All patients who have been successfully treated for a sleep-related breathing disorder should be seen periodically for follow-up visits in the office and, if indicated, in the laboratory to ensure that symptoms of the disorder have not returned and that there is no impairment in daytime alertness or functioning.

POLYSOMNOGRAPHIC EQUIPMENT USED IN THE EVALUATION OF SNORING AND SLEEP-RELATED BREATHING DISORDERS

Conventional Recording Equipment

Since the development of the EEG machine in 1928 (62), the measurement of mammalian sleep has been associated with the recording of brain electrical activity. Adopted as a tool for the evaluation of sleep disorders in the 1950s, the EEG machine is now considered to be the single most important piece of equipment used in the recording of human sleep, and it is essential to the execution of complete clinical diagnostic recordings. It is remarkable that the state of the art in sleep recording continues to include technology and methods that were developed so many years ago. It is perhaps even more remarkable that the EEG apparatus remains central and essential to the diagnosis of sleep disorders.

The EEG machine is typically composed of several alternating current channels that enable the simultaneous recording of multiple sites of brain electrical activity. The data collected from EEG machine recordings are sufficient to identify brain states associated with relaxed wakefulness and the five stages of sleep. However, because EEG machines used in a sleep laboratory setting are often employed to record many physiologic signals, such as the electro-oculographic (EOG) and electromyographic (EMG) signals, conventional EEG machines have come to be known as polygraph or polysomnograph machines. These terms are especially appropriate when identifying machines that are used for clinical purposes. Such machines are commonly equipped with a combination of alternating current and direct current channels that are configured to record a variety of physiologic variables during sleep, including ECG activity, air flow, respiratory effort, and oxygen saturation. A minimum of three channels is required for the scoring of the sleep EEG (at least one channel each of EEG, EOG, and chin EMG); however, most polysomnographic studies are performed using at least four or five channels that incorporate one or two EEG channels, two EOG channels, and one chin EMG channel. Clinical recordings that include additional measures require at least 7 channels, but are frequently made using more than 10.

Each channel of the polygraph machine is composed of an electrical input, amplifier, and electrical output. The input accepts signals that are obtained from a recording sensor, transducer, or other device. Human EEG activity is recorded by placing gold or silver cup electrodes at designated points on the surface of the scalp, and connecting these leads via an electrode board to the polygraph inputs. The signals that are received by the amplifier are modified by the amplifier controls. These controls typically consist of sensitivity controls, a low-frequency filter, a high-frequency filter, a 60-Hz rejection filter, and an electrical baseline adjustment. These serve to determine the degree of signal amplification as well as the height and frequency of the waveforms that will be sent to the output. The output of each channel is usually connected to a chart recorder. The chart recorder consists of a series of ink writing galvanometers that produce output on paper that is driven by a chart drive moving at a speed of 10 mm/sec (the standard paper speed for recording the sleep EEG).

A polygraph machine that is used for clinical sleep recordings is likely to be configured to have one to four alternating current channels dedicated to EEG recording, one or two dedicated to EOG recording, one channel dedicated to chin EMG recording, one or two channels dedicated to left and right anterior tibialis muscle recording, one channel dedicated to ECG recording, one or two channels dedicated to airflow recording, one or two channels dedicated to respiratory effort recording, and one channel dedicated to oxygen saturation recording. Additional channels may also be dedicated to the recording of other important variables such as snoring and body position. These channels may be assembled together in many ways. Table 3 provides an example of a common polygraph channel configuration and amplifier settings.

Clinical sleep recordings depend on specialized sensors or ancillary equipment used in the recording of respiration and oxygen saturation. These devices interface with the polygraph machine, providing input that can be processed through the polygraph amplifiers. Perhaps the most important specialized sensors are those used to measure air flow and respiratory effort. Air flow is traditionally measured with the use of thermistors or thermocouplers that are placed at the apertures of

TABLE 3. *Polygraph Amplifier Configuration*

Channel	Variable	½ Low Amplitude	½ High Amplitude	Sensitivity
1	Left EOG	0.3 Hz	30 Hz	5 μV/mm
2	Right EOG	0.3 Hz	30 Hz	5 μV/mm
3	EEG C_3–A_2	0.3 Hz	30 Hz	5 μV/mm
4	EEG C_4–A_1	0.3 Hz	30 Hz	5 μV/mm
5	EEG O_1–A_2	0.3 Hz	30 Hz	5 μV/mm
6	EEG O_2–A_1	0.3 Hz	30 Hz	5 μV/mm
7	Chin EMG	10 Hz	90 Hz	–
8	ECG	–	–	–
9	Left anterior tibialis	10 Hz	90 Hz	–
10	Right anterior tibialis	10 Hz	90 Hz	–
11	Nasal air flow	–	–	–
12	Oral air flow	–	–	–
13	Snoring microphone	–	–	–
14	Thoracic effort	–	–	–
15	Abdominal effort	–	–	–
16	SaO_2	+	+	+

–Indicates that these recordings are not typically calibrated or that no specific amplifer settings are commonly used.

+Signals are calibrated to oximeter voltage output.

the nose and mouth. These devices indirectly measure air flow by responding to changes in temperature as air passes over the sensors during inspiration and expiration. Air flow is also measured by air pressure transducers. These devices are a veridical measure of flow pressure. They measure the pressure and thereby the flow of expired air, usually at the nose.

Respiratory effort is measured with transducers that are built into belts placed around the thorax and abdomen. These transducers are sensitive to the changes in the circumference of the belts that occur with breathing. Expansion and contraction of the thoracic and abdominal walls result in changes in transducer conductivity that reflect respiratory effort. Respiratory effort can be measured with transducers that can be calibrated. An advantage of this is that one is able to determine the approximate volume of airflow that corresponds with the value of transducer change. The use of both thoracic and abdominal transducers also enables the identification of paradoxical breathing, which can be an indication of upper airway obstruction.

SaO_2 is recorded with the use of a pulse oximeter. This device typically uses the principles of spectrophotometry and plethysmography to determine arterial oxygen saturation. The oximeter consists of two low-voltage light-emitting diodes. One emits a red light, and the other infrared light. A photodetector determines the amount of hemoglobin that is saturated with oxygen by determining the absorption of red and infrared light as it passes through the sensor site. The oximeter is usually connected directly to the polygraph machine so that transient changes in SaO_2 (desaturation) can be observed in relation to respiratory events.

Conventions exist for electrode and sensor placement for clinical sleep recordings. Figure 3 provides a graphic illustration of common placements of EEG, EOG, and chin EMG electrodes. EEG electrodes are placed in accordance with the international 10/20 system (63). The electrode placements required for sleep stage scoring are the C_3–A_2 or C_4–A_1 placements (left and right parietal lobe electrodes referenced to the contralateral mastoids). Either one of these placements provides information that is sufficient to score sleep according to the currently accepted standardized methods. Many clinical sleep recordings include the application of electrodes placed at the O_1–A_2 or O_2–A_1 positions (left and right oc-

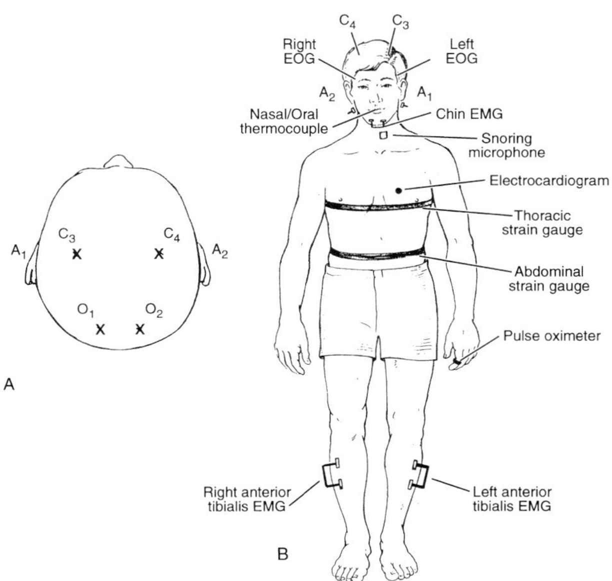

FIG. 3. A. Electroencephalographic electrode placements commonly used for polysomnographic recording. The C_3 or C_4 placements, referenced to the contralateral ear, are typically used for sleep stage scoring. The O_1 and O_2 placements are not used for scoring, but help to detect alpha activity, which helps to discriminate transitions between wakefulness and sleep. **B.** Illustration of sensor placements commonly used for polysomnographic recording.

cipital lobe placements referenced to the contralateral mastoids). These placements facilitate the visualization of alpha activity, which is useful in determining sleep onset, and some sleep stage transitions that occur during the sleep period. EOG electrodes are placed at the outer canthus of each eye and referenced to one mastoid (either the A_1 or A_2 placement). When this is done, the corneal surface of the eye, which is positively charged, and the retinal surface of the eye, which is negatively charged, produce opposite charges to the electrodes with conjugate eye movements. These can be easily visualized on the polygraph tracing. Chin EMG electrodes are typically placed underneath or on the chin. This provides a general measure of submental muscle tone, although these sensors can be sensitive to the presence of movement, gross abnormal movements during sleep, and specific movements such as those produced in cases of sleep-related bruxism.

Computerized Recording Equipment

Computerization of polysomnography has many benefits over analog devices. These benefits continue to grow as technology evolves. The ongoing challenge of computerized sleep systems manufacturers is to develop systems affording improvements in clinical efficiency over standard polysomnography. This efficiency must be accomplished from the full-featured computerized sleep system to the portable home device. Clinical efficiency is achieved when a computerized system provides increased flexibility and efficiency for the operator, and significant monetary and time savings for the sleep laboratory. One of the most obvious monetary savings occurs with the elimination of paper records. By storing the sleep record on magnetic or comparable storage media, a laboratory can realize thousands of dollars of savings annually. The elimination of paper records also frees the sleep laboratory from managing increasing paper storage costs.

Time savings of a sleep laboratory can best be achieved by reducing the record scoring and reporting time. Since the mid-1980s, manufacturers of computerized sleep systems have attempted to expedite sleep scoring by providing various levels of automated or semi-automated sleep staging and respiratory analysis algorithms. Validation studies of automated sleep staging have shown various ranges of success when correlating computerized sleep system staging and manual sleep staging. The primary difficulty in achieving a high degree of validity through computer systems lies in the attempt to develop algorithms that match the definition of the sleep stages as outlined by Rechtschaffen and Kales (60). Automated respiratory analysis typically reaches a higher range of correlation between automated and manual scoring because quantification of respiratory events is more precise. Although it is recognized that computerized automation of sleep scoring is not perfected, automated sleep scoring does represent a significant improvement in time effectiveness compared with manually scoring the paper record.

Efficiencies are also realized through the computer's ability to report multiple sleep stage and respiratory event statistics more quickly than can be calculated manually. Once identified, sleep stages and associations to significant events are trivial computations resulting in nearly instantaneous statistics and reports. Color graphic representations summarizing multiple channel types over an 8-hour study provide powerful overviews of the sleep record. The ability to export data files to external database packages allows the operator to format report statistics into customized tables not provided by the manufacturer. The types of calculations provided automatically on a computer are not feasible or time-effective for a technologist to generate from a paper record, making the computerized sleep system a valuable data management tool.

The full-functioning computerized sleep system may include many hardware options (Fig. 4). At a minimum, a computerized sleep system includes a processor, high-resolution monitor, data acquisition hardware, data archive device, keyboard, mouse, and printer. Typically, one computerized sleep system can manage data from two beds at one time. Data can be brought in from polygraph amplifiers or through a custom-designed amplifier by the system manufacturer. Nearly any analog signal can be accommodated on a computerized system. As data are acquired, they are digitized and stored directly to the hard drive or archival device. Once analyzed, data are formatted into a report and sent to the computer printer. On many manufactured systems, data can be output to a polygraph for printing a polygraph recording during or after data acquisition. Other options may include networking for communications among various sleep systems or portable devices, a modem for communications to the manufacturer or other systems, and synchronized video between a videocassette recorder and the digitized data.

Software options are specific to the system design dictated by the manufacturer. For example, manufacturers may separate the automated sleep scoring and respiratory analysis from the primary software application, to be purchased as options. Other software options may include specific data analysis packages such as arousal, ECG, or periodic limb movement identification. Some manufacturers offer research-based software options including

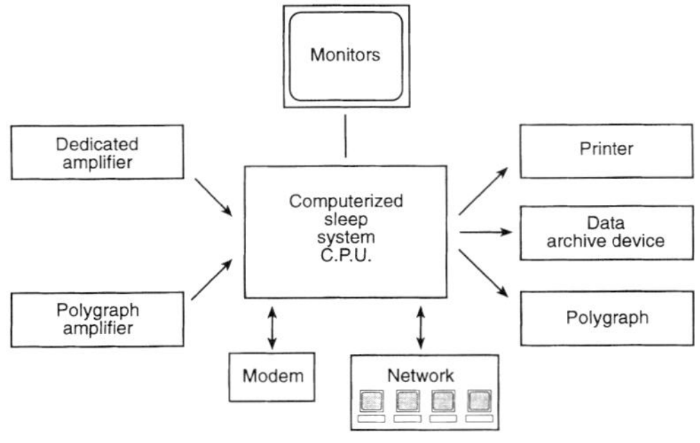

FIG. 4. Computerized polysomnography employs either dedicated or polygraph amplifier to acquire polygraphic signals, which are then sent to the central processing unit for display and analysis. The raw data may be forwarded directly to a polygraph machine for analog output. The raw or processed data may also be submitted to a printer or data archive device. Users of computerized systems may interact with data acquired at remote sites via modem or network.

access to the data format and computerized data analysis for downloading to mainframes or other research-oriented software packages.

The true advantages of a full-functioning computerized sleep system are realized at every level of operation. During the data acquisition phase of a sleep study, the computerized system will display the raw data and allow the operator to control many aspects of the recording and analysis. Systems with digitally controlled amplifiers allow the operator to change electrode connections through software, eliminating the need to manually change electrode jack connections or reconnect electrodes, which can potentially disturb the patient's sleep. Digital amplifiers maximize the operator's control of sensitivity and filtering during the night, while minimizing noise contamination of the data that can occur with analog amplifiers. Some of the most sophisticated computerized sleep systems allow data to be acquired from multiple beds while scoring data from all beds during acquisition. Automated scoring during the night's recording allows the operator to monitor the sleep staging and view the gestalt of results of the sleep study as it progresses. The operator's ability to override the automated scoring at night and manually score the record offers a significant time savings for the sleep laboratory, minimizing or eliminating the scoring normally required after the study is finished. Immediate on-line viewing of direct current signal types, such as SaO_2 or esophageal pressure, also maximizes the operator's information on patient state. Finally, the printing of data samples during acquisition enables the operator to share this information with a supervisor or colleague via fax modem for consultation.

After data acquisition, the benefits of a computerized system are many. Data can usually be displayed in any order on the screen. Individual channel display gains can be adjusted for critical visual analysis. Time displays extend beyond the typical 30-second epochs. Displays of 10-second epochs are useful for examining the EEG channels at a typical EEG time base. Collapsing the display to 3- or 5-minute epochs, while obscuring the high-frequency channels, more readily displays trends in respiratory and near-direct current channels. One of the most powerful computerized functions of these systems is the ability to highlight significant events such as arousals, periodic limb movements, or respiratory events. Color-coding of these highlights allows for fast identification of those events. Many systems allow an event to be selected with on-screen analysis of it. For example, the frequency of a sleep spindle or the duration of a hypopnea can be displayed immediately. A computer system may also allow an automatic search within the sleep record to identify user-specified events, patterns, or comments.

For most systems, the computer provides user control of the algorithms used for data analysis. Some systems provide different algorithms for different patient populations or allow the creation of a new set of rules by the user. The rules for event identification or sleep staging can be modified and reapplied to the same set of data to improve accuracy or to provide feedback to the user on personal scoring criteria. Some systems provide teaching tools such as an epoch-by-epoch matrix comparison of sleep staging. The matrix comparison can be used to compare sleep staging between two computer algorithms, between two human scorers, or between the computer and a human scorer.

Ambulatory Recording Equipment

Ambulatory recording equipment enables polysomnographic measurement to be obtained outside of the laboratory environment. This equipment is typically used to make home or hospital bedside recordings, which may have advantages over in-laboratory studies. Equipment that used ultraslow FM tape drives to record analog data was available as early as the mid-1970s. Manufacturers have since capitalized on advances in technology to create digital systems that can record physiologic measures and then interface (via hardwire connection or modem) with computerized data analysis systems. Therefore, ambulatory recording equipment increases flexibility in data acquisition and enables the user to take advantage of computerized analysis.

An ambulatory sleep recording device for use in the home or off-site location requires far less hardware options than a full system. The hardware requirements of the ambulatory device, however, are no less challenging. By the nature of the portability requirement, the device must be small enough to be easily transported. Because of its frequent transport, the device must be durable and be able to sustain impact. Ambulatory devices must meet the challenge of collecting and storing a full night's data. The more channels of data collected, the greater the demands on the data types, data storage capacity, and power supply. Ambulatory devices must also address safety issues such as patient isolation. Devices that offer battery-driven power are optimal as they address patient isolation as well as remove uncontrolled wiring variables that can occur in home settings. Devices that plug into the wall must include patient isolation at the power supply.

Ambulatory devices must be designed to address different levels of operation. Typically, an ambulatory device can be operated at two levels: by the patient in the patient's home or by the technologist at the patient's bedside. Any device that is taken home by the patient must be user friendly. It is unreasonable to expect patients to operate a complex instrument on their own. Consequently, the set-up and operation must be simple. Devices used by a technologist have more flexibility in system operation and level of control.

Analysis of data acquired on an ambulatory device can be managed independently of a computer or be interfaced to one. Ambulatory devices that are stand-alone units typically use a printer or data output to facilitate data review and analysis. Devices that interface to computer systems take advantage of data archiving, automated scoring, and reporting features found on the computer system. In this scenario, time for data transfer and conversion at the computer must be taken into consideration. Some of these devices also offer on-line monitoring capabilities through a modem, allowing a periodic "snapshot" of the patient data to be sent back to a clinical monitoring site such as a hospital sleep laboratory. The modem option allows the data monitoring to assess data integrity and state of the patient.

Although advances in technology have made many types of ambulatory recording possible, it should be emphasized that there are minimum acceptable standards for clinical polysomnography. We believe that standard level I polysomnography or its equivalent (ambulatory level IA) must be employed for the evaluation of snoring and sleep-related breathing disorders (see Table 2). Unattended portable recording (levels II and III polysomnography) offers convenience and accessibility, and may be available at less cost than standard polysomnography. However, these types of recording have not been adequately validated, and their potential advantages must be weighed against the possibility of missed or inaccurate diagnoses (64). This is especially true in patients with mild, moderate, or atypical sleep-related respiratory disturbances that may not be detected by levels II or III polysomnography. The American Sleep Disorders Association Standards of Practice Committee currently recommends that portable systems not be used for loud snoring or the routine assessment of obstructive sleep apnea (65).

It must be also emphasized that snoring and sleep-related breathing disorders cannot be reliably evaluated using some common alternative techniques. These techniques include daytime nap or abbreviated night-time studies. Such studies may be useful in detecting some severe cases, but may fail to detect mild to moderate cases. Neither provides a clear indication of the severity of the disorder or its impact on night-time sleep. Overnight oximetry is not considered a sufficient measure, as apneic and hypopneic events commonly occur without desaturation or with minimal (<4%) desaturation, and the diagnosis may be missed. Audiotape cannot be used to discriminate between normal breathing, snoring, and sleep apnea because breath or snoring sounds may persist during periods of hypopnea or upper airway resistance, yielding a false-negative result. It is unwise to use any of these measures as part of a screening process prior to polysomnography or as a follow-up after treatment. They may yield misleading information that shapes the physician's impression of the patient, leading to a deviation from appropriate diagnostic or treatment procedures.

CONCLUSION

The development and wide use of new laser-assisted surgical techniques for the treatment of snoring and sleep-related breathing disorders has led to the need for otolaryngologists to obtain pre- and postoperative sleep laboratory evaluation of their patients. Careful evaluation includes history and physical examination, as well as clinical polysomnography. Polysomnography can be performed using conventional recording equipment and methods, and is now possible through the use of computerized and ambulatory recording equipment. The appropriate use of polysomnography and the integration of new technologies into sound clinical practice will contribute to the safe and appropriate application of surgical procedures, reliable measures of treatment outcome, and the identification of patients who may require mechanical or other treatments for sleep-related breathing disorders.

ACKNOWLEDGMENT

The authors thank Sigurd H. Ackerman, M.D., for reviewing sections of the manuscript.

REFERENCES

1. Haraldson PO, Carenfelt C: Laser uvulopalatoplasty in local anaesthesia: A safe approach in the treatment of habitual snoring. *Rhinology* 28:65–66, 1990.
2. Kamami YV: Laser CO$_2$ for snoring: Preliminary results. *Acta Otorhinolaryngol Belg* 44:451–456, 1990.
3. Lugaresi E, Cirignotta F, Coccagna G, Piana C: Some epidemiological data on snoring and cardiocirculatory disorders. *Sleep* 3:221–224, 1980.
4. Kauffman F, Annesi I, Neukirch F et al: The relation between snoring and smoking, body mass index, age, alcohol consumption and respiratory symptoms. *Eur Respir J* 2:599–603, 1989.
5. Bloom JW, Kaltenborn WT, Quan SF: Risk factors in a

general population for snoring. Importance of cigarette smoking and obesity. *Chest* 93:678–683, 1989.

6. Lugaresi E, Cirignotta F, Montagna P, Sforza E: Snoring: pathogenic, clinical, and therapeutic aspects. In: Kryger MH, Roth T, Dement WD, eds. *Principles and practice of sleep medicine.* Philadelphia: WB Saunders, 1994:621–629.

7. Skatrud JB, Dempsey JA: Airway resistance and respiratory muscle function in snorers during NREM sleep. *J Appl Physiol* 59:328–335, 1985.

8. Issa FG, Sullivan CE: Upper airway closing pressure in snorers. *J Appl Physiol* 57:528–535, 1984.

9. Jan MA, Marshall I, Douglas NJ: Effect of posture on upper airway dimensions in normal human. *Am J Respir Crit Care Med* 149:145–148, 1994.

10. Cartwright RD, Lloyd S, Lilie J, Kravitz H: Sleep position training as a treatment for sleep apnea syndrome: A preliminary study. *Sleep* 8:87–94, 1985.

11. Sanders M: Medical therapy for sleep apnea. In: Kryger MH, Roth T, Dement WD, eds. *Principles and practice of sleep medicine.* Philadelphia: WB Saunders, 1994: 678–693.

12. Fairbanks DNF: Snoring: An overview with historical perspectives. In: Fairbanks DNF, Fujita S, Ikematsu T, Simons FB, eds. *Snoring and obstructive sleep apnea.* New York: Raven Press, 1987:1–18.

13. Issa FG, Sullivan CE: Alcohol, snoring, and sleep apnea. *J Neurol Neurosurg Psychiatry* 115:353–359, 1982.

14. Jennum P, Schultz-Larsen K, Christensen N: Snoring, sympathetic activity and cardiovascular risk factors in a 70 year old population. *Eur J Epidemiol* 9:477–482, 1993.

15. Jennum P, Sjol A: Snoring, sleep apnoea and cardiovascular risk factors: The MONICA II study. *Int J Epidemiol* 22: 439–444, 1993.

16. American Sleep Disorders Association: *The international classification of sleep disorders.* Lawrence, Kansas: Allen Press, 1990:195–197.

17. Partinen M: Cerebrovascular disorders and sleep. In: Thorpy MJ, ed. *Handbook of sleep disorders.* New York: Marcel Dekker, 1990:693–702.

18. Jennum P, Hein HO, Suadicani P, Gyntelberg F: Cardiovascular risk factors in snorers. A cross-sectional study of 3,323 men aged 54 to 74 years: The Copenhagen Male Study. *Chest* 102:1371–1376, 1992.

19. Hoffstein V, Mateika JH, Mateika S: Snoring and sleep architecture. *Am Rev Respir Dis* 143:92–96, 1991.

20. Gislason T, Benediktsdottir B, Björnsson J. Snoring, hypertension, and the sleep apnea syndrome. An epidemiologic survey of middle-aged women. *Chest* 103:1147–1151, 1993.

21. Koskenvuo M, Kaprio J, Telakivi T et al: Snoring as a risk factor for ischaemic heart disease and stroke in men. BMJ 294: 16–19, 1987.

22. Smirne S, Palazzi S, Zucconi M et al: Habitual snoring as a risk factor for acute vascular disease. *Eur Respir J* 6:1357–1361, 1993.

23. Palomaki H: Snoring and the risk of ischemic brain infarction. *Stroke* 22:1021–1025, 1991.

24. Spriggs DA, French JM, Murdy JM et al: Snoring increases the risk of stroke and adversely affects prognosis. *QJM* 83:555–562, 1992.

25. Partinen M, Palomaki H: Snoring and cerebral infarction. *Lancet* 2:1325–1326, 1985.

26. Guilleminault C, Stoohs R, Duncan S: Snoring. I. Daytime sleepiness in regular heavy snorers. *Chest* 99:40–48, 1991.

27. Stradling JR, Crosby JH, Payne CD: Self reported snoring and daytime sleepiness in men aged 35–65 years. *Thorax* 46:807–810, 1991.

28. Kapunuiai LE, Andrew DJ, Crowell DH, Pearle JW: Estimated prevalence of sleep apnea in adults based on self report survey apnea scores. *Sleep Research* 14:175, 1985.

29. Lavie P: Incidence of sleep apnea in a presumably healthy working population: A significant relationship with excessive daytime sleepiness. *Sleep* 6:312–318, 1983.

30. Peter JH, Siegrist J, Podszus T et al: Prevalence of sleep apnea in healthy industrial workers. *Klin Wochenschr* 63:807, 1985.

31. Young T, Palta M, Dempsey J et al: The occurrence of sleep-disordered breathing among middle-aged adults. *N Engl J Med* 328:1230–1235, 1993.

32. Coleman RM, Roffwarg HP, Kennedy SJ et al: Sleep wake disorders based on polysomnographic diagnosis: A national cooperative study. *JAMA* 247:997–1003, 1982.

33. Ancoli-Israel S, Kripke DF, Klauber MR et al: Sleep disordered breathing in community-dwelling elderly. *Sleep* 14:486–495, 1991.

34. Rubenstein I, Colapinto N, Rotstein LE et al: Improvement in upper airway function after weight loss in patients with obstructive sleep apnea. *Am Rev Respir Dis* 138:1192–1195, 1988.

35. Guilleminault C: Clinical features and evaluation of obstructive sleep apnea. In: Kryger MH, Roth T, Dement WC, eds. *Principles and practice of sleep medicine.* Philadelphia: WB Saunders, 1989:552–558.

36. Keidar A, Zammit GK, Krespi YP: The relationship between polysomnographic findings and self-reported symptoms in laser assisted uvulopalatoplasty (LAUP) candidates. *Sleep Research* 23:271, 1994.

37. Krieger J: Obstructive sleep apnea: Clinical manifestations and pathophysiology. In: Thorpy MJ, ed. *Handbook of sleep disorders.* New York: Marcel Dekker, 1990; 259–284.

38. Guilleminault C, Stoohs R: The upper airway resistance syndrome. *Sleep Research* 20:250, 1991.

39. Guilleminault C, Stoohs R, Clerk A et al: A cause of excessive daytime sleepiness: The upper airway resistance syndrome. *Chest* 104:781–787, 1993.

40. Guilleminault C, van den Hoed J, Mitler MM: Clinical overview of the sleep apnea syndromes. In: Guilleminault C, Dement WC, eds. *Sleep apnea syndromes.* New York: Alan R. Liss, 1978:1–12.

41 Wittig RM, Romaker A, Zorick FJ et al: Night-to-night consistency of apneas during sleep. *Am Rev Respir Dis* 129:244–246, 1984.

42. Stepanski E, Lamphere J, Roehrs T et al: Experimental sleep fragmentation in normal subjects. *Int J Neurosci* 33:207–214, 1987.

43. Stepanski E, Lamphere J, Badia P et al: Sleep fragmentation and daytime sleepiness. *Sleep* 7:18–26, 1984.

44. Roehrs T, Zorick F, Wittig R et al: Predictors of objective level of daytime sleepiness in patients with sleep-related breathing disorders. *Chest* 95:1202–1206, 1989.

45. Kribbs NB, Getsy JE, Dinges D: Investigation and management of daytime sleepiness in sleep apnea. In: Saunders NA, Sullivan CE, eds. *Sleep and breathing,* 2nd ed. New York: Marcel Dekker, 1994:575–604.

46. Guilleminault C, Billiard M, Montplasir J, Dement WC: Altered states of consciousness in disorders of daytime sleepiness. *J Neurol Sci* 26:377–393, 1975.

47. Roth T, Hartse KM, Zorick F, Conway W: Multiple naps and the evaluation of daytime sleepiness in patients with upper airway sleep apnea. *Sleep* 3:425–439, 1980.

48. Westbrook PR: Sleep disorders and upper airway obstruction in adults. *Otolaryngol Clin North Am* 23: 727–743, 1990.

49. Findley LJ, Unverzagt ME, Suratt PM: Automobile accidents involving patients with obstructive sleep apnea. *Am Rev Respir Dis* 138:337–340, 1988.

50. Findley LJ, Fabrizio MJ, Knight H et al: Driving simulator performance in patients with sleep apnea. *Am Rev Respir Dis* 140:529–530, 1989.

51. Podszus T, Greenburg H, Scharf SM: Influence of sleep state and sleep-disordered breathing on cardiovascular function. In: Saunders NA, Sullivan CE, eds. *Sleep and breathing*. New York: Marcel Dekker, 1994:257–310.

52. Burack B, Pollak C, Borowiecki B, Weitzman E: The hypersomnia-sleep apnea syndrome (HSA): A reversible major cardiovascular hazard. *Circulation* 56: 111–117, 1977.

53. Millman RP, Redline S, Randall C et al: The relationship between nocturnal sleep events and daytime hypertension in a population of patients with obstructive sleep apnea. *Chest* 99:861–866, 1991.

54. Partinen M, Jamieson A, Guilleminault C: Long-term outcome for obstructive sleep apnea syndrome patients (mortality). *Chest* 94:1200–1204, 1988.

55. Shepard JW Jr, Garrison MW, Grither DA, Dolan GF: Relationship of ventricular ectopy to oxyhemoglobin desaturation in patients with obstructive sleep apnea. *Chest* 88:335–340, 1985.

56. Scharf SM, Garshick E, Brown R et al: Screening for subclinical sleep-disordered breathing. *Sleep* 13: 344–353, 1990.

57. Guilleminault C, Connolly S, Winkle R: Cardiac arrythmia during sleep in 400 patients with sleep apnea syndrome. *Am J Cardiol* 52:490–494, 1983.

58. Seppala T, Partinen M, Pentilla A et al: Sudden death and sleeping history among Finnish men. *J Intern Med* 229:23–28, 1991.

59. He J, Kryger MH, Zorick FJ et al: Mortality and apnea index in obstructive sleep apnea. *Chest* 94:9–14, 1988.

60. Rechtschaffen A, Kales A: *A manual of standardized terminology, techniques, and scoring system for sleep stages of human sleep subjects*. Washington, DC: US Government Printing Office, 1968.

61. Carskadon MA, Dement WC, Mitler MM et al: Guidelines for the multiple sleep latency test: A standard measure of sleepiness. *Sleep* 9:519–524, 1986.

62. Hobson JA: *The dreaming brain*. New York: Basic Books, 1988:114–116.

63. Tyner FS, Knott JR, Brem Mayer W Jr: *Fundamentals of EEG technology*. New York: Raven Press, 1983:136–145.

64. Ferber R, Millman R, Coppola M et al: Portable recording in the assessment of obstructive sleep apnea. *Sleep* 17:378–392, 1994.

65. American Sleep Disorders Association, Standards of Practice Committee: Practice parameters for the use of portable recording in the assessment of obstructive sleep apnea. *Sleep* 17:372–377, 1994.

Office-Based Surgery of the Head and Neck
Edited by Yosef P. Krespi, MD
Lippincott–Raven Publishers, Philadelphia © 1998

7

Guidelines and Procedures Used in the Assessment of Laser-Assisted Uvulopalatoplasty Patients

Anat Keidar

SPEECH AND VOICE CONSIDERATIONS

Although laser-assisted uvulopalatoplasty (LAUP) is a procedure designed primarily to attenuate or eliminate snoring, approximately 90% of patients seeking surgical intervention for snoring have sleep apnea (1). Preliminary studies and clinical observations suggest that speech and swallowing disorders are more prevalent among sleep apnea patients than among the nonapnea population (2). Over the past decade, only a handful of reports on speech following the traditional uvulopalatopharyngoplasty (UPPP) procedure have been published (3–7). Some reported no changes in speech. Others noted no changes in nasality, but changes in voice quality, resolving over time. Articulatory difficulties involving certain uvular and pharyngeal consonants were also reported, but overall, most findings pertained to nonspeech problems, such as swallowing difficulties, nasal regurgitation, choking, gagging, altered sensations, dryness, and postnasal irritation, lasting for several months after surgery. Salas-Provance and Kuehn (7) found more phonatory (voice) and articulatory problems among 20 postsurgical UPPP test subjects than their 15 non-UPPP age-matched control subjects. However, resonance problems (specifically hypernasality) were not identified among the UPPP group. With the exception of the above study, little or no information has been provided by other au-

thors regarding methodologic approach, subject selection, measurement parameters, assessment tasks, perceptual criteria, and analysis techniques. It should also be noted that in the absence of published studies comparing pre- and post-UPPP speech status, there is no evidence linking the observed or reported changes to the surgery. As indicated by Monoson and Fox, "pre-existing" speech problems may be more common in the apnea population (2).

Because LAUP is a relatively new procedure, there are no published scientific studies examining the effects of LAUP on speech. Performed in a stage-wise fashion, LAUP allows for greater flexibility on the part of the surgeon, and greater adaptation and "plasticity" on the part of the patient. From a speech or voice production vantage point, this is a significant advantage over UPPP. Preliminary analyses of selected voice, articulation, and resonance parameters derived from 78 consecutive patients seen in our office between 1992 and 1994 (preoperatively, prior to each stage, and following the last treatment) suggest that LAUP is a relatively safe procedure, provided that strict guidelines are followed to prevent iatrogenic effects on speech. Our protocol has been useful in identifying persons who are:

1. Unsuitable
2. Marginally suitable and at high risk of developing complications

3. Suitable, but must be treated with caution
4. Suitable for LAUP

The collaboration between the speech-language pathologist, the surgeon, and the patient has enabled us to weigh the potential risks and benefits of LAUP (including whether or not to perform the procedure, when to perform it, and how much should be anatomically altered) and to learn from experience.

The Velopharyngeal Mechanism

One of the most important considerations in LAUP is the maintenance of adequate partitioning between the oropharynx and nasopharynx through a sphincter-like action that sufficiently reduces the proximity between the soft palate and the posterior and lateral pharyngeal walls. Although velopharyngeal (VP) valving exists primarily for vegetative functions (such as middle ear ventilation, deglutition, swallowing, sucking, and blowing), one of its key functions is to valve the airstream during speech and enable the production of nonnasal vowels and consonants (8–10). Hence, when assessing the suitability of a patient for LAUP, it is necessary both to ascertain that VP function for nonspeech and speech tasks is intact presurgically and to predict how that mechanism will function postsurgically.

Although LAUP patients share several common tendencies, such as obesity, hypertension, and sleep apnea (1), on personal, social, and vocational levels, they appear to be a heterogeneous group. Inherent in this diversity is a clinical challenge for the management team.

As will be noted in the next section, whereas ordinary anatomic or physiologic considerations may render certain candidates suitable for treatment, other, task-specific factors may place them at risk of incurring side effects. The parameters found critical in evaluating our population are surveyed below.

Linguistic Constraints

Unlike French or Portuguese, which are languages rich in nasal phonemes, in only three sounds of the English language is it acceptable for the VP port to remain open: / m /, / n /, and / η / (as in ri*ng*). All other English sounds (vowels and consonants) are produced with the VP port closed and virtually no contact between the oral and nasal cavities. VP manipulation is a dynamic event involving precise timing and sequencing. In running speech or singing, certain consonants in particular (such as / p /, / t /, and / k /) or consonant blends (such as / spl /, / str /, or / skr /) require a significant build-up of intraoral air pressure (3–7 cm H_2O) and a VP port constriction of ≤ 0.02 cm^2 over a very short time frame. If the VP mechanism does not operate properly (owing to structural, neuromuscular, functional, or psychogenic defects), the air leaks through the nose, resulting in a nasal resonatory disorder. A resonatory disorder may include hypo- or hypernasal resonance, nasal air emissions, articulatory distortions and substitutions, and perceived dysphonia. The palate, in combination with the posterior pharyngeal wall and/or the tongue is involved in the production of numerous consonants found in other languages (such as the uvular trilled / r /, or the pharyngeal fricative / x /). Speech patterns may vary across geographic regions, and cultural, ethnic, and linguistic environments. If the patient habitually communicates in languages other than English, it is recommended that a sample of that language be obtained and analyzed so that the patient can be appropriately counseled presurgically and carefully monitored after each LAUP procedure.

It is important to keep in mind that whether objective or subjective, any assessment of speech and voice attributes must take into account each individual's dialectal, phonologic, and linguistic background. One should also remember that the primary purpose of assessing LAUP candidates' speech is to obtain baseline data (to which follow-up data can be compared), detect and document problems prior to surgery, and monitor and interpret changes within (rather than between) patients after each operative stage. Comparing LAUP subjects, as a group, with non-LAUP controls may also prove interesting, but in practices not funded through federal grants or affiliated with academic institutions, clinical efficacy must take priority and focus on intra-subject variability.

Professional Voice Users and Vocal Performers

Professional singers use their palate to manipulate the timbre and loudness of their voices (11,12). Trained singers, in particular, (ie, classical or operatic) typically tend to "cover" the sound by raising the soft palate on production of all cardinal vowels. The right amount of palatal lifting (in combination with other important technical parameters) corresponds to refinement of tone production, and to enhancement of vocal efficiency, intensity, and projection (13). Therefore, singers, actors, and other professionals whose livelihood depends on vocal versatility, stability, and projection should be carefully evaluated. Professional singers must undergo a comprehensive vocal capability battery, administered by a qualified singing specialist. Such assessment typically comprises a wide variety of vocal tasks and includes samples of sung repertoire. For singers with voice teachers, it is highly recommended that the teachers assume an active role in the decision-making process, and, if treated, in the ongoing evaluation and post-surgical adjustments of the patient.

Structural Defects

Patients who exhibit congenital structural or maxillofacial deviations (such as submucous cleft, bi-fid uvula, short palate, large nasopharynx, large tongue, and micrognathia), or alterations due to injury, disease, trauma, or neurologic involvement should be handled with extreme caution, and, in some cases, discouraged from pursuing LAUP treatment. (For more information, see references 9,14–17.) It is important to document these pre-existing problems, preferably through high-resolution still or dynamic imaging, and to explain to the patient the implications of the findings. Some

of the patients in our clinic chose to be treated despite minor structural defects. With mindful approach and surgical modifications, LAUP reportedly brought about satisfactory results for this group.

Neurologic Dysfunction

Patients with myoneural, upper, or lower motor neuron dysfunction, and movement disorders affecting the speech musculature should be identified in advance, and, in some cases, dissuaded from surgery. Preoperative manifestation of flaccid, spastic, ataxic, mixed, hyperkinetic or hypokinetic dysarthria, or speech apraxia should be documented. After thorough evaluation and effective counseling, patients should be considered on a case-by-case basis, and treated only if the benefits outweigh the risks. The same applies to patients with expressive aphasia affecting speech. For patients in moderate or advanced stages of degenerative neurologic diseases, such as Parkinson's disease, amyotrophic lateral sclerosis, multiple sclerosis, supranuclear degeneration (with bulbar involvement), and Alzheimer's disease, LAUP is not a recommended procedure. (For more information on the signs, symptoms, etiology, epidemiology, diagnosis, and treatment of neurogenic communicative disorders, see references 18–23.)

Speech Disorders

When evaluating LAUP candidates, special attention must be given to pre-existing disorders of articulation, fluency, resonance, and voice. We have questioned all our patients about their speech and language development, including any history of speech or voice problems, whether they have ever had speech therapy or required surgery to correct a problem with their speech or voice, and whether any remarks by family members, friends, acquaintances, and business associates were ever made regarding unusual speech or voice characteristics. Among our patients, we have found a relatively large subgroup of stutterers (≈4%). Although the onset of stuttering is typically during early childhood, many stutterers engage in avoidance behaviors and try to conceal their dysfluencies. When questioned about their stuttering, most patients were surprised to have been exposed after years of cover-up attempts. Letting these patients know that we have documented their stuttering as a pre-existing condition certainly discouraged them from attributing any future dysfluent "outbursts" to the LAUP procedure. Likewise, patients with articulation or voice disorders should be well documented, and should be informed about the presence, nature, and severity of their problem. However, unless the speech or voice disturbance interferes with intelligibility or communicative effectiveness, most such patients qualify as LAUP candidates provided that they are treated with caution. (For more information, see references 9, 24.)

OTHER CONSIDERATIONS

Woodwind and Brass Instrumentalists

The consequences of VP insufficiency can be disastrous for wind and brass players (25, 26), who use their VP mechanism extensively to control and valve supraglottal airflow and to assist in tone articulation. Such instrumentalists should not be automatically disqualified, but they must be rigorously evaluated, thoroughly educated, and treated with extreme caution. (Added to that category are other professionals, such as glass blowers.) In our practice, we have treated several professional brass players whose evaluation included a practical analysis of airflow management while playing their instruments. As is the case with singers, the amount and manner of tissue removal at each LAUP stage should be conservative for brass and wind players, and the time interval between successive stages should be sufficiently prolonged to allow complete healing and functional modifications to take place.

Psychogenic, Cognitive, and Interpersonal Factors

Overt manifestation of hostility, depression, or anxiety on the part of patients should be interpreted as prohibitive to surgery. To allow the surgeon to proceed without trepidation and to ensure a sound patient-doctor relationship, surgical treatment of such patients should be deferred until they are adequately managed for these problems. Patients prone to extreme forms of somatization (27) should also be targeted, and preferably ruled out as LAUP candidates. Such patients are likely to develop a host of reactions and complications that will ultimately consume tremendous time and effort postsurgically. Cognitive dysfunction warrants serious investigation and extreme caution. Patients who exhibit memory deficits, poor judgment, difficulty comprehending language, and impulse control problems due to dementia, traumatic brain injury, stroke, disease, or congenital causes may not be suitable for LAUP.

On a final note, be aware that snoring constitutes convenient grounds for interpersonal alienation and sexual denial among couples. Hence, prior to treatment, presence, loudness, and duration of snoring should be established not only through the bed partner's allegations, but preferably, confirmed through sleep laboratory documentation. All too often, the act of snoring or the snorer personally is blamed for lack of intimacy and physical closeness when, upon probing, a variety of factors (other than snoring) underlying marital discord or relationship disintegration can be uncovered. A clear warning signal is a spouse who announces: "I have had it! This is his last chance! If this surgery does not work, I am divorcing him!" In all likelihood, she will divorce him with or without LAUP. Do not let the patient be bullied into undergoing this procedure if there is no clear evidence to support habitual snoring and if the patient conveys a notion that resolution of the snoring problem holds the key to a gratifying interpersonal and sexual future. Based on many couples' testimony, reduction or elimination of snoring enabled them to share a bed or bedroom again. Nevertheless, it is clear that LAUP is not a panacea for rejuvenation of sexual attraction, romance, and intimacy. Whether trapped in a fragile relationship, scarred by past rejections, or attempting to escape from the grip of loneliness, a candidate's unrealistic expectations can lead to bitter disappointments.

ESSENTIAL COMPONENTS FOR ASSESSMENT OF LAUP CANDIDATES

Questionnaires

Each patient should fill out an initial questionnaire and a final questionnaire (1–3 months following the final procedure). Most of the items require forced choice responses (yes or no); checking one or several items in an array; or rating (using a five-point equally appearing interval scale). Although comprehensive, the questionnaires tap into many areas that have been linked to snoring and sleep apnea and may, therefore, affect the suitability, compliance, and outcome of each patient. The assigned responses or numerical values constitute an extractable data base for statistical analyses, which allow comparisons between pre- and post-LAUP findings and between patients' and clinicians' assessments of results. Such analyses may also be useful in formulating and refining the criteria for patient selection and evaluation of success. Such analyses may enable the investigators to detect, cluster, and prioritize factors that justify the application of LAUP versus those factors that caution against the use of this particular technique or lead to further modification of the technique.

The initial encounter form covers background information (vital statistics); complaints and symptoms; onset, progression, possible correlates, contributing factors, and consequences of the problem; subjective rating of severity and impact of the problem, management of the problem by other professionals or means; medical history and current mental or physical health status; intake habits and patterns (food, alcohol, and so forth); prescription, over-the-counter, and recreational drug use; professional or occupational aspirations and demands; communicative utility and drive; linguistic factors; personality and emotionality factors; common symptoms associated with sleep apnea and management thereof; and goals for improvement and desired outcome. (See questionnaire developed by Anat Keidar and Yosef Krespi in 1993, contained in Appendix 1.)

The final follow-up questionnaire addresses presence, severity, and type of discomfort secondary to LAUP; the effect of LAUP on snoring, sleep patterns, and routine daily functioning thus far; the degree of improvement or satisfaction following the procedure; and the patient's perception of his or her speech. Numerous items submitted in the initial questionnaire are repeated to allow for comparison and *post hoc* analysis. In addition, this questionnaire also solicits retrospective opinions from the patients on whether they would have done anything differently (and if so, what?), and on ways in which the management of their problems could have been improved. (See questionnaire developed by Anat Keidar and Yosef Krespi in 1994, contained in Appendix 2.)

Clinical Interview

A clinical interview should follow the completion of each initial questionnaire. The interview is often fragmented, starting before and ending after the physical, polysomnographic, and speech or voice evaluation. Audio or video recordings of portions pertaining to the patient's speech and other information considered critical should be obtained using high-quality apparatus. Such recordings are useful for retention of specific information that might otherwise be unretrievable, as well as for legal purposes. Questions that the patient might have should be answered. In addition to information exchange, the interview also serves as a format for counseling and medical or behavioral management. Patients whose written answers or oral testimony reveal factors that are likely contributors to their problem (eg, significant weight gain, smoking, habitual bedtime intake of alcohol, consumption of sleep medication or tranquilizers) and who wish to fortify their standing as candidates for LAUP should receive education or counseling (supplemented by medical intervention as needed) aimed at minimizing or even eliminating the potential adverse effect(s) of such factors on their problem. It should be expected that these patients would demonstrate reasonable compliance with the recommendations given. However, it is the responsibility of the management team to follow them up to determine whether, and to what extent, alleviation of symptoms will have resulted from adherence to the prescribed measures.

Based on clinical experience, we have compiled a few guidelines for the physician conducting the preoperative interview:

1. Always keep in mind that while you are interviewing the patient, the patient is interviewing you. Listen and communicate effectively.
2. Avoid making any definitive prognostic statements until you have acquired *recent, reliable* polysomnographic data, and have concluded your examination protocol.
3. Be truthful and cautious about a candidate's prognosis, and avoid quoting "cure rate" statistics (especially if you have little or no follow-up data to support your own track record). Rather, advise the patient that despite your competence as a surgeon and your overall belief in the benefits of LAUP, there appears to be a continuum of success, ranging from outstanding to (occasional) disappointing results. Discuss both favorable and unfavorable prognostic indicators pertaining to the individual being interviewed, keeping in mind that it is sensible for you, as well as for the patient, to defer a decision in order to gather more information and to consider the pros and cons of the procedure.
4. *Do not* minimize the level and duration of pain and discomfort following LAUP surgery (especially after the first stage). You are better off preparing patients for the worst, while reassuring them that you and your staff will help to make their recovery as comfortable as possible. As is the case with any painful procedure, you should be prepared to keep your word and personally engage in some form of hand holding and comforting.

Structural, Auditory-Perceptual, and Aerodynamic Evaluation

A short evaluation (emphasizing resonance, articulation, and voice parameters) should be conducted by a trained speech-language pathologist preoperatively. It is recommended that the patient be reassessed prior to each subsequent LAUP stage and at least 1 month following the final stage. Each evaluation should be recorded on high-quality apparatus (audio or video) for documentation and further analysis, and should include:

1. A simple oral mechanism examination (including physical probing for submucous cleft). A basic oral mechanism assessment, such as the protocol outlined by Darley et al. (18), is recommended to detect structural, neurologic, and functional abnormalities affecting phonation, articulation, and resonance.
2. Airflow assessment. A useful screening test of nasal air emission is the mirror fogging test. It is carried out by placing a small reflector mirror in front of each nostril (while holding the other nostril closed) and having the patient perform a variety of speech tasks. Fogging of the mirror on vowels and nonnasal sounds is a simple but reliable way to determine whether air escapes through the nose. It can also provide useful information on insufficient nasal airflow if the mirror does not fog during production of nasal sounds. Nasality can be rated on a 0–3 equally appearing interval scale (EAI) as indicated in Appendix 3. Another simple but useful device is the See-Scape, which involves placing a nasal button in one nostril while occluding the other. The button is connected via a flexible plastic tube to a rigid Plexiglas tube that contains a Styrofoam ball. The ball rises as airflow in the tube increases,

thus allowing for visual tracking and rating of nasal airflow. For most patients in most clinical settings, one of these techniques will suffice. For research purposes, a variety of instruments and measurement techniques are available to provide precise information on oral and nasal pressure or flow profiles, such as the Nasometer (developed by Kay Elemetrics), and other marketed or specially developed software (28–30).

3. Perceptual rating of voice, articulation, and overall acceptability of spoken utterances.
4. Inventory of speech tasks (to be used as needed with above-listed procedures 1–3; see also Appendices 3 and 4):

   a. A sample of spontaneous speech, including commentary by the patient reflecting personal perception of his or her own speech, voice, and resonance on the date of the evaluation and in general; other people's reactions to or comments about his or her voice and speech; a brief history of voice and speech development and problems (if any); and the reasons for seeking this type of intervention.
   b. A reading passage.
   c. Prolongation of sustained vowels / a /, / i /, and / u / at comfortable loudness and pitch.
   d. Diadochokinetic tasks (rapid, repetitive production) of pressure consonants /p /, / k /, and / t /.
   e. Diadochokinetic and other speech tasks targeting nasal consonants /m / and / n /.
   f. A list of ≥10 sentences that do not contain nasal phonemes.
   g. A list of ≥10 sentences that do contain nasal phonemes.

Dynamic Imaging Techniques

Nasal-Pharyngeal-Laryngeal Videoendoscopy

Fiberoptic endoscopy should be used to rule out nasal and tongue base obstruction (as possible contributors to snoring and apnea) and to examine carefully the structure, timing, and function of the VP mechanism during speech and nonspeech activities. This procedure is effective in detecting structural deviations as well as insufficient valving. It also allows the surgeon to examine movement of the tongue and the posterior and lateral pharyngeal walls while the patient performs a variety of tasks. The acoustic and video signals should be recorded simultaneously on separate channels for further analysis. Because phonatory disorders have been reported to be higher among apnea patients (2,7), it is also important to assess overall phonatory function in terms of vocal fold mobility and mucosal status. If laryngeal pathology is detected using a flexible fiberoptic endoscope, it is strongly recommended that the surgeon obtain video documentation using a rigid laryngeal telescope (70° or 90°) and stroboscopic illumination.

Video-Fluoroscopy (Dynamic Cephalometry)

Video-fluoroscopic imaging is not routinely incorporated into the assessment battery of LAUP candidates in our institution. We recommend that this type of imaging (implementing lateral and basal views, as suggested by Okamoto and Fujito [31]) be used only in special cases: those wherein maxillofacial anomalies are manifested or suspected; those wherein the obstruction sites are not easily discernible; or where possible complications of VP insufficiency, dysphagia, and dysarthria are either present or anticipated. This procedure, which supplements fiberoptic endoscopic information, further defines the upper airway configurations, tongue and jaw movement, and velar and pharyngeal function at rest or during swallowing, sucking, blowing, snorting, and selected speech (nasal and nonnasal) tasks. The radiographic video portion of the speech tasks should be recorded simultaneously with the audio portion of the corresponding acoustic signals for *post hoc* analysis by the management team.

Overall Suitability Rating by the Management Team

In an ideal setting, patients should be managed by a multidisciplinary team headed by the otolaryngologist. Other members may include a sleep specialist, a nurse who follows the patient from the initial encounter to recovery, and a speech-language pathologist. Apart from the surgeon, it is recommended that at least one other team member review the input in each patient's file to formulate an independent preoperative suitability rating (see Appendix 5). Integrating the information at hand (using EAI rating scales), each LAUP candidate should be considered in terms of the severity of the problem (as perceived by the healthcare professional as well as by the patient), the presence, nature and influence of complicating factors, the patient's likelihood to benefit from LAUP, the patient's overall long-term prognosis, the physician's expected outcome of the procedure, and the patient's expected satisfaction with the results. Pooled ratings and grouping of patients generally leads to a more coherent clinical outlook. Candidates whose combined suitability ratings are indicative of successful results should be treated with fewer reservations, whereas those who appear least likely to benefit from LAUP should be reevaluated, reconsidered, counseled carefully, or withdrawn from the procedure at any given stage.

CONCLUSION

It is recommended that all patients be evaluated preoperatively, preferably within a team framework involving a speech-language pathologist and an otolaryngologist. Those patients who qualify as candidates for LAUP intervention should be reassessed prior to each stage. Regardless of the number of stages required, it is recommended that patients be thoroughly evaluated following the last procedure. Patients whose linguistic inventory requires abundant productions of palatopharyngeal or linguopalatal consonants, or who are professional voice users, wind or brass instrumentalists, or glass blowers should be handled with extreme caution. Patients with relatively mild, unrelated speech-language disturbances, or mild neurogenic or structural dysfunction of the palate, pharynx, or larynx also deserve special consideration.

Finally, LAUP may not be advisable for patients with significant psychogenic findings (primarily extreme forms of somatization), patients with serious cognitive deficits, and patients in advanced stages of systemic degenerative diseases. With each additional procedure, the examiner must become more vigilant in detecting, documenting, and, if necessary, communicating to the patient any measured, observed, or perceived warning signs. A final reminder: Before "seeing the light at the end of the tunnel," the typical LAUP patient must go through an agonizing journey. It starts with the social, interpersonal, or sexual humiliation brought about by snoring and ends with the pain brought about by surgery. It is important that all healthcare professionals involved in scheduling, evaluating, and treating LAUP patients work in close collaboration, be fully accountable, and deal with the patients with the utmost patience, respect, and compassion.

REFERENCES

1. Keidar A, Khosh M, Krespi Y, Zammit G: *The relationship between self-reported symptoms and polysomnographic findings in LAUP candidates.* Presented at the American Academy of Otolaryngology, Anaheim, CA, 1994.
2. Monoson P, Fox A: Preliminary observation of speech disorder in obstructive and mixed sleep apnea. *Chest* 92:670–675, 1987.
3. Gislason T, Lindblom C, Almqvist M et al: Uvulopalatoplasty in the sleep apnea syndrome. *Arch Otolaryngol Head Neck Surg* 114:45–51, 1988.
4. Poole M, Postma D, Pillsbury H et al: Obstructive sleep apnea: Recognition, evaluation, and treatment. *N C Med J* 47:768–771, 1986.
5. Dickson R, Blockmanis A: Treatment of obstructive sleep apnea by uvulopalatopharyngoplasty. *Laryngoscope* 97:1054–1059, 1987.
6. Zohar Y, Finkelstein Y, Talmi Y: Surgical concepts in uvulopalatopharyngoplasty: Complications and sequelae. In: Chouard C, ed: *Chronic rhynchpathy.* John Libby Eurotext, 1988;363–367.
7. Salas-Provance M, Kuehn D: Speech status following uvulopalatoplasty. *Chest* 97:111–117, 1990.

8. Shprintzen R, McCall G, Skolnick M, Lencione R: Selective movements of the lateral aspects of the pharyngeal walls during velopharyngeal closure for speech, blowing, and whistling in normals. *J Speech Hear Res* 18:308–318, 1975.

9. Aronson A: *Clinical voice disorders: An interdisciplinary approach*, 3rd ed. New York: Thieme Inc, 1990.

10. Kent R, Vorperian H: *Development of the craniofacial-oral-laryngeal anatomy: A review*. San Diego: Singular Publishing Group, 1995.

11. Pershall K, Boone D: Supraglottic contribution to voice quality. *J Voice* 1:186–190, 1987.

12. Damste H: Shortness of the palate: A cause of problems in singing. *J Voice* 2:96–98, 1988.

13. Sundberg J: Supralaryngeal contributions to vocal loudness and projection. In Lawrence VL, ed: *Transcripts of the 13th symposium: Care of the professional voice.* New York: The Voice Foundation.

14. Crysdale W: Otorhinolaryngologic problems in patients with craniofacial anomalies. *Otolaryngol Clin North Am* 14:145–155, 1981.

15. Shprintzen R: Palatal and pharyngeal anomalies in craniofacial syndromes. *Birth Defects* 18:53–78, 1982.

16. Peterson-Falzone SJ: Resonance disorders in structural defects. In: Lass N, McReynolds L, Northern J, Yoder D, eds: *Speech and language*. Philadelphia: WB Saunders, 1982.

17. Berkowitz S: *Cleft lip and palate: Perspectives in management with an introduction to craniofacial anomalies.* (vol. I and II). San Diego: Singular Publishing Group, 1996.

18. Darley F, Aronson A, Brown J: *Motor speech disorders*. Philadelphia: WB Saunders, 1975.

19. Wertz R, LaPointe L, Rosenbek J: *Apraxia of speech in adults: The disorder and its management.* San Diego: Singular Publishing Group, 1991.

20. Murdoch B: *Acquired speech and language disorders: A neuroanatomical and functional neurological approach*. Melbourne, Australia: Chapman & Hall, 1990.

21. Hartman D, Dworkin J: *Aphasia, apraxia of speech, and dysarthria samples: Audiotape, manual, and test manual*. San Diego: Singular Publishing Group, 1993.

22. Dworkin J, Hartman D: *Cases in neurogenic communicative disorders: A workbook*, 2nd ed. San Diego: Singular Publishing Group, 1993.

23. Murdoch B, Chenery H: *Dysarthria: A physiological approach*. San Diego: Singular Publishing Group, 1997.

24. Tomblin B, Morris H, Spriestersbach D: *Diagnosis in speech language pathology*. San Diego: Singular Publishing Group, 1994.

25. Weber J, Chase R: Stress velopharyngeal incompetence in an oboe player. *Cleft Palate J* 7:858–861, 1970.

26. Shanks J: Velopharyngeal incompetence manifested initially in playing a musical instrument. *J Voice* 4:169–171, 1990.

27. Lipowski Z: Somatization: The concept and its clinical application. *Am J Psychiatry* 145:1353–1368, 1988.

28. Orlikoff R, Baken R: *Clinical speech and voice measurement*. San Diego: Singular Publishing Group, 1993.

29. Baken R: *Clinical measurement of speech and voice*. Boston: College-Hill Press, 1987.

30. Grunwell P: *Analyzing cleft palate speech*. San Diego: Singular Publishing Group, 1993.

31. Okamoto M, Fujita S: Role of dynamic cephalometry in upper airway evaluation of obstructive sleep apnea syndrome. In: Togawa K, Katayama S, Hishikawa Y et al., eds: *Sleep apnea and rhonchopathy*. Basel: Karger, 1993.

Initial Questionnaire for LAUP Candidates

Developed by Anat Keidar, Ph.D., CCC-SLP and Yosef P. Krespi, M.D.

(Copyright © 1993)

Head & Neck Surgical Group
Department of Otolaryngology, Head & Neck Surgery
St. Luke's-Roosevelt Hospital Center
New York, NY

Instructions: Please read each item carefully and answer **all** questions. For some questions you will be asked to choose one or more answers. If you are asked to provide specific information in writing, use the blank space following the question. If a certain question does not apply to your case, please indicate so by writing 'N/A.'

I. Personal Data

Name: Last_________________________/ First_____________________________/ M.I.____________

Home Address: Street & #____

City, State & Zip Code____

Home Phone: ( )________-__________   **Work Phone:** ( )________-__________

Main Occupation:____

Additional Occupation:____

Age:____ / **Date of Birth:** Month____/ Day____/ Year_____/ **Country of Birth:**____________

Sex: (circle) Male Female

Race: (circle) Asian Black Caucasian Hispanic Other (specify)_________________

Height: ________ft. ________inches

Weight: _________lbs.

Marital Status: (circle) Single Engaged Married Separated Divorced Widowed

Language(s) Routinely <u>Spoken</u>: (list in order from most used to least used) _________________

____

Are you a **vocal performer?** (check one)   yes_______ no_______

If **yes**, are you a (circle) Singer Actor Announcer Clergy Other (specify)____________

Are you a **wind instrument player?** (check one)   yes_______ no_______

II. Background Information

1. Who referred you to this office? (circle)   Self   Spouse   Mate   Parent (s)   Child(ren)
Friend(s)   Physician (specify)_______________   Other(s) (specify)_________________________

2. In Your own words, describe precisely the *nature* and *severity of your problem*, and why you
came here____
____
____
____

3. How long have you had this problem? (specify) ____

4. Did your problem start: (circle)   Suddenly   Gradually   Intermittently (off & on)
Other (specify)____

5. In your opinion, what *caused* your problem? (explain)_______________________________________
____

6. Are you primarily concerned with: (circle)   Snoring   Disturbed Sleep   Sleep Apnea
Other (specify)____

7. On a scale of 0 to 5, where **0 = no effect, 1 = mildly negative, 3 = moderately negative,** and **5
= extremely negative,** please rate the *effect* of your problem *on your personal life.*

no effect	mildly negative	_	moderately negative	_	extremely negative
0	1	2	3	4	5

8. On a scale of 0 to 5, where **0 = no effect, 1 = mildly negative, 3 = moderately negative,** and **5
= extremely negative,** please rate the *effect* of your problem *on your job performance.*

no effect	mildly negative	_	moderately negative	_	extremely negative
0	1	2	3	4	5

9. Explain your treatment goals (i.e., what you wish to accomplish after having received medical treatment
in this facility)____
____
____

III. Snoring

1. On a scale of 0 to 5, where **0 = no problem, 1 = mild** problem, **3 = moderate** problem, and
5 = severe problem, please rate *your overall perception of your snoring problem.*

no problem	mild problem	_	moderate problem	_	severe problem
0	1	2	3	4	5

2. On a scale of **0** to **5**, where **0 = no** problem, **1 = mild** problem, **3 = moderate** problem, and **5 = severe** problem, please rate *other people's perception of your snoring problem.*

no problem	mild problem		moderate problem		severe problem
0	1	2	3	4	5

3. On a scale of **1** to **5**, where **1 = much worse**, **3 = no change**, and **5 = much better**, please rate the *condition of your snoring* since the onset of the first symptoms.

much worse		no change		much improved
1	2	3	4	5

4. On a scale of **0** to **5**, where **0 = inaudible,** **1 = extremely soft**, **3 = moderately loud**, and **5 = extremely loud**, please rate the *loudness level of your snoring.*

inaudible	extremely soft		moderately loud		extremely loud
0	1	2	3	4	5

5. On a scale of **0** to **5**, where **0 = never**, **1 = rarely**,   **3 = occasionally**, and **5 = always,** please rate the *frequency of your snoring.*

never	rarely		occasionally		always
0	1	2	3	4	5

6. On a scale of **1** to **5**, where **1 = significantly worse**, **3 = no change**, and **5 = significantly improved**, please rate *your relationship(s) with your 'significant other(s)'* since the onset of symptoms.

significantly worse		no change		significantly improved
1	2	3	4	5

7. On a scale of **0** to **5**, where **0 = not bothersome**, **1 = mildly bothersome**, **3 = moderately bothersome**, and **5 = extremely bothersome**, please rate the *extent to which your snoring bothers (an)other person(s) who share(s) a bed / bedroom with you.*

not bothersome	mildly bothersome		moderately bothersome		extremely bothersome
0	1	2	3	4	5

8. Have you ever:
    a. *Been 'evicted' from your* Bed / Bedroom / Adjacent Part of the House *because of your snoring?* (check one)   yes_______   no_______
    b. *Lost the companionship of a* Bed / Bedroom *partner because of your snoring?* (check one)   yes_______   no_______

9. Have you ever been *treated for snoring*? (check one)   yes______   no______

If **no**, skip to question **11.**   If **yes**, were you treated: (check appropriate response(s))

________**a.** with a device (Examples: CPAP, Dental Appliance, Snore Ball, Pillow, Nasal Dilators)

________**b.** surgically (Examples: Tonsillectomy, Nasal Surgery, Palatal Surgery, Jaw Surgery)

________**c.** medically (Examples: Drugs Such As Progesterone Agents, Protriptyline, Others...)

Describe the type(s) and course(s) of treatment_______________________________________

____

When and for how long? (provide dates)____

By whom? (physician name / specialty / or self) ____

Where? (clinic / institution)____

Have any of the snoring remedies you tried been *effective*? (check one) yes______   no______

10. On a scale of **1** to **5**, where **1 = much worse**, **3 = no change**, and **5 = much improved**, please
rate the *condition of your snoring problem following snoring treatment.*

	much worse		no change		much improved
	1	2	3	4	5

11. On a scale of **0** to **5**, where **0 = unmotivated**, **1 = mildly motivated**, **3 = moderately motivated**,
and **5 = very motivated**, please rate the *degree of your motivation* to alleviate your **snoring**
problem.

	not motivated	mildly motivated		moderately motivated		very motivated
	0	1	2	3	4	5

IV.   Sleep

1. Do you have (a) *preferred sleep position(s)*? (check one)   yes______   no______

If **yes**, circle favored position(s): Supine (Back)   Prone (Stomach)   Right Side   Left Side   Other______

Explain your preference____

2. Have you ever undergone a *sleep study*? (check one)   yes______   no______

If **no**, skip to question **3.**   If **yes**, when? (month / year)_______________________

Where? (clinic / institution)____

By whom? (physician name / specialty) ____

Was it a *full night polysomnography* in a sleep lab? (check one)   yes______   no______

If **no**, explain *how you were tested* (circle one): MSLT (Nap Study)   Split Night Study   Home Study

Other (specify)_____________________________

3. Have you ever been *diagnosed with sleep apnea*? (check one)   yes______   no______

If **no**, skip to the **next section.**   If **yes**, is your *sleep apnea clearly associated*
with snoring? (check one)   yes______   no______

4. Have you ever been *treated for sleep apnea*? (check one)   yes______   no______
If **no**, skip to the **next section.**   If yes, when? (month / year)__________________
Where? (clinic / institution)____
By whom? (physician name / specialty) ____
How? (describe type and course of treatment)____
____

5. Did you *comply with the sleep apnea treatment prescribed*? (check one) yes______ no______
If **not**, why? (explain) ____

6. If On a scale of **1 to 5**, where **1** = very dissatisfied, **3**= neutral, and **5** = very satisfied,
please rate *your* *degree of satisfaction with the sleep apnea treatment* you received
thus far.

very dissatisfied	_	neutral	_	very satisfied
1	2	3	4	5

V. General Health

1. Do you have, or have you had any of the following health problems? [In the space to the left of
each item, please check the appropriate response (**N = No, Y = Yes, P = Past, C = Current**)
Provide additional information (specify) in the line provided following each item.]

N__ Y__ (P__ C__)   **a.** Cardiac (heart):____
N__ Y__ (P__ C__)   **b.** Blood Pressure: (high)____/ (low)____/ ________________________
N__ Y__ (P__ C__)   **c.** Stroke: (CVA)____/ (TIA) ____/ ____________________________
N__ Y__ (P__ C__)   **d.** Cancer:____
N__ Y__ (P__ C__)   **e.** Pulmonary / Respiratory:____________________________________
N__ Y__ (P__ C__)   **f.** Diabetes / Hypoglycemia:___________________________________
N__ Y__ (P__ C__)   **g.** Gastro-Intestinal:____
N__ Y__ (P__ C__)   **h.** Bleeding:____
N__ Y__ (P__ C__)   **i.** Neurologic:____
N__ Y__ (P__ C__)   **j.** Thyroid: (hyper)____/ (hypo)____/ __________________________
N__ Y__ (P__ C__)   **k.** Allergies:____
N__ Y__ (P__ C__)   **l.** Endocrinal / Hormonal:____________________________________
N__ Y__ (P__ C__)   **m.** Emotional:____
N__ Y__ (P__ C__)   **n.** Nose / Sinus:____
N__ Y__ (P__ C__)   **o.** Throat / Voice:____
N__ Y__ (P__ C__)   **p.** Hearing / Balance:_______________________________________
N__ Y__ (P__ C__)   **q.** Language / Articulation / Voice / Resonance:_____________________
N__ Y__ (P__ C__)   **r.** Other:____

2. Are you currently *on any medication* (prescription or over the counter)?
(check one)   yes______   no______

If **no**, skip to question **3.**   If **yes**, please **list by name** each medicine you are taking, **dose per day,** the **date** you began taking it, and the **reason(s)** for taking the medication.

   a. Medicine:________________/ Dose / Day:__________/ Beginning Date:____/____/____
       Reason:____
   b. Medicine:________________/ Dose / Day:__________/ Beginning Date:____/____/____
       Reason:____
   c. Medicine:________________/ Dose / Day:__________/ Beginning Date:____/____/____
       Reason:____
   d. Medicine:________________/ Dose / Day:__________/ Beginning Date:____/____/____
       Reason:____
   e. Medicine:________________/ Dose / Day:__________/ Beginning Date:____/____/____
       Reason:____

3. Have you *ever had surgery*? (check one)   yes______   no______
If **no**, skip to question **4.**   If **yes**, please list each surgery, and **when** and **why** it was performed.

   a. Surgery:____ Date:____/____/____
       Reason:____
   b. Surgery:____ Date:____/____/____
       Reason:____
   c. Surgery:____ Date:____/____/____
       Reason:____

4. Do you *exercise*? (check one)   yes______   no______
If **no**, skip to question **5.**   If **yes**, what type of activity? (specify)________________________
How often? (circle)   Rarely   Occasionally $\frac{1}{2}$ the time   Frequently   Always   Other (specify)_______

5. Do you *currently smoke*? (check one)   yes______   no______
If **no**, skip to question **6.**   If **yes**, How long have been smoking? (specify)_________ Years
How many cigarettes per day? (specify)_________ Cigarettes

6. If you do not smoke now, have you *ever smoked* in the past? (check one) yes______   no______
If **no**, skip to question **7.**   If **yes**, How long have you smoked? (specify)_________ Years
How many cigarettes per day? (specify)_________ Cigarettes
When did you quit smoking? (specify) Month:_________ / Year:_________

7. Are you *exposed to cigarette smoke*:

   a. At home? (check one)   yes______   no______
   b. At work? (check one)   yes______   no______

8. Do you consume *alcoholic beverages* (beer / wine / liquor)? (check one)   yes______   no______
If **no**, skip to question **9**.   If **yes**, what type(s)? (specify)__________________________________
When you have a drink, is it usually *in the evening or before bedtime*?
(check one)   yes______   no______
How frequently do you have an alcoholic drink? (check appropriate response(s))

________**a.** At least one a day
________**b.** Four or more a week
________**c.** Two or more a week
________**d.** Only on weekends
________**e.** Only on rare occasions
________**f.** Other (explain) ____

9. Do you take *sleep medication, tranquilizers, or other substances* to help you 'relax' / fall asleep
before bedtime? (check one)   yes______   no______
If **no**, skip to question **10**.   If **yes**, what type(s)? (specify)_________________________________
How often? (circle)   Rarely   Occasionally $1/2$ the time   Frequently   Always   Other (specify)______

10. Have you recently:

a. *Gained* weight? (check one)   yes______   no______
If **yes**, over what period of time? (specify)_______ Years / _______ Months
How many pounds? (specify)_________   Have you tried to lose it again?   yes______   no______

b. *Lost* weight? (check one)   yes______   no______
If **yes**, over what period of time? (specify)_______ Years / _______ Months
How many pounds? (specify)_________   Did you try to lose it on purpose?   yes______   no______

c. Been *on a diet* to lose weight? (check one)   yes______   no______

11. Based on your current height and weight, do you consider yourself to be: (check one)
within normal weight range   overweight   Obese

12. On a scale of 1 to 5, where **1 = poor**, **2 = fair**, **3 = average**, **4 = good**, and **5 = excellent**, please
rate your current *overall health status*.

poor	_	average	_	excellent
1	2	3	4	5

13. On a scale of 1 to 5, where **1 = extremely low**, **2 = fairly low** (below average), **3 = average**,
4 = fairly high (above average), and **5 = extremely high**, please rate your current *energy level.*

extremely low	_	average	_	extremely high
1	2	3	4	5

VI. Miscellaneous

1. On a scale of **0** to **5**, where **0** = no problem, **1** = **mild** problem, **2** = **mild to moderate** problem, **3** = **moderate** problem, **4** = **moderate to severe** problem, and **5** = **severe** problem, please rate the **presence / severity** of the following symptoms as they apply to you *in the present.* (Circle only **one number** which best corresponds to your condition.)

		no problem	mild problem	-	moderate problem	-	severe problem
a.	difficulty falling asleep at night	0	1	2	3	4	5
b.	difficulty staying asleep	0	1	2	3	4	5
c.	difficulty waking up (feeling tired / unrested in the morning)	0	1	2	3	4	5
d.	difficulty staying awake during the day	0	1	2	3	4	5
e.	tendency to fall asleep involuntarily during active hours	0	1	2	3	4	5
f.	frequent morning headaches	0	1	2	3	4	5
g.	frequent napping during the day	0	1	2	3	4	5
h.	difficulty concentrating	0	1	2	3	4	5
i.	difficulty remembering things	0	1	2	3	4	5
j.	difficulty staying on task (or following through with projects)	0	1	2	3	4	5
k.	difficulty in overall daily functioning	0	1	2	3	4	5
l.	difficulty staying alert when driving	0	1	2	3	4	5
m.	tendency to tire quickly (feel physically weak / easily fatigued)	0	1	2	3	4	5
n.	difficulty in moderate physical activity	0	1	2	3	4	5
o.	difficulty / reduction in sexual activity	0	1	2	3	4	5
p.	difficulty in motor coordination / control	0	1	2	3	4	5
q.	tendency to feel frustrated, irritable, impatient & "moody.	0	1	2	3	4	5
r.	tendency to become apathetic, withdrawn, uninvolved	0	1	2	3	4	5
s.	tendency to feel depressed, "down," or "sad"	0	1	2	3	4	5
t.	tendency to feel anxious, restless, nervous, worried	0	1	2	3	4	5
u.	tendency to feel unattractive, undesirable, rejected	0	1	2	3	4	5
v.	tendency to respond emotionally, "snap" at people, argue, or over-react to what they say or do	0	1	2	3	4	5
w.	tendency to cry easily or laugh about little (trivial) things	0	1	2	3	4	5
x.	difficulty breathing (shortness of breath) during the day	0	1	2	3	4	5
y.	difficulty breathing (shortness of breath) at night	0	1	2	3	4	5
z.	sensation of choking / gasping for air during sleep	0	1	2	3	4	5
aa.	tendency to awaken suddenly with heart pounding	0	1	2	3	4	5
bb.	sensation of tightness / fullness in the throat	0	1	2	3	4	5
cc.	difficulty breathing through your nose when asleep	0	1	2	3	4	5
dd.	sensation of tightness or pressure in the chest	0	1	2	3	4	5
ee.	dizzy spells or problems with balance	0	1	2	3	4	5
ff.	tremor (shakiness) in your hands or other body parts	0	1	2	3	4	5
gg.	numbness / weakness of arms / legs / other body parts	0	1	2	3	4	5

You have reached the end of the questionnaire. Thank you for your participation

Follow-up Questionnaire for LAUP Patients

Developed by Anat Keidar, Ph.D., CCC-SLP and Yosef P. Krespi, M.D.

(Copyright © 1993)

**Head & Neck Surgical Group
Department of Otolaryngology, Head & Neck Surgery
St. Luke's-Roosevelt Hospital Center
New York, NY**

In order to assess the efficacy of the LAUP procedure, we must obtain information from each patient who has been treated in our medical facility. By completing this questionnaire, you will be contirubuting valuable data which will enable us to compare between pre- & post-operative conditions. Be assured that the information disclosed here will be held in strict confidence.
Your cooperation is greatly appreciated.

Instructions: Please read each item carefully and answer **all** questions. For some questions you will be asked to choose one or more answers. If you are asked to provide specific information in writing, use the blank space following the question. If a certain question does not apply to your case, please indicate so by writing 'N/A.'

Today's Date: ______/______/______
　　　　　　　　　　　　month　　day　　year

I. Personal Data

Name: Last________________________/　First__________________________/　M.I.__________

Have there been *any changes* in your **address, telephone number, occupation,** or **marital status** since you filled out your initial questionnaire ? (check one)　　　　　yes______　no______

If **yes**, please provide current information____

II. LAUP Procedure

1. How many **LAUP** *treatments* have you had? (circle one)

1   2   3   4   5   6   7   8   9

2. Date of *first* procedure_____/_____/_____,   Date of *last* procedure______/______/_____
                  month day   year   month day   year

3. Have **all** your LAUP procedures been performed *in the office*?(check one) yes_____ no______
    If **no**, have you received **all** or **part** of your treatment in a(n): (check appropriate response (s))
    a._________ Hospital operating room
    b._________ Ambulatory surgery facility

4. On a scale of **0** to **5**, where **0 = none**, **1 = mild**, **3 = moderate**, and **5 = severe**, please rate the
    pain / discomfort which **you typically experienced** following each LAUP procedure.

none	mild pain / discomfort		moderate pain / discomfort		severe pain / discomfort
0	1	2	3	4	5

If your response to question **4.** (above) was **0** (none), skip to question **7.**

5. Typically, on which day after each LAUP procedure did the **pain reach its peak?** (circle one)

1   2   3   4   5   6   7   8   9   10   11   12   13   14   15   16   17   18   19   20   21

6. Typically, on which day after each LAUP procedure did the **pain completely subside?** (circle one)

1 2 3 4 5 6 7 8 9 10 11 12 13 14 15 16 17 18 19 20 21 22 23 24 25 26 27 28 29 30

7. In conjunction with LAUP, have you undergone any of the following: (check appropriate response(s))
    a._____Correction of deviated septum   **d.**_____Lingual tonsillectomy
    b._____Turbinectomy (__with / ___ without laser)   **e.**_____Adenoidectomy
    c._____Tonsillectomy (__with / ___ without laser)   **f.**_____other (specify)_________________

8. Have **you** noticed any *changes in your speech / resonance / voice* following LAUP treatment?
    (check one)   yes_____ no______
    If **yes**, describe____

9. Has **anyone else** noticed or commented on any *changes in your speech / resonance / voice*
    following LAUP treatment? (check one)   yes_____ no______
    If **yes**, describe____

III. Snoring

1. On a scale of **0** to **7**, where **0 = no** problem, **1 = mild** problem, **4 = moderate** problem, and **7 = severe** problem, please rate *your overall perception of your snoring problem* following LAUP treatment.

no problem	mild problem	_	moderate problem	_	severe problem
0	1	2	3	4	5

2. On a scale of **0** to **5**, where **0 = no** problem, **1 = mild** problem, **3 = moderate** problem, and **5 = severe** problem, please rate *other people's perception of your snoring problem* following LAUP treatment.

no problem	mild problem	_	moderate problem	_	severe problem
0	1	2	3	4	5

3. On a scale of **0** to **5**, where **0 = inaudible**, **1 = extremely soft**, **3 = moderately loud**, and **5 = extremely loud**, please rate the *loudness level of your snoring* following LAUP treatment.

inaudible	extremely soft	_	moderately loud	_	extremely loud
0	1	2	3	4	5

4. On a scale of **0** to **5**, where **0 = never**, **1 = rarely**, **3 = occasionally**, and **5 = always**, please rate the *frequency of your snoring* following LAUP treatment.

never	rarely	_	occasionally	_	always
0	1	2	3	4	5

5. On a scale of **0** to **5**, where **0 = not bothersome**, **1 = mildly bothersome**, **3 = moderately bothersome**, and **5 = extremely bothersome**, please rate the *extent to which your snoring bothers* (an)other person(s) who share(s) a bed / bedroom with you following LAUP treatment.

not bothersome	mildly bothersome	_	moderately bothersome	_	extremely bothersome
0	1	2	3	4	5

6. On a scale of **1** to **5**, where **1 = extremely negative**, **3 = no effect**, and **5 = extremely positive**, please rate the *effect* of LAUP treatment *on your job performance.*

extremely negative	_	no effect	_	extremely positive
1	2	3	4	5

7. On a scale of **1** to **5**, where **1 = extremely negative**, **3 = no effect**, and **5 = extremely positive**, please rate the *effect* of LAUP treatment *on your personal life.*

extremely negative	_	no effect	_	extremely positive
1	2	3	4	5

8. On a scale of **1** to **5**, where **1 = significantly worse**, **3 = no change**, and **5 = significantly improved**, please rate *your relationship with your 'significant other'* following LAUP treatment.

significantly worse		no change		significantly improved
	_		_	
1	2	3	4	5

IV.   Sleep

1. Since your *first consultation* with a physician in our office regarding your candidacy for LAUP, have you been *advised* to undergo a *sleep study*? (check one)   yes________ no________

If **no**, skip to question **2.**   If **yes**, have you actually undergone a sleep study since then?

(check one)   yes________ no________

When? (date) ___/___/___ Where? (clinic / institution) _______________________________

By whom? (physician name / specialty) ____

If **no**, why not? (explain)____

2. Have you **ever** been *diagnosed with sleep apnea*? (check one)   yes______ no________

If **no**, skip to question **3.**

If **yes**, were you diagnosed **prior to** your initial consultation?(check one) yes______ no________

If you have been diagnosed **after** your initial LAUP consultation, was the diagnosis based on a *full night of polysomnography*? (check one)   yes______ no______

If **no**, explain *how you were tested* (circle one): MSLT (Nap Study)   Split Night Study   Home Study

Other (specify)____________________________

3. Since receiving LAUP treatment, have you noticed any changes in your *sleep patterns*?

(check one)   yes________ no________

4. On a scale of **1** to **5**, where **1 = markedly deteriorated**, **3 = no change**, and **5 = markedly improved**, please rate the *quality of your sleep* following LAUP treatment.

markedly deteriorated		no change		markedly improved
	_		_	
1	2	3	4	5

5. Since receiving LAUP treatment, have you experienced *daytime sleepiness*?

(check one)   yes______ no________

6. On a scale of **1** to **5**, where **1 = significantly increased**, **3 = no change**, and **5 = significantly decreased**, please rate *your daytime sleepiness* following LAUP treatment.

significantly increased		no change		significantly decreased
	_		_	
1	2	3	4	5

V. General Health

1. On a scale of **1** to **5**, where **1 = poor, 2 = fair, 3 = average, 4 = good,** and **5 = excellent,** please rate your *overall health status* since your last LAUP treatment.

poor	_	average	_	excellent
1	2	3	4	5

2. On a scale of **1** to **5**, where **1 = extremely low, 2 = fairly low** (below average), **3 = average, 4 = fairly high** (above average), and **5 = extremely high,** please rate your *energy level* since your last LAUP treatment.

extremely low	_	average	_	extremely high
1	2	3	4	5

3. Do you *currently smoke*? (check one)   yes_______ no_______

If **no**, skip to question **4.**   If **yes**, How long have been smoking? (specify)__________________
How many cigarettes / packs per day? (specify)____
Have you tried to quit smoking since your initial LAUP consultation? (check one) yes______ no_______

4.   Since your last LAUP treatment, have you been *consuming alcoholic beverages* (beer / wine / liquor)? (check one)   yes_______ no_______
If **no**, skip to question **5.**   If **yes**, what type(s)? (specify)_________________________________
When you have a drink, is it typically *in the evening or before bedtime?*
(check one)   yes_______ no______
How frequently do you have an alcoholic drink? (check appropriate response(s))

________**a.** At least one a day	________**d.** Only on weekends
________**b.** Four or more a week	________**e.** Only on rare occasions
________**c.** Two or more a week	________**f.** Other (explain)_________________

5. Since your last LAUP treatment, have you been *taking sleep medication, tranquilizers, or other substances* to help you 'relax' / fall asleep before bedtime? (check one)   yes______ no_______
If **no**, skip to question **6.**   If **yes**, what type(s)? (specify)_________________________________
How often? (circle)   rarely   occasionally   ¹/₂ the time   frequently   always   other (specify)_______

6. Since your last LAUP treatment, have you:

a. *Gained* weight? (check one)   yes_____ no______
How many pounds? (specify)____________

b. *Lost* weight? (check one)   yes_____ no______
How many pounds? (specify)____________

c. Been *on a diet* to lose weight?   yes_____ no______

7. Do you have hypertension [high blood pressure]? (check one)   yes_____ no______
If **yes**, since receiving LAUP treatment, has your hypertension condition: (circle one)
worsened   remained unchanged   improved   other (specify)_________________

VI. Miscellaneous

1. On a scale of **0** to **5**, where **0 = no** problem, **1 = mild** problem, **2 = mild to moderate** problem, **3 = moderate** problem, **4 = moderate to severe** problem, and **5 = severe** problem, please rate the **presence / severity** of the following symptoms as they apply to you *in the present* , i.e., following LAUP treatment. (Circle only **one number** which best corresponds to your condition.)

	no problem	mild problem	-	moderate problem	-	severe problem
a. difficulty falling asleep at night	0	1	2	3	4	5
b. difficulty staying asleep	0	1	2	3	4	5
c. difficulty waking up (feeling tired / unrested in the morning)	0	1	2	3	4	5
d. difficulty staying awake during the day	0	1	2	3	4	5
e. tendency to fall asleep involuntarily during active hours	0	1	2	3	4	5
f. frequent morning headaches	0	1	2	3	4	5
g. frequent napping during the day	0	1	2	3	4	5
h. difficulty concentrating	0	1	2	3	4	5
i. difficulty remembering things	0	1	2	3	4	5
j. difficulty staying on task (or following through with projects)	0	1	2	3	4	5
k. difficulty in overall daily functioning	0	1	2	3	4	5
l. difficulty staying alert when driving	0	1	2	3	4	5
m. tendency to tire quickly (feel physically weak / easily fatigued)	0	1	2	3	4	5
n. difficulty in moderate physical activity	0	1	2	3	4	5
o. difficulty / reduction in sexual activity	0	1	2	3	4	5
p. difficulty in motor coordination / control	0	1	2	3	4	5
q. tendency to feel frustrated, irritable, impatient & "moody.	0	1	2	3	4	5
r. tendency to become apathetic, withdrawn, uninvolved	0	1	2	3	4	5
s. tendency to feel depressed, "down," or "sad"	0	1	2	3	4	5
t. tendency to feel anxious, restless, nervous, worried	0	1	2	3	4	5
u. tendency to feel unattractive, undesirable, rejected	0	1	2	3	4	5
v. tendency to respond emotionally, "snap" at people, argue, or over-react to what they say or do	0	1	2	3	4	5
w. tendency to cry easily or laugh about little (trivial) things	0	1	2	3	4	5
x. difficulty breathing (shortness of breath) during the day	0	1	2	3	4	5
y. difficulty breathing (shortness of breath) at night	0	1	2	3	4	5
z. sensation of choking / gasping for air during sleep	0	1	2	3	4	5
aa. tendency to awaken suddenly with heart pounding	0	1	2	3	4	5
bb. sensation of tightness / fullness in the throat	0	1	2	3	4	5
cc. difficulty breathing through your nose when asleep	0	1	2	3	4	5
dd. sensation of tightness or pressure in the chest	0	1	2	3	4	5
ee. dizzy spells or problems with balance	0	1	2	3	4	5
ff. tremor (shakiness) in your hands or other body parts	0	1	2	3	4	5
gg. numbness / weakness of arms / legs / other body parts	0	1	2	3	4	5

2. If On a scale of 1 to **5**, where **1** = **very dissatisfied**, **3**= **neutral**, and **5** = **very satisfied,** please rate *your overall satisfaction **with the LA UP treatment*** you received in our facility for snoring and / or (an)other associated problem(s).

very dissatisfied	_	neutral	_	very satisfied
1	2	3	4	5

3. On a scale of **1** to **5**, where **1** = **strongly discourage**, **3** = **neutral**, and **5** = **strongly encourage,** please rate the ***extent to which you will recommend*** LAUP treatment to others with problems similar to yours.

strongly discourage	_	neutral	_	strongly encourage
1	2	3	4	5

4. If you have any ***comments*** or ***suggestions*** related to your experience with the LAUP procedure please write them below:

____

____

____

____

____

____

____

You have reached the end of the questionnaire.   Thank you for your participation.

Appendix 3
Reading Passage

Man's First Boat

Long ago, men found that it was easier to travel on water than on land. They needed a cleared path or road when traveling on land. But on water, a log of wood or any large object that would float became a man's boat. It served to carry him across a stream or down a river.

The earliest boats were probably made by fastening three or four logs of wood together. Such a boat we call a "raft." A long pole was used by the man on the raft to help guide it across the water. The pole was also useful if the raft got stuck in the mud.

Instructions: Place a small reflector mirror underneath the nostril while holding the other closed. (Present each task twice; once to each nostril.) On a scale of **0 - 3**, where **0 = no flow** (i.e., complete occlusion, no fogging), **1 = slight flow**, **2 = moderate flow**, and **3 = extensive flow**, rate the observed nasal air flow, as depicted by the amount of fogging on the reflector mirror. Make **comments** if you perceive resonance to be unusual, aberrant, hyper- or hypo-nasal.

Sustained Vowels

"Say these sounds and hold them for as long as you can."

a. "Say <u>ah</u> and hold it as long as you can.": L _____ R_____ Comment:__________________
b. "Say <u>ee</u> and hold it as long as you can.": L _____ R_____ Comment:__________________
c. "Say <u>oo</u> and hold it as long as you can.": L _____ R_____ Comment:__________________

Diadochokinetic Tasks Involving Pressure Consonants

"Now I will ask you to say some other sounds. This time repeat them as quickly and as precisely as you can."

a. "Say puh-puh-puh-puh-puh-puh..."   L _____ R_____ Comment:__________________
b. "Say tuh-tuh-tuh-tuh-tuh-tuh..."   L _____ R_____ Comment:__________________
c. "Say kuh-kuh-kuh-kuh-kuh-kuh..."   L _____ R_____ Comment:__________________
d. "Now take the three sound --puh, tuh, and kuh-- and put them together."
   "Like this, puh-tuh-kuh-puh-tuh-kuh..." L _____ R_____ Comment:__________________

Nasal Consonants

"Now I want you to say different sounds. First say them slowly and then as quickly and as precisely as you can."

a. "Say mommi-mommi-mommi-mommi..." L _____ R_____ Comment:__________________
b. "Say no-no-no-no-no-no..."   L _____ R_____ Comment:__________________
c. "Say fun sun fun sun fun sun..." L _____ R_____ Comment:__________________
d. "Say hamper -- hamper -- hamper..." L _____ R_____ Comment:__________________
e. "Now hum as long as you can."
   "Like this, mmmmmmmmmmmmmmm..." L _____ R_____ Comment:__________________

Appendix 4

Simple Sentences **Containing** Nasal Consonants

1. I saw Mickey and Minnie Mouse.
2. Make me a fancy airplane.
3. My uncle's name is Tom.
4. Nancy painted the window green.
5. Mom made him lunch and dinner.
6. The monkey likes bananas.
7. Ben enjoys eating in McDonalds.
8. Make time for brunch on Sunday.
9. It's fun to munch on jelly-bean candy.
10. A man who makes miracles is a magician.

More complex Sentences Containing **No Nasal** Sounds

1. I will purchase the vegetables for supper.
2. You are requested to stay right here.
3. The subway fire caused great fright.
4. East coast dwellers appreciate good seafood.
5. The holidays passed altogether too quickly.
6. Who will give us the gist of the topic?
7. She had to go back to law school today.
8. I saw her go out to greet Peter.
9. The celebrity happily received the key to the city.
10. The letter gave her a severe shock.
11. He greatly appreciates this gesture of good will..
12. The food served at the hotel had little variety.
13. The crawl stroke is easy to execute.
14. The parcel was delivered to the correct address.
15. The liberal arts college is located close by.
16. Bad weather prevailed throughout their voyage.
17. Are the people just rescued seriously hurt?
18. The subdued lights cast shadows about the hall..
19. Basketball develops superb athletic skills.
20. Will you give this girl a piece of paper?
21. Proper posture is a requisite for proper speech.
22. Powerful political parties forget earlier pledges.
23. Library clerks are typically polite.
24. Read your essay aloud to the whole group.
25. Debby graduated at the top of her class.
26. The propeller accelerated as the aircraft took off.
27. His law school professor prepared a hard quiz.
28. Last quarter's profits were difficult to predict.
29. The doctor's secretary will schedule your visit.
30. The tribal rituals extricated the evil curse.

Simple Sentences Which **Do Not** Contain Nasal Consonants

1. Today I will visit the park.
2. Please, cut the birthday cake.
3. Chocolate fudge is tasty.
4. Popeye is a brave sailor.
5. He is just a little baby.
6. Give Billy a big hug.
7. Do you prefer cats or dogs?
8. The dog has two cute puppies.
9. The fur is as soft as silk.
10. Will you play quietly?
11. They threw rocks at the truck.
12. It is terribly cold outside.
13. Margaret goes to church.
14. Yesterday we took the bus.
15. Did you wash your feet?
16. The teacher told us a story.
17. Black pepper is a spice.
18. Everybody is very excited.
20. Where do you wish to go?
21. Pull the tugboat ashore!
22. Bob argued with his coach.
23. Her older sister is pretty.
24. The tie costs twelve dollars.
25. I will get back to you later.
26. Always respect your elders.
27. Jill saw a beautiful butterfly.
28. Joe traded his baseball card.
29. She gave the cab driver a tip.
30. Pay this bill before it is due.
31. Startreck is a popular series.
32. The TV show starts at eight.
33. He quickly solved the puzzle.
34. The strike lasted four weeks.
35. O.K., lets close the deal!
36. Brush your teeth regularly.
37. I received a registered letter.
38. Yellow is a bold bright color.
39. Edward caught a huge fish.
40. Dick Tracy was a detective.
41. Her father will arrive shortly.
42. What subject was discussed?
43. Tell the judge the whole truth.
44. The house was built years ago.
45. Society rewards good deeds.

Appendix 5

Suitability Rating & Treatment Recommendation Summary Sheet for LAUP Patients

Patient Name: ______________________   Date: ___/___/_____

Recommended Treatment (check one):

------------ LAUP (in office)
------------ LAUP (hospital)
------------ SMR
------------ Turbinectomy
------------ LAST (Laser Assisted Serial Tonsillectomy)
------------ Laser Lingual Tonsillectomy
------------ FESS
------------ Other   (specify)_______________________________

____

On a scale of **0** to **5** where **0** is unsuitable, **1** is marginally suitable, **3** is
moderately suitable, and **5** is highly suitable, please rate the *patient's
suitability* for LAUP.

     0   **1**   **2**   **3**   **4**   **5**

If $\leq$ 2, explain   reservations:____________________________
____
____
____
____
____

Comments:

____
____
____
____

Office-Based Surgery of the Head and Neck
Edited by Yosef P. Krespi, MD
Lippincott–Raven Publishers, Philadelphia © 1998

8

Palatal Flutter Snoring

Pathogenesis, Diagnosis and Possible Office Treatments

Peter D. M. Ellis, S. James Quinn, and Niall J. Daly

EARLY WORK

In the latter half of the 1980s, uvulopalato-pharyngoplasty (UPPP) was the standard treatment for snoring (1–3). We became dissatisfied with this operation on account of its radical nature, associated complications, and uncertain results (4–7). We thought it unlikely that we could design treatment improvements unless we understood the precise pathogenesis of the snoring noise in individual patients. Because the fundamental problem is one of noise and noise control we formed a research group consisting of acoustic engineers and otolaryngologists. The acoustic engineers designed laboratory snoring models that have allowed evaluation both of how the snoring noise is produced and how it can be controlled (8,9). The otolaryngologists have investigated human snoring both with sleep nasendoscopy (10) and with sound analysis (11). The information we have derived from these investigations has allowed us to design a treatment program with some scientific basis.

LABORATORY EXPERIMENTAL WORK IN THE DEPARTMENT OF ACOUSTIC ENGINEERING, UNIVERSITY OF CAMBRIDGE, UNITED KINGDOM

Two laboratory experiments were needed to simulate the events taking place at the palatal level in human subjects.

The first experiment consisted of a wind tunnel with air drawn simultaneously above and below a flexible membrane that simulated the soft palate (Fig. 1A). When the wind speed was raised to a certain critical level, the flexible membrane began to flutter (Fig. 1B) and a snoring noise was produced. It was now possible to alter various parameters in the experimental model and find out which alterations most effectively controlled the flutter. The most effective alterations were:

1. Reduction of wind speed
2. Shortening of the membrane
3. Stiffening of the membrane by a longitudinal strut or struts. These alterations were more effective when running the whole length of the membrane, and two struts were found to be more effective than one (Fig. 2).

The second experiment consisted of a length of rubber tubing through which air was drawn by a pump attached to one end (Fig. 3). As the air speed increased, a central portion of the tube began a rapid cycle of collapsing and opening, and this produced a snoring noise. The collapsing and opening were recorded by a video camera placed at one end of the tube as shown in Figure 3. Alterations that controlled the collapsing-opening cycle were:

1. Reduction of wind speed
2. Stiffening of the rubber tube

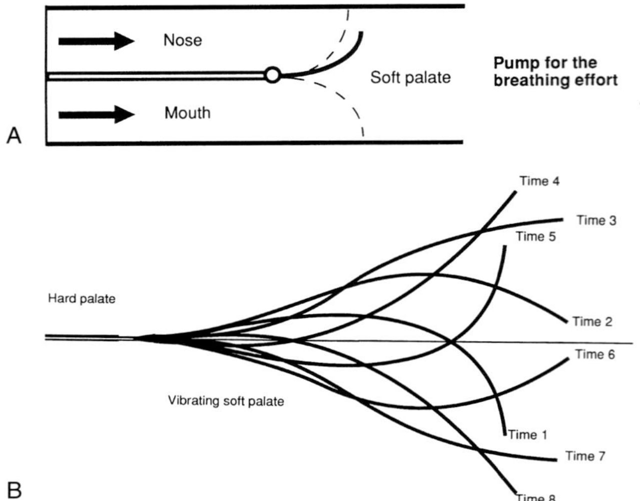

FIG. 1. **(A)** First experimental model. Air is drawn simultaneously above and below a flexible membrane that simulates the soft palate. **(B)** Position of the soft palate at eight consecutive stages of the vibration period. (Reprinted with permission from Ellis PDM, Ffowcs Williams JE, Shneerson JM: Surgical relief of snoring due to palatal flutter: A preliminary report. *Ann R Coll Surg Engl* 75:286–290, 1993.)

HUMAN INVESTIGATIONS

The ideal way to define the pathogenesis of snoring in individual patients would be direct observation of the palate and pharynx during natural sleep. The difficulties involved in such a technique are obvious, although a miniaturized camera placed in the nasopharynx may eventually provide a solution. Cine magnetic resonance imaging and cine computed tomography are attractive possibilities, but, again, the practical difficulties of obtaining these images at night with the patient asleep are clear. The loss of muscle tone in the sleeping patient means that the dynamic events in the pharynx may be very different from those occurring while the patient is awake. For this reason, we place little value on dynamic investigations carried out on awake patients. To try to overcome these problems, we have used nasendoscopy under light anesthesia (sleep nasendo-scopy) and sound analysis of the patient's night-time snoring noise. Both techniques have been useful, but light anesthesia does not necessarily mimic natural sleep and for this and other reasons discussed below we prefer sound analysis in the clinical setting.

In 1991, Croft and Pringle described the technique of sleep nasendoscopy (12). This technique involves the administration of an intravenous hypnotic agent titrated until the subject falls asleep. Once the subject is asleep, the pharynx is examined nasally with a fiberoptic nasendoscope. Sleep nasendoscopy offers the opportunity to directly visualize the dynamic events occurring in the pharynx during sleep-like conditions. Pringle and Croft (13) originally used their technique to observe the sites of obstruction in the pharynx during sleep nasendoscopy in a group of obstructive sleep apnea patients. We have since used their technique to observe the sites of vibration of the

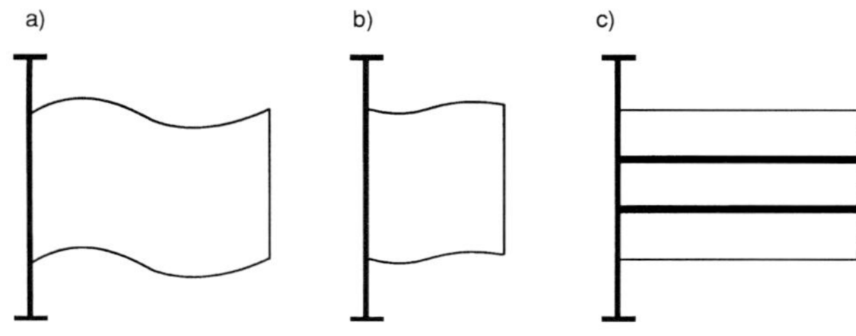

FIG. 2. Control of palatal flutter. **(a)** Fluttering membrane. **(b)** Control by shortening. **(c)** Control by longitudinal rods.

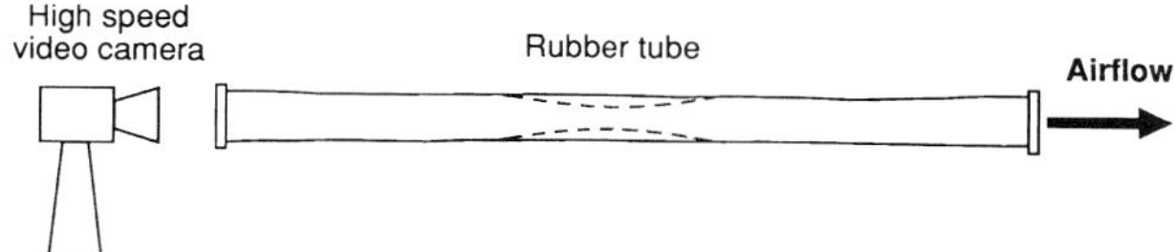

FIG. 3. Second experimental model. Rapid collapsing and opening of rubber tube causes a snoring noise.

pharynx in a group of heavy snorers who did not suffer from obstructive sleep apnea (10). We found several mechanisms of snoring noise production.

In the awake subject asked to simulate snoring, air is drawn through the mouth and nose and then over the upper and lower surfaces of the soft palate. This leads to instability in the airflow over the palate, and the soft palate starts to flap back and forth, intermittently obstructing the nasal and oral airways (Fig. 4). This mechanism is very close to our laboratory experiment illustrated in Figure 1A. During the sleeplike conditions of sleep nasendoscopy, however, a different pattern appeared. The most common form of snoring noise production involved a closed oral airway. Air was drawn through the nose, and narrowing of the airway at the nasopharyngeal isthmus was followed by intermittent obstruction of the airway as the palate and pharyngeal walls rhythmically collapsed together (Fig. 5). This mechanism closely resembles our second laboratory experiment illustrated in Figure 3. In our group of heavy snorers, 90% displayed evidence of palatal level snoring. However, 20% also displayed evidence of snoring noise production at a second site. This most commonly involved the epiglottis (10%), with either the epiglottis flapping rhythmically against the posterior pharyngeal wall or the supraglottis rhythmically collapsing in upon itself (Fig. 6). In 8%, the tonsils were seen to vibrate together (Fig. 7), and in 2%, there was evidence of palatal and tongue base snoring. Of the remaining 10% who did not show any evidence of palatal snoring, nearly all were tongue base snorers (Fig. 8).

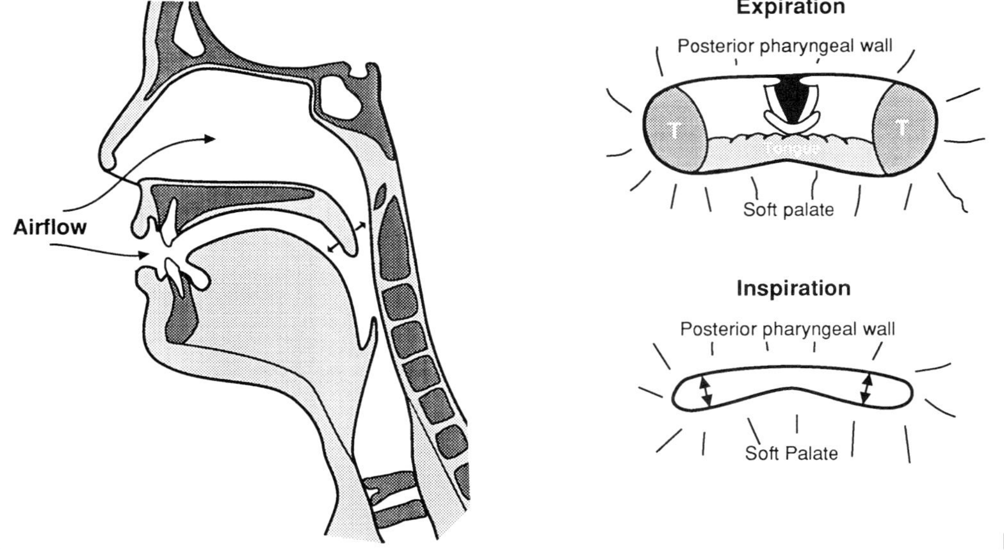

FIG. 4. Simulated snoring. (**A**) Sagittal view. (**B**) Nasendoscopic views. (Reprinted with permission from Quinn SJ, Daly N, Ellis PDM: Observation of the mechanism of snoring using sleep nasendoscopy. *Clin Otolaryngol* 20:360–364, 1995.)

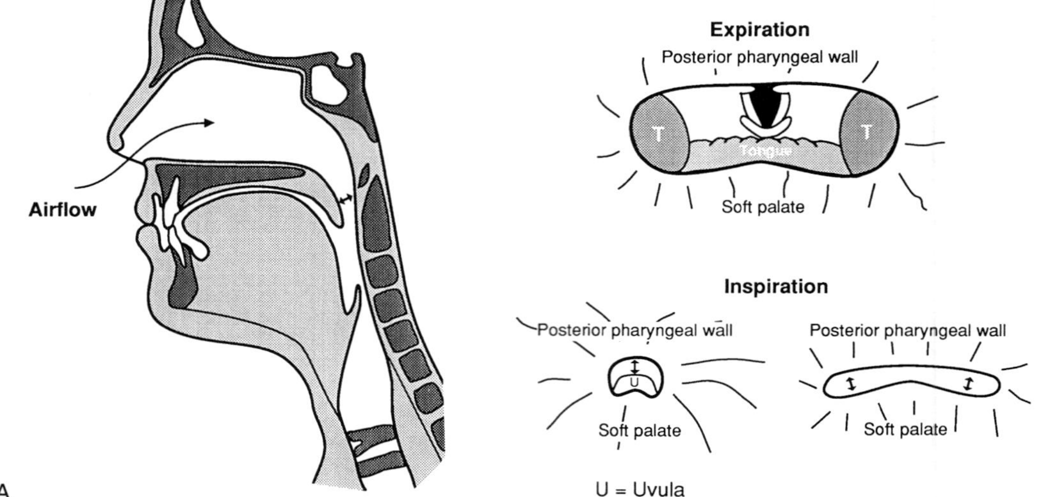

FIG. 5. Palatal snoring. (**A**) Sagittal view. (**B**) Nasendoscopic views. (Reprinted with permission from Quinn SJ, Daly N, Ellis PDM: Observation of the mechanism of snoring using sleep nasendoscopy. *Clin Otolaryngol* 20:360–364, 1995.)

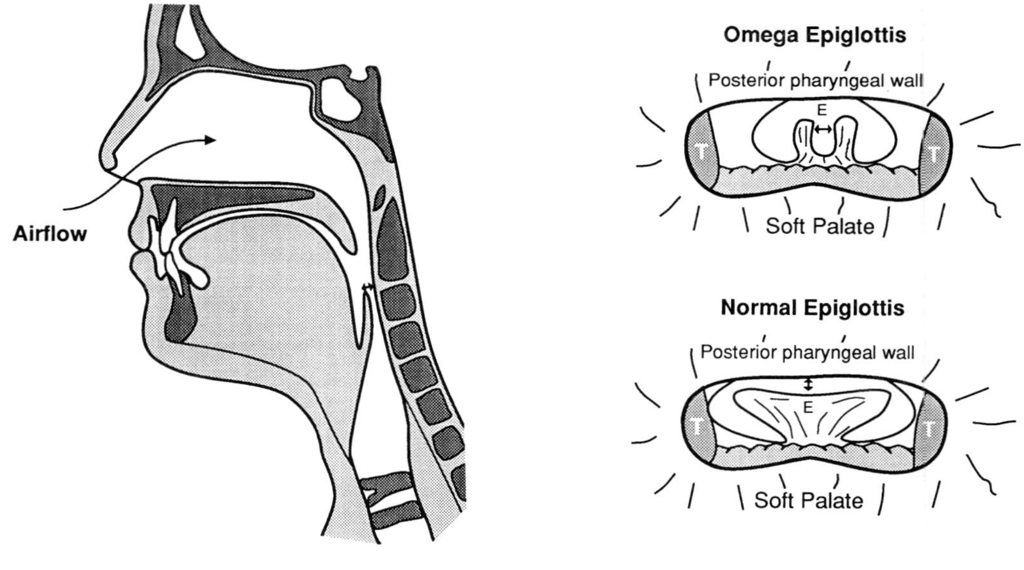

FIG. 6. Epiglottic snoring. (**A**) Sagittal view. (**B**) Nasendoscopic views. (Reprinted with permission from Quinn SJ, Daly N, Ellis PDM: Observation of the mechanism of snoring using sleep nasendoscopy. *Clin Otolaryngol* 20:360–364, 1995.)

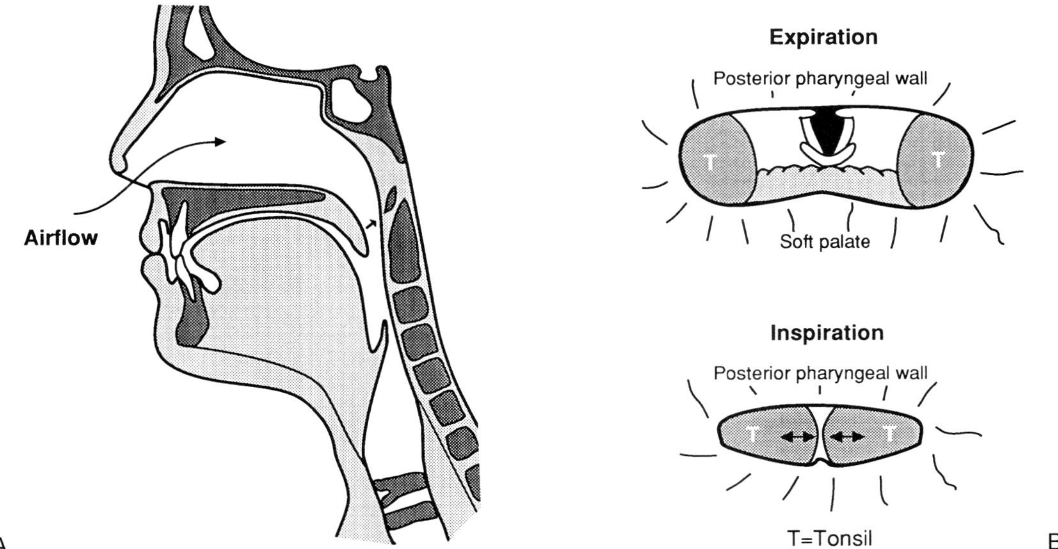

FIG. 7. Tonsillar snoring. (**A**) Sagittal view. (**B**) Nasendoscopic views. (Reprinted with permission from Quinn SJ, Daly N, Ellis PDM: Observation of the mechanism of snoring using sleep nasendoscopy. *Clin Otolaryngol* 20:360–364, 1995.)

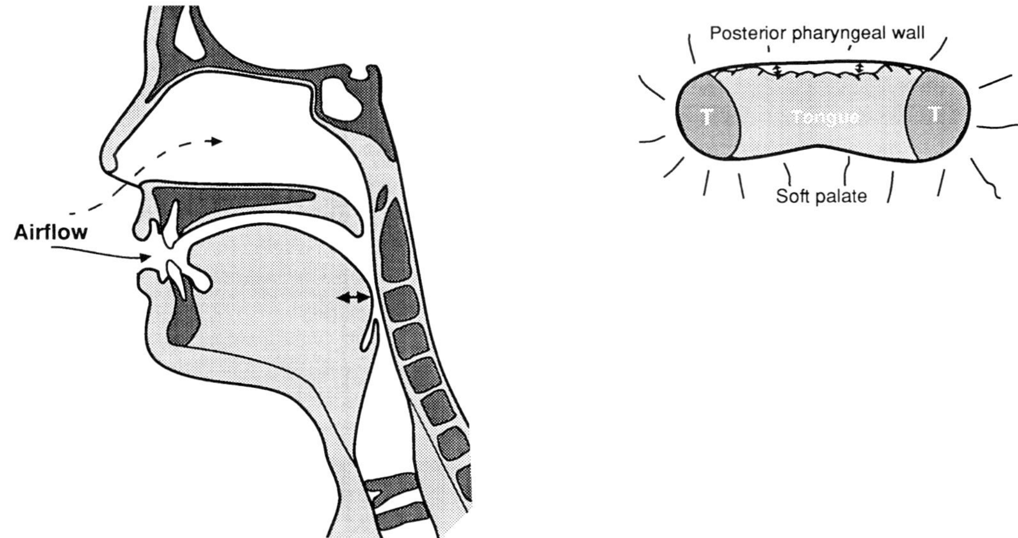

FIG. 8. Tongue base snoring. (**A**) Sagittal view. (**B**) Nasendoscopic view. (Reprinted with permission from Quinn SJ, Daly N, Ellis PDM: Observation of the mechanism of snoring using sleep nasendoscopy. *Clin Otolaryngol* 20:360–364, 1995.)

The tongue base snorers comprise an interesting subgroup because they appear to be separate from the rest. First, 80% of them showed no evidence of palatal flutter snoring; second, they tended to breathe through an oral or oronasal airway, whereas the palatal snorers tended to breathe through a nasal airway. Finally, tongue base snoring sounded different from that of palatal snoring. We investigated this last finding by recording the sound made by four tongue base and six palatal snorers (11). Using a computer, the sound was analyzed for waveform pattern and frequency range. We found that palatal snoring is characterized by repeated impulses in the waveform occurring every 10–31 ms (Fig. 9). These impulses correspond to the rhythmic obstruction of the nasopharyngeal airway seen during sleep nasendoscopy. The peak frequency of palatal snoring is low, averaging 285 Hz in our group (Fig. 10). Tongue base snoring, by comparison, had a chaotic waveform pattern without the repeated impulses seen with palatal snoring (Fig. 9). Furthermore, the peak frequency was higher, averaging 885 Hz (Fig. 10). The difference between the two types of snoring appears to be that during palatal snoring the airway is intermittently obstructed, whereas during tongue base snoring the airway is severely narrowed, but not obstructed,

WAVEFORM

PALATAL SNORING

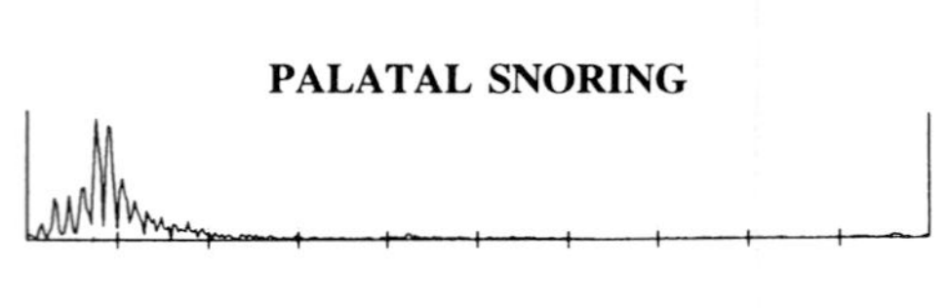

TONGUE BASE SNORING

FIG. 9. Examples of the sound waveform patterns of palatal and tongue base snoring.

FREQUENCY SPECTRUM

PALATAL SNORING

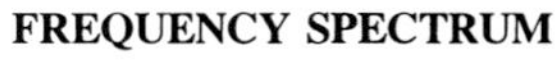

TONGUE BASE SNORING

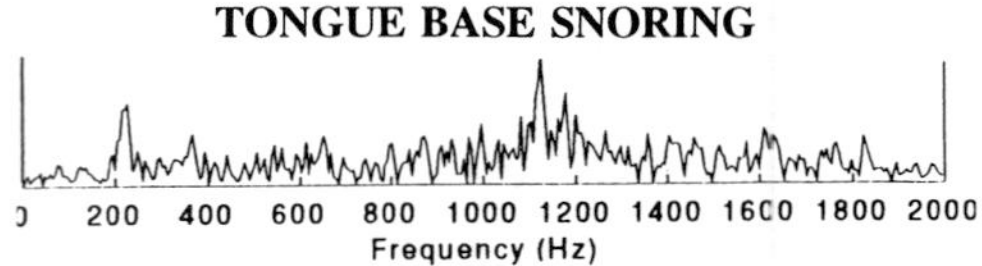

FIG. 10. Examples of the frequency spectra of palatal and tongue base snoring.

producing turbulent, noisy airflow. The human ear can also easily detect the difference between palatal snoring (a flapping noise) and tongue base snoring (a noise similar to inspiratory stridor). The otolaryngologist, therefore, can differentiate between palatal and tongue base snoring by listening to a recording of the noise made. Whether sound analysis can be used to differentiate other types of snoring remains to be seen, but it will certainly be harder because the other snoring types are usually associated with simultaneous palatal snoring.

Sleep nasendoscopy appears to be able to differentiate different types of snoring mechanisms and it is likely that this information would be helpful in formulating a logical surgical treatment plan. However, the technique is somewhat time-consuming and, because of the potential danger of airway obstruction and hypoxia, requires the presence of trained nursing staff, an anesthesiologist, and full monitoring and resuscitation equipment. This makes the technique relatively expensive to perform. Human ear sound analysis, on the other hand, is easy and inexpensive to perform, but it is less precise, probably offering differentiation only between palatal and tongue base snorers.

SURGICAL TECHNIQUES SUITABLE FOR THE OFFICE

According to our experimental work, an effective technique for palatal flutter snoring should either shorten or longitudinally stiffen the soft palate. Although we accept that a minor degree of shortening is likely to be risk-free, we prefer the concept of stiffening as the safer alternative. Over the past 5–10 years, a number of groups, including ours, have been developing appropriate office techniques under local anesthesia, and we now propose to analyze these and define our current practice. [The reader will note that most of these techniques involve the use of lasers. We wish to stress that, although the laser is an elegant surgical tool, there is no evidence that snoring control with laser use is any better accomplished than what might be achieved with the cutting diathermy or even a simple surgical knife.]

Removal of Uvula and Rim of Soft Palate

This is accomplished by electrocautery (14) (Fig. 11). This operation is simply the palatal part of UPPP and relies wholly on shortening the soft palate. Both success and complication rates are likely to be related to the amount of palate resected.

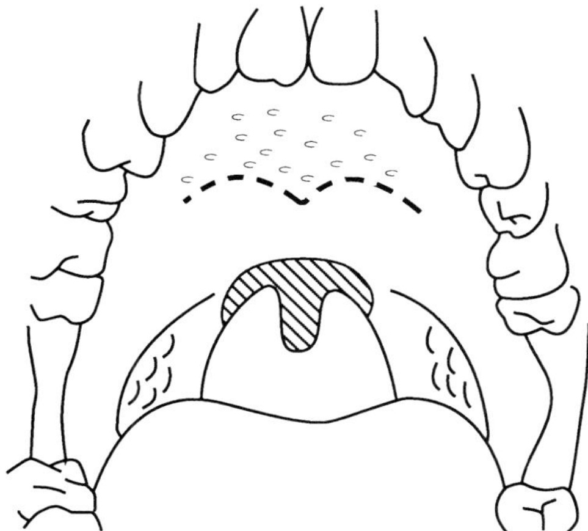

FIG. 11. Removal of uvula and a rim of soft palate. *Curved dotted line* indicates junction of hard and soft palate. Uvula and ring of soft palate have been removed. *Cross-hatched area* indicates resected area.

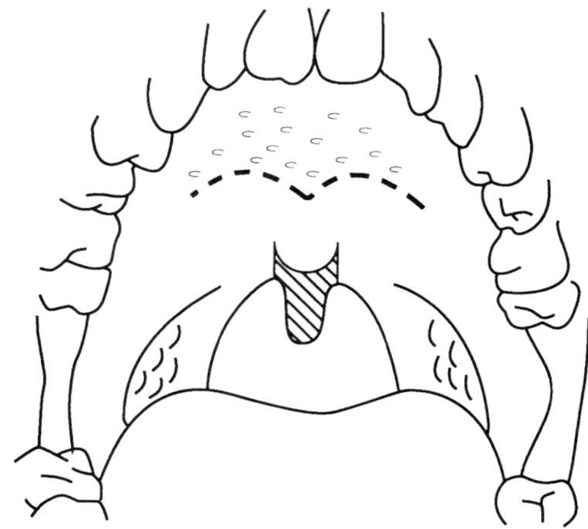

FIG. 12. Kamami type 1 operation. *Curved dotted line* indicates junction of hard and soft palate. Two vertical incisions have been made. The uvula has been shortened. *Cross-hatched area* indicates resected area.

Kamami Type 1 Operation

The Kamami type 1 operation done with a carbon dioxide (CO_2) laser (15) (Fig. 12) is fundamentally a shortening of the soft palate (as in electrocautery) accompanied by some limited stiffening. Because of the indentations in the excision line, longitudinal scar tissue will form on either side of the uvula. These longitudinal scars, however, will be short, and our experimental work suggests that they will be relatively ineffective. We are, therefore, not surprised that further palatal resections are often needed. The difficulty is that the greater the palatal resection, the greater the likelihood of palatal incompetence.

Kamami Type 2 Operation

Following dissatisfaction with the need for multiple procedures, Kamami has described his one-stage technique (Fig. 13) with the CO_2 laser as follows: Two paramedial vertical incisions . . . lateral to the root of the uvula and up to the junction of the soft and the hard palate . . . The new uvula hangs at the back-

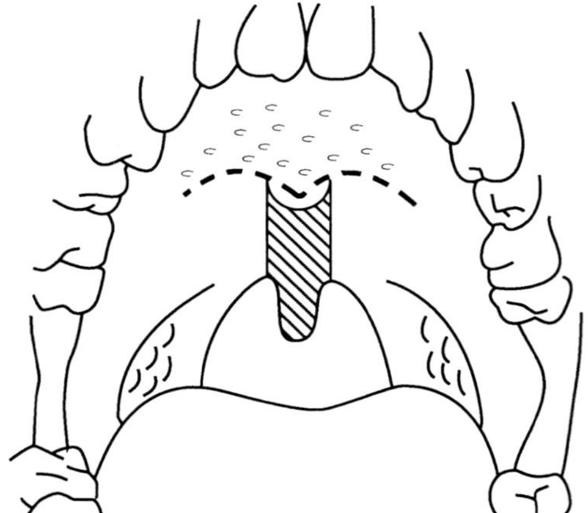

FIG. 13. Kamami type 2 operation. *Curved dotted line* indicates junction of hard and soft palate. Two vertical incisions to junction of hard and soft palate have been made; a 5-mm new uvula is left hanging on hard palate. *Cross-hatched area* indicates resected area.

side of the hard palate, approximately 5 mm under the junction joint between hard and soft palate . . . (15). Figure 13 shows the amount of palatal tissue to be resected in this technique. To reduce the central part of the soft palate to a mere 5 mm seems quite radical and we wonder if this is really what is done. Perhaps it is difficult to be certain of the exact anatomy of the palate when operations are being carried out under local anesthesia.

Ellis Type 1 Operation

This operation (Fig. 14) was our first attempt to introduce longitudinal stiffening into the palate (16). A central longitudinal strip of mucosa was removed from the oral surface of the whole length of the soft palate; the strip was 1.5 cm wide and ran from the junction of the hard and soft palates to the uvula. This was done with an Nd:YAG (Neodymium-Yttrium Aluminium Garnet) contact laser at a power of 10 W. The ulcer was made of sufficient depth to expose part of the palatal aponeurosis and tensor palati muscle, as we

believed that such exposure would lead to maximal fibrosis. We also removed the uvula, as our studies with sleep nasendoscopy showed that the uvula frequently played a major part in palatal level snoring.

Ellis Type 2 Operation

Although our early results with the Ellis type 1 operation were good (16), we began to notice that relapse was common (see below). At the same time we became aware of Kamami's operations and were impressed with the concept of introducing two longitudinal rods rather than one. Our current operation, also using the Nd:YAG laser (Fig. 15), combines the concept of two stiffening rods and some shortening of the soft palate.

RESULTS

The snorer has two main questions. First, will the operation stop the snoring? And second, are there any complications? These are legitimate questions, especially when the pa-

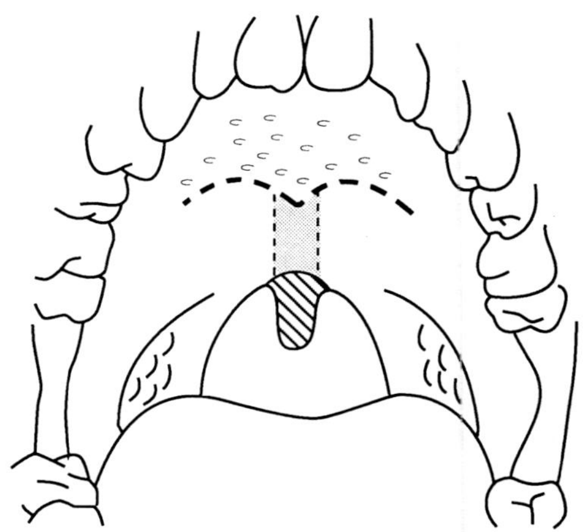

FIG. 14. Ellis type 1 operation. *Curved dotted line* indicates junction of hard and soft palate. Longitudinal ulcer created in midline as indicated by *stippled area*. Uvula is removed. *Cross-hatched area* indicates resected area.

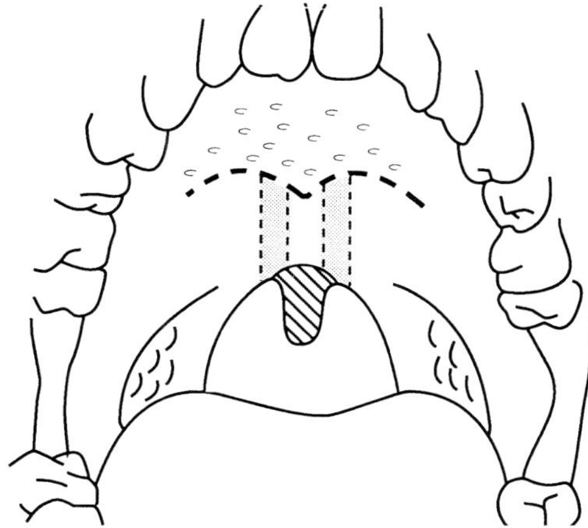

FIG. 15. Ellis type 2 operation. *Curved dotted line* indicates junction of hard and soft palate. Two longitudinal ulcers created as indicated by *stippled area*. Uvula is removed. This may be extended to include an appropriate rim of soft palate depending on the length and degree of redundancy of the soft palate. *Cross-hatched area* indicates resected area.

tient is considering undergoing an operation for someone else's benefit.

Will the operation stop the snoring? It might be supposed that this would be a simple question to answer. It is not. Most surgeons reporting results of their palatal operations rely on questioning the sleeping partner by face-to-face interview, by mailed questionnaire, or by telephone. By making overnight sound recordings Stradling (17) and Miljeteig et al. (18) have shown how misleading such responses can be. The severity of snoring reported by the sleeping partner often bore little or no relation to the actual noise recorded, either before or after palatal surgery. In reviewing our results of the Ellis type 1 operation, we used a mailed questionnaire (Fig. 16) and visual analogue scales (VAS), a methodology that at least removed the possibility of bias by an interviewer and also allowed a numerical assessment of snoring severity. The average preoperative VAS was 9.7, indicating severe snoring in our patients. Postoperatively, we have taken a VAS of 0–4 as a good result, 5–7 as an intermediate result, and 8–10 as a bad

result. These are arbitrary separations, but we think they fairly reflect the perceptions of our patients. Additionally, the questionnaire actively sought the occurrence of side effects and complications. Table 1 shows our good early results and how many of these cases subsequently relapsed. Table 2 shows the incidence of side effects. Various throat symptoms comprised most of the common problems. These varied from globus type symptoms to feelings of dryness or tightness or excess mucus in the throat. One of the functions of the soft palate is to act as a windscreen wiper, wiping mucus down the posterior pharyngeal wall, and it is probably loss of this function that is responsible for these throat symptoms. We believe that various minor throat symptoms will be seen in all types of palatoplasty so far described. We do not yet have adequate data on whether the Ellis type 2 operation will give better results and whether or not human ear sound analysis is of value in selecting those patients liable to respond to palatal surgery. However, we do have some evidence that the use of sleep nasendoscopy has increased our success rate.

CONCLUSION AND CURRENT PRACTICE

There is now little doubt that limited operations on the soft palate can reduce or even abolish snoring in the short term. It is likely that numerous different techniques will be described, but it will be some years before adequate evidence of a best technique is available. In the meantime, difficulties remain in differentiating palatal and nonpalatal snorers (human ear sound analysis may help), and there is insufficient evidence to show that one technique is necessarily more effective and trouble-free than another.

Our current management of snoring patients begins with a full history and clinical examination. This examination obviously centers on the nose and throat, but the general medical state of the patient should not be forgotten. For example, acromegaly can present

DEPARTMENT OF OTOLARYNGOLOGY

NAME AND ADDRESS

Addenbrooke's Hospital
Cambridge
United Kingdom

....

....

....

January 1995

Please return this form to me in the enclosed stamped addressed envelope.

Before my operation my snoring was

____

Now my snoring is

____

AFTER YOUR OPERATION:

Have you any swallowing difficulties?   Yes/No*
(e.g. does your food or drink come back
down your nose)

If yes, what are they? ....

Has there been any change in your voice?   Yes/No*

If yes, what change? ....

Has there been any change in your taste?   Yes/No*

If yes, what change?...

Does your throat feel any different?   Yes/No*

If yes, in what way?...

*** Delete as appropriate**

Peter DM Ellis FRCS
Consultant Otolaryngologist
Addenbrooke's Hospital

FIG. 16. The Cambridge Snoring Form.

as snoring or sleep apnea. Appropriate advice is given about weight loss, reduction of alcohol and tobacco consumption, and the inadvisability of taking sedative or hypnotic medication. Relief of nasal obstruction, either medical or surgical, can help some patients. In our own series, nasal polypectomy was particularly effective in this regard (19). If the tonsils are grossly enlarged, then a simple tonsillectomy may be sufficient.

All our patients undergo an overnight sleep study to look for sleep apnea. The results of UPPP for sleep apnea, which are well documented, are not always encouraging (2,20,21). There is no reason to suppose that limited palatal surgery of any kind will be any more effective than a full UPPP. For this reason, most of our patients with sleep apnea are referred to a respiratory sleep physician for possible continuous positive airway pressure

TABLE 1. *Results of Ellis Type 1 Operation*

Postoperative VAS	3–12 Months Follow-up (%)	12–34 Months Follow-up (%)
0–4	87	60
5–7	13	14
8–10	0	26

Sixty-three patients with a median age of 48 years. Preoperative VAS was 9.7.
VAS, visual analogue scale.

management. Only a very few are offered one or another of the more aggressive maxillofacial surgical options that are available (22–25).

Those patients without sleep apnea are asked to provide a recording of their snoring for human ear sound analysis and are then offered the Ellis type 2 operation under local anesthesia. They are given the following information.

1. The early effect is likely to be good, but may not be maintained; after 2 or 3 years, only approximately two thirds of patients are likely to retain a good result.
2. The operative site is painful for up to 2 weeks.
3. Approximately one half of patients experience long-term throat symptoms, such as dryness, a catarrhal feeling or globus type symptoms.

We firmly believe that the efficacy of these operations should not be exaggerated. Unfortunate publicity and commercial pressures have given rise to wholly unrealistic patient expectations, and we find that one of the most difficult aspects of our work is to bring down a patient's hopes to a reasonable level.

TABLE 2. *Side Effects of Ellis Type 1 Operation*

46% Various throat symptoms
3% Temporary taste alteration
3% Inability to roll 'R'
3% Occasional nasal regurgitation

Sixty-three patients with a median age of 48 years. Follow-up period ranged from 3 to 34 months.

REFERENCES

1. Fujita S, Conway W, Zorick F, Roth T: Surgical correction of anatomic abnormalities in obstructive sleep apnea syndrome: Uvulopalatopharyngoplasty. *Otolaryngol Head Neck Surg* 89:923–934, 1981.
2. Sharp JF, Jalaludin M, Murray JAM, Maran AGD: The uvulopalatopharyngoplasty operation: The Edinburgh experience. *J R Soc Med* 83:569–570, 1990.
3. Blair Simmons F, Guilleminault C, Miles LE: The palatopharyngoplasty operation for snoring and sleep apnea: An interim report. *Otolaryngol Head Neck Surg* 92:375–380, 1984.
4. Croft CB, Golding-Wood DG: Uses and complications of uvulopalatoplasty. *J Laryngol Otol* 104:871–875, 1990.
5. Fairbanks DNF: Uvulopalatopharyngoplasty complications and avoidance strategies. *Otolaryngol Head Neck Surg* 102:239–245, 1990.
6. Levin BC, Becker GD: Uvulopalatophayrngoplasty for snoring: Long-term results. *Laryngoscope* 104:1150–1152, 1994.
7. Haavisto L, Suonpää J: Complications of uvulopalatopharyngoplasty. *Clin Otolaryngol* 19:243–247, 1994.
8. Huang L: *Acoustic control for men and machines.* PhD thesis, University of Cambridge, Cambridge, 1992.
9. Huang L, Quinn SJ, Ellis PDM, Ffowcs Williams JE: Biomechanics of snoring. *Endeavour* 96–100, 1995.
10. Quinn SJ, Daly N, Ellis PDM: Observation of the mechanism of snoring using sleep nasendoscopy. *Clin Otolaryngol* 20:360–364, 1995.
11. Quinn SJ, Huang L, Ffowcs Williams JE, Ellis PDM: The differentiation of snoring mechanisms using sound analysis. *Clin Otolaryngol* 21:119–123, 1996.
12. Croft CB, Pringle MB: Sleep nasendoscopy: A technique of assessment in snoring and obstructive sleep apnea. *Clin Otolaryngol* 16:504–509, 1991.
13. Pringle MB, Croft CB: A grading system for patients with obstructive sleep apnea based on sleep nasendoscopy. *Clin Otolaryngol* 18:480–484, 1993.
14. Blythe WR, Heinrich DE, Pillsbury HC: Outpatient uvuloplasty: An inexpensive, single-staged procedure for the relief of symptomatic snoring. *Otolaryngol Head Neck Surg* 113:1–4, 1995.
15. Kamami Y-V: Outpatient treatment for snoring with CO_2 laser: Laser-assisted UPPP. *J Otolaryngol* 23:391–394, 1994.
16. Ellis PDM, Ffowcs Williams JE, Shneerson JM: Surgical relief of snoring due to palatal flutter: A preliminary report. *Ann R Coll Surg Engl* 75:286–290, 1993.
17. Stradling JR: *Handbook of sleep-related breathing disorders.* Oxford: Oxford University Press, 1993.
18. Miljeteig H, Mateika S, Haight JS et al: Subjective and objective assessment of uvulopalatopharyngolplasty for treatment of snoring and obstructive sleep apnea. *Am J Respir Crit Care Med* 150:1286–1290, 1994.
19. Ellis PDM, Harries ML, Ffowcs Williams JE, Shneerson JM: The relief of snoring by nasal surgery. *Clin Otolaryngol* 17:525–527, 1992.
20. Petri N, Suadicani P, Wildschiodtz G, Bjorn-Jorgensen J: Predictive value of Müller maneuver, cephalometry and clinical features for the outcome of uvulopalatopharyngoplasty. *Acta Otolaryngol* (Stockh) 114:565–571, 1994.

21. Larsson LH, Carlsson-Nordlander B, Svanborg E: Four-year follow-up after uvulopalatopharyngoplasty in 50 unselected patients with obstructive sleep apnea syndrome. *Laryngoscope* 104:1362–1368, 1994.
22. Metes A, Hoffstein V, Mateika S et al: Site of airway obstruction in patients with obstructive sleep apnea before and after uvulopalatopharyngoplasty. *Laryngoscope* 101:1102–1108, 1991.
23. Riley RW, Powell NB, Guilleminault C: Inferior mandibular osteotomy and hyoid myotomy suspension for obstructive sleep apnea: A review of 55 patients. *J Oral Maxillofac Surg* 47:159–164, 1989.
24. Waite PD, Wooten V, Lachner J, Guyette RF: Maxillomandibular advancement surgery in 23 patients with obstructive sleep apnea syndrome. *J Oral Maxillofac Surg* 47:1256–1261, 1989.
25. Riley RW, Powell NB, Guilleminault C: Maxillofacial surgery and nasal CPAP: A comparison of treatment for obstructive sleep apnea syndrome. *Chest* 98: 1421–1425, 1990.

Office-Based Surgery of the Head and Neck
Edited by Yosef P. Krespi, MD
Lippincott–Raven Publishers, Philadelphia © 1998

9

Laser-Assisted Uvulopalatoplasty for Snoring

Yosef P. Krespi

Snoring has long been described as a socially disturbing problem. Only relatively recently have the adverse medical effects of snoring and its association with obstructive sleep apnea (OSA) (1,2) and upper airway resistance syndrome (UARS) (3) been recognized. Various methods have been utilized to alleviate snoring and OSA. They include behavior modification, sleep positioning, continuous positive airway pressure, and uvulopalatopharyngoplasty (UPPP) (4). Laser-assisted uvulopalatoplasty (LAUP) allows treatment of snoring and mild OSA in an office or ambulatory setting under local or topical anesthesia (5–7).

Snoring is a loud, recurrent breath sound, with variable intensity and frequency, that occurs upon inspiration during sleep. It is generated by the vibration of the soft tissue structures in the pharynx. Snoring (snorting) from the palatal origin can be characterized as a rhythmic sound in the low frequencies as opposed to snoring from the hypopharynx, which is a nonrhythmic sound in the mid frequency. OSA is the most severe end of the sleep disturbance continuum. It is characterized by periodic apneas and hypopneas that produce asphyxia, sleep fragmentation, and arousal from sleep. Diagnosis of OSA is confirmed by polysomnography. OSA can be classified according to the apnea hypopnea index (AHI) and oxygen desaturation. The diagnosis of snoring is made primarily by history, much of which can be obtained from the patient's bed partner. The character and consistency of the snoring are examined to determine its severity and possible presence of OSA. Frequent episodes of breathing cessa-

tion followed by sudden and intensified snoring is a strong indication of OSA. Management of OSA is discussed further in Chapter 10. A detailed survey that explores the snorer's medical condition, sleeping position, alcohol and sedative intake, weight changes, and daytime performance is an important part of the history. The use of questionnaires designed for this disorder provides the health care provider the ability to obtain a complete history (see Chapter 7) (8,9).

Physical examination should include complete evaluation of the upper airway, including nose, nasopharynx, oral cavity, oropharynx, hypopharynx, and larynx. Flexible fiberoptic nasolaryngoscopy completes this examination. Much time is spent in the nasopharynx to visually analyze the velum. The area is observed for anatomic and functional abnormalities. The soft palate is also observed in motion. The patient is asked to breathe regularly from the nose, then to swallow. The nasopharyngeal closure is observed. Findings such as hypertrophy of the adenoids, retention cysts, or other lesions of the nasopharynx must be documented. Muscle hypertrophy, muscle weakness, or lack of muscle causing functional abnormalities of the velum need to be identified. Then the patient is asked to snort voluntarily and the vibrations of the velum are observed (Fig. 1). Pressure can be applied to the center portion of the soft palate and uvula by curving the nasopharyngoscope forward; this may eliminate or reduce the voluntary snorting, which we consider a strong diagnostic sign for palatal snoring. The Müller maneuver is also performed; it consists of inhaling against a closed mouth and nose to create

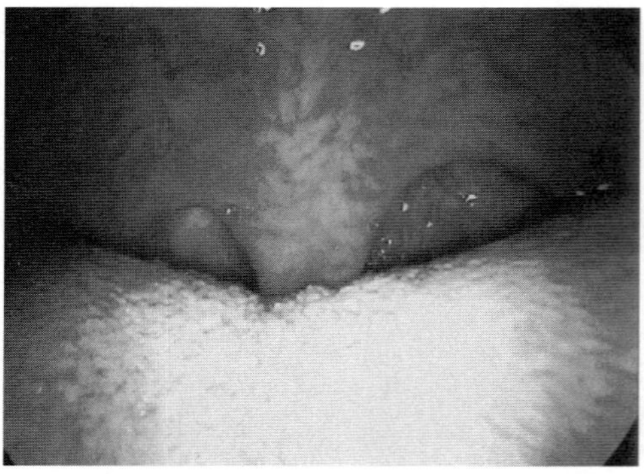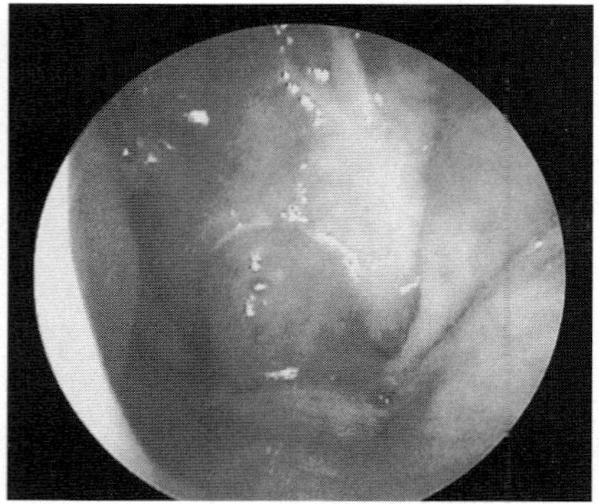

FIG. 1. **(A)** Transoral and **(B)** transnasal examination of the velum with endoscopes. Note the elongated uvula prolapsing into the nasopharynx during voluntary snorting.

maximal negative pressure in the upper airway. This maneuver aids in the detection of any collapsing site in the pharynx, and is an important part of the examination in understanding the site and the pathophysiology of the pharyngeal obstruction. It is repeated at the tongue base level as well.

Snoring may originate from vibration of the soft tissue structures in the pharynx, including the soft palate, uvula, tonsils, tonsillar pillars, tongue base, and posterior and lateral walls of the pharynx. These vibrations occur because of airflow turbulence in the sleeper's pharynx, originating either in the nose (ie, due to turbinate enlargement or septal deviation) or in the oropharynx. The turbulent airflow produces a flutter-valve effect in the collapsible pharyngeal tissues. OSA results from the collapse of the pharyngeal walls in response to negative inspiratory pressure in the upper airway. Pharyngeal musculature hypotonicity allows upper airway collapse at more modest negative inspiratory pressures. This facilitates pharyngeal collapse or soft tissue flutter, leading to apnea or snoring.

The physical examination must be extended to the mesopharynx and the hypopharynx. Observation of the palate and the entire length of the uvula in motion is very important. Depressing the tongue base and stimulating the patient for gag reflex provides an opportunity to select the proper candidates for LAUP under local anesthesia.

The palatine and lingual tonsils are examined. The size and position of the tongue base in relation to the pharyngeal airway is observed and documented. The hypopharynx is examined with flexible and rigid scopes. During this phase the patient is asked to protrude the tongue, and the presence of a vallecula space is observed. Those patients who are unable to demonstrate vallecula and those with persistent vertical pharyngeal folds are considered poor candidates for LAUP because of obstruction at the hypopharynx that cannot be improved with palatal surgery.

NONSURGICAL MANAGEMENT

Surgical procedures to address snoring entail certain minor risks and discomfort. It is therefore prudent to attempt medical intervention or behavioral modification in appropriate circumstances. Sleep positioning may be sufficient in grade I snoring. Nasal allergies should be treated when present. Elimination of tranquilizers and sleeping pills, avoidance of alcohol prior to sleep, weight reduction using strict dietary measures, and daily exercise are imperative. Exposure to upper airway irritants, such as smoke and fumes, must be eliminated.

Because both medical and behavioral management require prolonged follow-up and adherence to a restrictive lifestyle, not all patients are able to comply. Additionally, many patients do not respond to conservative treatment measures. Surgical management is generally preferred by young and middle-aged individuals (8–10).

SURGICAL PROCEDURE

LAUP is a technique developed by Kamami in France in the late 1980s (8). It was introduced in the United States as a treatment for snoring without apnea in 1992. The procedure is designed to improve the airway obstruction and soft tissue vibration at the level of the soft palate by reducing, reshaping, and stiffening the tissues of the velum and the uvula (5–7).

Contraindications

Absolute contraindications to LAUP in an office setting are relatively few. They include significant obstructive sleep apnea (AHI >30), uncontrolled hypertension, trismus, submucus cleft of the palate, pre-existing velopharyngeal insufficiency or soft palate weakness (paresis), uncooperative patients and patients with severe gag reflex, or an anatomic source of snoring other than the soft palate (Fig. 2).

Caution should be exercised in patients who use their voice professionally or play wind instruments. Linguistic constraints for certain languages that use the soft palate or the uvula extensively (eg, Arabic, Russian, French, Hebrew, and Farsi) may also be a consideration. Patients with allergies to local anesthetics and a hyperactive gag reflex can be treated under general anesthesia.

Procedure

LAUP is performed in an upright sitting position in an otolaryngology examination chair. The patients report to the office on an empty stomach without premedication. A topical anesthetic such as benzocaine 20% (Hurricane, Beutlich Pharmaceuticals, Niles, IL) is sprayed in the posterior oral cavity over the soft palate, tonsils, and uvula. After 3 minutes, a 1.0-mL mixture of 2% lidocaine with 1:100,000 epinephrine and 0.5 mL of 0.5% bupivicaine is injected into the junction of the soft palate and the uvula bilaterally and into the base of the uvula. A small-gauge needle is used; for best results, the injection must be given slowly into the muscle layer of the palate. If laser ablation of the tonsils and the tonsillar pillars is to be performed, injection is also given into the superior junction of the anterior and posterior pillars bilaterally.

Surgical use of the laser begins after allowing 10 minutes for the anesthetic to take effect and for vasoconstriction to occur. A carbon dioxide (CO_2) laser is preferred, owing to its

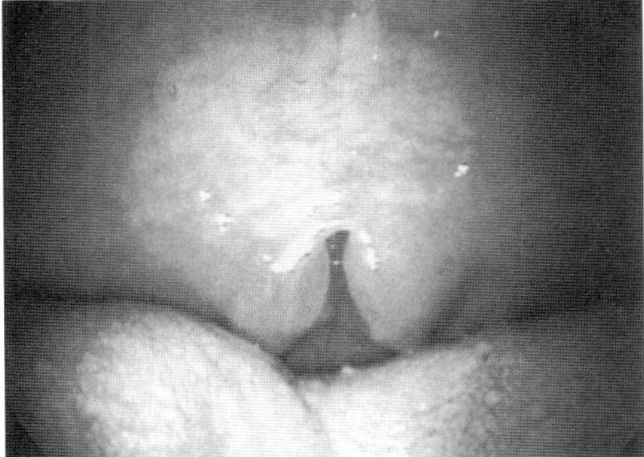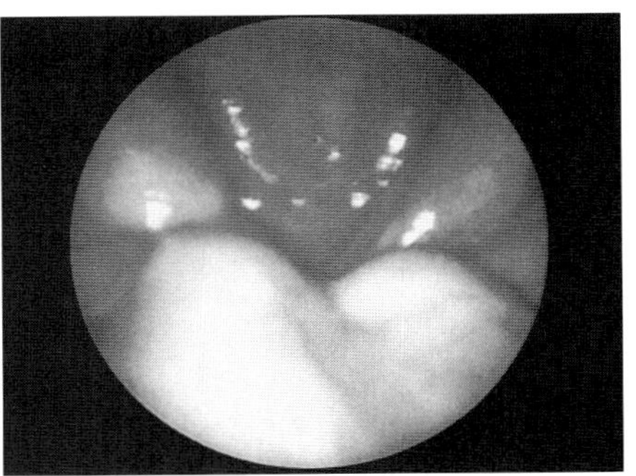

FIG. 2. (A) Transoral and **(B)** transnasal examination of soft palate with bifid uvula and submucus cleft.

wide availability and ease of use. The CO_2 laser with its scanning attachments can adequately coagulate the small-diameter vessels encountered in this procedure. The following description outlines LAUP performance with the CO_2 laser.

The patient and staff are equipped with protective goggles, and laser safety rules are followed. Power is set at 18–20 W in the continuous mode. For optimal laser tissue interaction, a scanning device (SwiftLase or SurgiTouch, Sharplan Lasers, Inc., Allendale, NJ) is activated. The scanning device provides surface ablation of a large surface (2–4 mm) in the focus mode. This method provides char-free ablation, without raising the temperature in tissue to extreme levels of 300°C–400°C. The tongue is depressed inferiorly with an ebonized tongue depressor, which has an integrated smoke evacuation channel. Through and through, full-thickness, vertical trenches measuring 1.0–1.5 cm are created on the free edge of the soft palate at either side of the uvula. These trenches are made using a focused beam with a scanning device to avoid charring and a special handpiece with a back-stop tip. The patient is asked to inhale first, and then the laser is activated during slow exhalation to avoid inhalation of the plume. Adequate and rapid smoke evacuation is mandatory to provide full patient comfort and to avoid nausea and cough.

Shortening and thinning of the uvula are carried out with the regular handpiece in the focused mode or with the SwiftLase flash-scanner. The uvula is reduced by 80%–90% from its original dimension by coring it in a cephalic direction. Overall, the goal is to reduce its length and bulk. Reshaping of the soft palate and uvula can be done with the back-stop handpiece. Care must be taken not to burn the mucosa covering of the soft palate and the uvula excessively. The uvula is shortened by ablating and thinning the muscle from within, creating a "fish-mouth" appearance of its tip, while preserving the mucosa of its base, and that of the nasal and oral surfaces. Light bleeding may occur during surgery when using other methods, such as laser amputation of the uvula; however, bleeding is easily controlled by applying silver nitrate.

INTERACTIVE LASER-ASSISTED UVULOPALATOPLASTY

Since January 1996 we have been using a new method called "interactive" LAUP under local anesthesia in an office setting. This technique requires full participation on the part of the patient during surgery. The uvula is trimmed and reduced in size, layer by layer, starting from its very tip upward toward the base. The CO_2 laser with conventional pharyngeal handpiece and scanning device is used to trim and reshape the uvula and open the palate arches, gradually and sequentially. However, the endpoint of the procedure is decided on by getting a sound input from the patient by a gradual reduction or elimination of the snorting sound. The patient's full participation is necessary during the procedure; therefore, preoperative or intraoperative sedation or narcotic medication is not used during interactive LAUP. The rhythmic vibrations of the uvula, which is the classic effect for palatal snoring, is documented prior to the procedure by allowing the patient to snort voluntarily. The cyclical vibrations from the movement of the uvula and the soft palate occur every 10–30 ms with an average frequency in the 300-Hz range. This sound is quite typical for snoring originating in the soft palate and can be easily distinguished from snoring originating from the nose, the tongue base, or the pharynx. The surgical goal is significant reduction or total elimination of the snorting sound. The interactive method of palate treatment allows us to reduce the number of LAUP sessions and achieve a cure usually after one session in most patients when the patients are properly selected. In addition, it eliminates excessive trimming of the soft palate and the uvula, which may cause significant postoperative dryness and a sensation of thick mucus in the back of the throat. It also retains one of the most important functions of the soft palate and the uvula, which is lubrication and sweeping of the retropharyngeal mucous. By using the interactive method, this common postoperative complication of sensation of thick mucus in the throat is practically eliminated.

"Interactive LAUP" allows the surgeon to achieve a success rate, probably in one session, and reduces or eliminates the most common postoperative discomfort, such as foreign body and thick mucus sensation in the back of the throat. A major advantage of UPPP performed with the laser as opposed to electrocautery is the ability to titrate the optimal trimming and reshaping of the soft palate and the uvula and to successfully eliminate the snoring sound without significant postoperative discomfort or complication (Figs. 3–6).

Postoperative Instructions

Patients may resume regular activities immediately following surgery. A soft, bland diet with avoidance of citrus products and spicy food is recommended. Aggressive hydration, humidification, and steam inhalation are emphasized. Dryness of the mucous membranes is thought to be an important source of postoperative pain and discomfort. Viscous Xylocaine gel (Astra, Westboro, MA) is used to relieve pain every 4 hours as needed or before meals. Gargling with diluted hydrogen peroxide or nonalcoholic mouthwash is recommended. Aloe vera juice swallowed periodically in small amounts has had a comforting effect on the healing palate. The need for analgesics varies according to each patient's tolerance. Various analgesics from acetaminophen, to acetaminophen with codeine, to oxycodone hydrochloride can be used. Prophylactic antibiotics are prescribed for every patient. Steroids, however, are not indicated in this group of patients unless a nasal procedure (eg, septoplasty or turbinate reduction) is performed in conjunction with LAUP.

Typically, LAUP requires two or three treatments spaced a minimum of 8–10 weeks

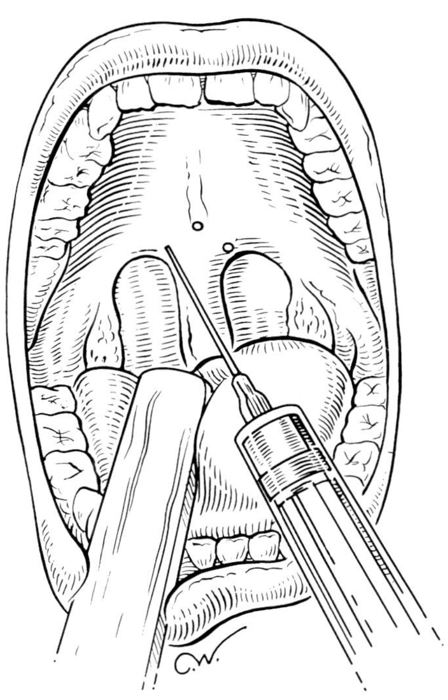

FIG. 3. Injection site for local anesthesia.

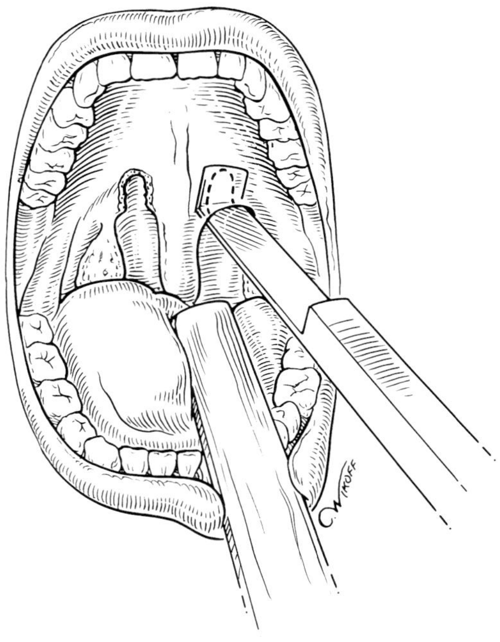

FIG. 4. Bilateral trenches on the free edge of the velum (inverted U shape) using a CO_2 laser with a scanning device.

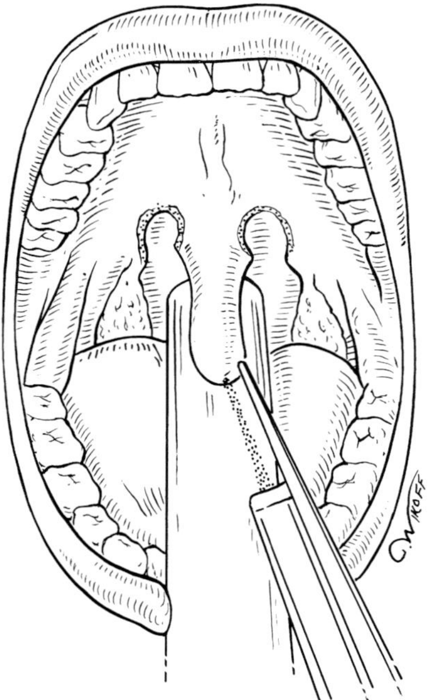

FIG. 5. Reduction and reshaping of the uvula with a scanning device. Note the tongue blade used as a backstop.

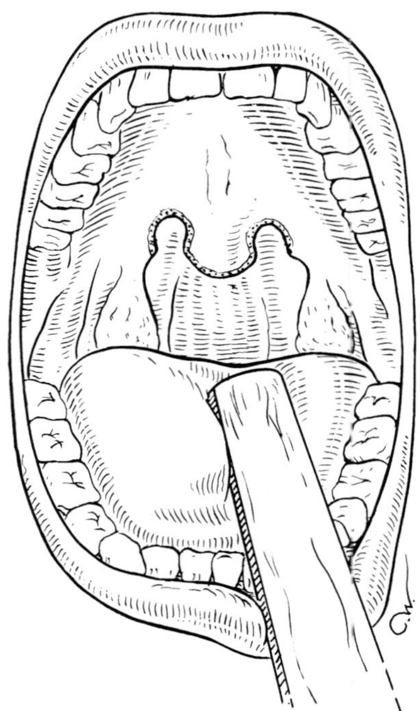

FIG. 6. Postoperative view after interactive laser-assisted uvulopalatoplasty. Note the fullness retained in the center of the soft palate. This structure may prevent postoperative dryness and foreign body sensation.

apart. Elapsed time between the procedures allows proper healing of the soft palate mucosa. The endpoint of LAUP is when snoring is significantly reduced or eliminated. Confirmation is obtained by history from the patient or the bed partner or by the inability of the patient to perform voluntary snoring.

Efficacy

Krespi et al. reviewed 280 patients who underwent LAUP in the office, with a 3-month to 2-year follow-up (6,7). They reported that 84% had snoring eliminated, and an additional 7% had a reduction in snoring. Carenfelt reported 85% total or near-total elimination of snoring during a short-term follow-up (duration not specified) of 60 patients. Kamami, in a review of 31 patients with a maximal follow-up of 18 months, reported 77% elimination or significant reduction of snor-

ing (5). Ellis et al. published the results of laser palatoplasty in 16 patients with 3–6-month follow-up. The surgical technique described by Ellis et al. was slightly different, in that only a central longitudinal strip of mucosa was removed from the surface of the soft palate (Figs. 7 and 8). This resulted in 85% elimination or significant reduction of snoring. Long-term results of LAUP treatment for snoring are not yet available owing to the novelty of the procedure. It is possible that prolonged follow-up will reveal more modest success for this operation.

Complications

The reported complications for LAUP are rare. Moderate to severe pain is the major side

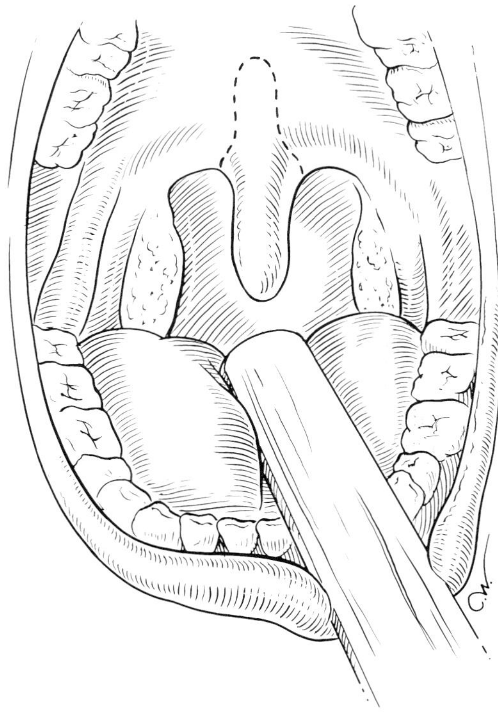

FIG. 7. Laser-assisted uvulopalatoplasty—British method. Area of ablation is outlined.

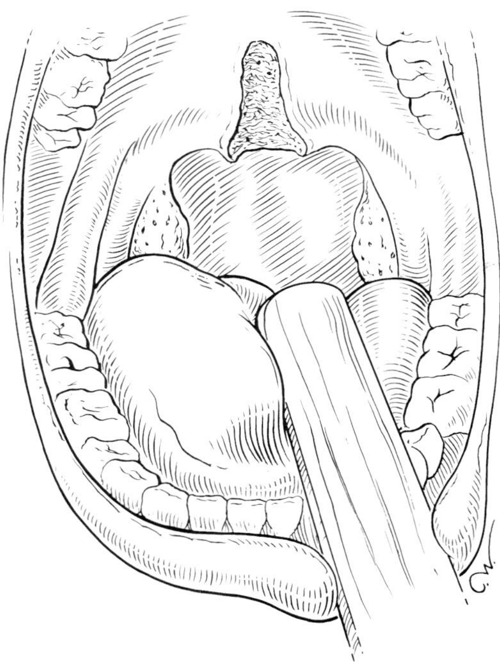

FIG. 8. Laser-assisted uvulopalatoplasty—British method. (Uvulectomy and laser ablation of center of palate, mucosa, and muscle only.)

effect of the procedure. Pain intensity reaches its peak 4 days postoperatively, with complete relief of symptoms in 8–10 days. Pain is usually well controlled with hydration, anesthetic gel, and oral analgesics. Most patients report some degree of weight loss, typically less than 10 pounds over the course of the postoperative healing. Healing occurs by formation of white eschar in 3–5 days following the procedure. Complete mucosal healing takes place following the slough of eschar in about 12–14 days.

Intraoperative bleeding occurs in about 3% of the patients. Bleeding is usually from the apex of the palate trench incision and is stopped with application of silver nitrate. No patients have required hospital admission or transfusion. Delayed bleeding is rare; we have encountered this in only one patient in our series. Krespi et al. reported two vasovagal episodes following injection of the local anesthetic in a review of 280 patients (6).

Velopharyngeal insufficiency, either temporary or permanent, has not been reported, probably due to the graded surgical approach. Nasopharyngeal stenosis has not been encountered because, by using the special handpiece with backstop to make the palatal incisions, the nasopharyngeal mucosa is protected from injury. Approximately 40% of patients may complain of a scratchy or "dry mucus" sensation in the throat. This is usually self-limited and resolves within 2 months.

CONCLUSION

LAUP is an effective method for treating patients with loud, habitual snoring, UARS, and mild OSA. LAUP offers several advantages to the classic UPPP, including reduced cost, decreased operative morbidity, diminished postoperative pain, and abbreviated convalescence period, as well as avoidance of general anesthesia.

LAUP or "interactive" LAUP as an office procedure, performed under local anesthesia, has proved to be a safe and effective method of alleviating bothersome snoring. The surgery may be undertaken in stages to allow titration of tissue removal with minimal risk of overcorrection. Patient selection requires a careful review of the medical history and a thorough physical evaluation. The nose, tongue base, and hypopharynx should be ruled out as the primary site of airway obstruction. Polysomnography is indicated in those patients at risk for OSA. LAUP, when performed in properly selected candidates, can result in excellent clinical outcome and patient satisfaction.

CASE REPORT OF A TYPICAL PATIENT WITH THICKENED UVULA AND HABITUAL SNORING

A 40-year-old man was seen for snoring. His wife had refused to sleep in the same bedroom for the previous 3 years owing to the intensity of his snoring. His wife denied episodes of breathing cessation. The patient did not smoke or consume alcohol or sedatives. The patient also reported mild daytime sleepiness.

Examination

The patient was mildly obese at 5'8" and 179 pounds (calculated body mass index = 27.4). Mild hypertension was present. Nasal examination did not demonstrate significant septal deviation or turbinate enlargement. Intraoral evaluation revealed a flat-appearing palate, an elongated thick uvula, and thick posterior pharyngeal folds. Fiberoptic nasopharyngoscopy showed that lingual tonsils were not enlarged, and there was no hypopharyngeal collapse on Müller maneuver. Polysomnography performed at the patient's home revealed mild apnea (apnea hypopnea index of 12) and no desaturation.

Diagnosis

Snoring due to mild obesity, thickened uvula, and redundant thick lateral pharyngeal folds.

Anesthesia

Topical benzocaine 20% spray applied to the posterior oral cavity, followed by injection of a mixture of 1.0 mL of 2% lidocaine with 1:100,000 epinephrine and 0.5 mL of 0.5% bupivicaine into the soft palate.

Procedure

LAUP was performed using the CO_2 laser with SurgiTouch scanner at 18-W continuous mode. Full-thickness vertical trenches measuring 1.0 cm were made on either side of the uvula with a focused beam. Thinning out of the uvula was performed with the scanner to reduce the uvula's size layer by layer with the patient's interactive participation. The uvula was trimmed by 80%.

Postoperative Results

The patient's snoring is now nearly inaudible and he is unable to perform a voluntary snort. The patient and his wife are again able to share a bed. The patient reports better quality of sleep, ability to dream, and reduced morning fatigue.

REFERENCES

1. Fairbanks DNF: Snoring: Surgical vs. non-surgical management. *Laryngoscope* 94:118, 1984.
2. Fairbanks DNF: Obstructive sleep breathing: Rhinology and the management of snoring. In: Goldman JL, ed. *The principles and practice of rhinology.* New York: John Wiley & Sons, 1987:753–759.
3. Guilleminault C, Stoohs R, Clerk A et al: A cause of excessive daytime sleepiness: The upper airway resistance syndrome. *Chest* 104:781–787, 1993.
4. Katsantonis GP, Friedman WH, Rosenblum BN, Walsh JK: The surgical treatment of snoring: A patient's perspective. *Laryngoscope* 100:138–140, 1990.

5. Kamami YV: Laser CO$_2$ for snoring: Preliminary results 1990. *Acto Otorhinolaryngological Belg* 44:451–456, 1990.
6. Krespi YP, Pearlman SJ, Keidar A et al: Laser assisted uvulapalatoplasty for snoring. *Insights in Otolaryngology* 9:1–8, 1994.
7. Krespi YP, Pearlman SJ, Keidar A: Laser assisted uvulo-palatoplasty for snoring. *J Otolaryngol* 23:328–334, 1994.
8. Lugaresi E, Cirignotta F, Cirignotta G, Piana D: Some epidemiological data on snoring and cardiocirculatory disturbances. *Sleep* 3:221–224, 1980.
9. Lugaresi E, Mondidi S, Zucconi M et al: Staging of heavy snorers disease: A proposal. *Bull Eur Physiopathol Respir Disorders* 19:590–594, 1983.
10. Ikematsu T: Study of snoring, 4th report: Therapy. *Nippon Jibiinkoka Gakkai Kaiho (J Otol Rhinol Laryngol Soc of Jpn)* 64:434–435, 1964.

Office-Based Surgery of the Head and Neck
Edited by Yosef P. Krespi, MD
Lippincott–Raven Publishers, Philadelphia © 1998

10

The Efficacy of Laser-Assisted Uvulopalatoplasty in the Management of Obstructive Sleep Apnea

Yosef P. Krespi and M. Morad Khosh

CLINICAL SIGNIFICANCE OF LOUD SNORING AND OSA

Snoring, as discussed in Chapter 9, is a multifaceted problem that is commonly graded on a scale of I to IV. Grades II and III apply to extremely loud snorers who can be heard throughout the entire household. These patients typically snore in all sleep positions. Such snoring is usually associated with upper airway resistance syndrome (UARS) or obstructive sleep apnea (OSA).

Chronic snorers often report restless sleep, morning headaches, or fatigue. They may demonstrate daytime listlessness and hypersomnolence. Other symptoms associated with OSA and UARS include memory difficulties, attention or concentration deficits, behavioral and affective changes, impotence, loss of alertness, and even sudden death due to cardiovascular complications.

Upper airway resistance may be a risk factor for hypertension, angina pectoris, cerebral infarction, pulmonary hypertension, and congestive heart failure (1–3), conditions thought to be more commonly associated with OSA (4). The incidence of OSA may be as high as 4% in the general population and 5%–10% in adult men (5,6). OSA is much more common in men and in obese patients. It is rarely found in premenopausal women.

It is well known that OSA is a multifactorial problem whose underlying constituents interact in a complex manner. Therefore, the management of OSA, be it medical, surgical, or behavioral, is complex and challenging. This syndrome requires a multidisciplinary team approach that includes several medical and surgical specialties. The most effective method used in the medical management of OSA is continuous positive airway pressure (CPAP). In addition, weight loss, body position training for sleep, and avoidance of alcohol and sedative medications must be behaviorally addressed. However, because medical and behavioral management requires ongoing, prolonged follow-up and adherence to the above-mentioned therapy regimens, not all patients are able to comply with these recommended treatment modalities. Surgical intervention becomes a more viable option for such patients. Surgical management appears more desirable, particularly to younger or middle-aged individuals who wish to overturn the harsh sentencing of nightly attachment to a CPAP machine for a long time, maybe for life.

Precise identification of each anatomic region of constriction is essential for accurate planning and sequencing of surgical intervention. Fujita et al. (1,7) proposed a classification of upper airway architecture that can be used to categorize the findings in the nasopharynx, oropharynx, and hypopharynx.

OSA is an ongoing, developing disease process, which makes it difficult to label a patient "cured" by any treatment modality without extensive follow-up. As patients with OSA modify their habits and activities during their lifetime, their apnea parameters change significantly. Hence, a combination of sequential surgeries with CPAP and ongoing behavioral management is strongly recommended. Proper follow-up of patients with severe OSA should include yearly polysomngraphic evaluation to adjust their treatment needs.

The surgical approach described by Powell and Riley (8,9) includes a protocol with two phases. Phase I surgery is reserved for patients with mild OSA and includes nasal reconstruction, uvulopalatopharyngoplasty (UPPP), and inferior mandibular osteotomy with geniohyoid advancement in selected patients. The cure rate of phase I surgery ranges from 62% to 67%. However, for more severe cases, phase II surgery primarily involves maxillary and mandibular osteotomies or tongue base surgery. According to their report, patients who could not reap satisfactory benefits from phase I surgery were often helped by phase II surgery, thereby increasing the cure rate to 90% (8,9).

In our treatment protocol, all patients are advised to use CPAP for 4–6 weeks prior to surgery, especially those with an apnea hypopnea index (AHI) >30 or mean oxygen desaturation of ≤80%. This period allows for adaptation and smooth transition to the device. Each patient is maintained on CPAP postoperatively starting the first day after surgery and continuing until polysomnography is obtained, approximately 3 months after surgery.

The failure of UPPP surgery to yield satisfactory results can be attributed to the preoccupation with one anatomic site and neglect of the nasal airway or tongue base. These potentially obstructive regions in the upper respiratory tract should always be examined. Most OSA patients who do not fully respond to UPPP may benefit from intranasal surgery or surgery that addresses hypertrophic lingual tonsils or an enlarged tongue base (Fig. 1).

Surgical techniques for tongue reduction have not been popular because of potential complications. Most historic tongue base procedures required tracheostomy, owing to edema and the subsequent airway compromise. The introduction of lasers in otolaryn-

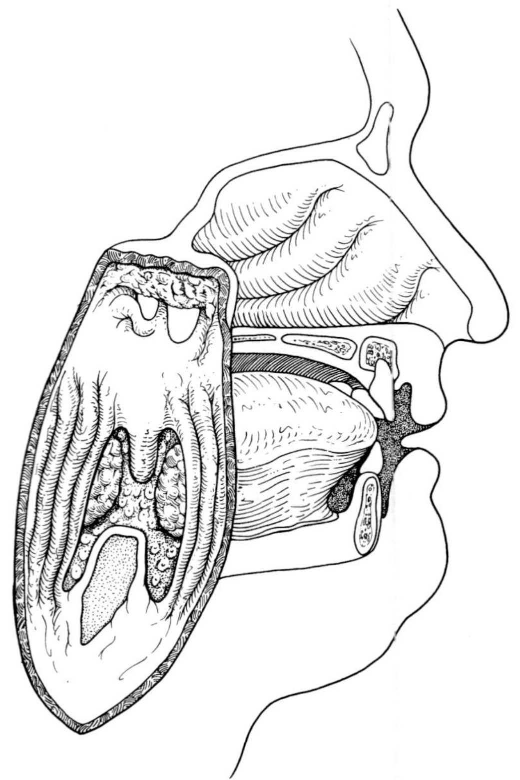

FIG. 1. Anatomy of a patient with obstructive sleep apnea may involve turbinate hypertrophy, partial nasopharyngeal obstruction due to adenoid enlargement, long uvula, low lying soft palate, large palatine tonsils, hypertrophic lingual tonsils, and thick vertical mucosal folds of the pharyngeal walls.

gology has markedly improved the ability to reduce tongue base volume, particularly hypertrophic lingual tonsils. Krespi et al. (10) reported laser lingual tonsillectomy in a series of 82 patients with successful results and minimal side effects. Fujita et al. (1,7) reported on 12 patients who received laser midline glossectomy. All but one of these patients had been incompletely treated by UPPP and all were considered to have hypopharyngeal obstruction. Further reduction in respiratory events was reported in 80% of these patients following laser glossectomy.

Contrary to Powell and Riley, we propose laser lingual tonsillectomy or laser midline glossectomy as a precursor to orthognathic surgery (8–10). In our series, we found that laser surgery on the tongue base can be easily performed in an outpatient setting. Generally, this procedure results in significant reduction of hypopharyngeal obstruction. In contrast to mandibular or maxillary advancement, reduction of soft tissues in the hypopharynx further improves patients' ability to breathe without compromising their airway. There is sufficient evidence that outpatient or ambulatory surgical care using lasers can advance the quality and efficacy of management of patients with OSA.

PATHOPHYSIOLOGY OF SNORING AND OSA

The actual noise associated with snoring is created by vibration of the uvula, the edges of the soft palate, and the tonsillar pillars. OSA is usually linked to collapse or suction of the structures surrounding the upper airway during inspiration. This collapse occurs when the negative pressure within the pharynx exceeds the ability of the pharyngeal musculature to resist collapse. In accordance with the Bernoulli effect, any narrowing along the upper airway increases volume velocity, which produces negative pressure perpendicular to the direction of the flow. This pressure consequently promotes further narrowing, further reducing intraluminal pressure. A redundant palate and elongated or thickened uvula can cause snoring from the rapid airflow created during inspiration and expiration. Anatomic narrowing or obstruction anywhere along the upper airway, as well as physiologic dysfunction of neuromuscular and respiratory control mechanisms, can cause OSA.

In an early stage of OSA, "continuous" snoring is present, which is an inspiratory noise associated with almost every breath. This snoring tends to sound the same, without gross fluctuations in amplitude. As the disease evolves, the appearance of "obstructive or pathologic snoring" is frequently reported when increased upper airway resistance reaches a threshold and esophageal pressure reaches a peak negative inspiratory level. Finally, in full-blown OSA, there is intermittent and cyclic snoring with waxing and waning intensity and frequent quiet intervals representing apneas.

Polysomnographic recordings in snorers disclose an increased negative endothoracic pressure with a concomitant increased activation of inspiratory muscles (11,12). This abnormal increase in negative endothoracic pressure creates a suction mechanism that triggers the downward traction of the laryngotracheobronchial tree and consequently the lengthening and narrowing of the oropharyngeal isthmus (Fig. 2). Total obstruction culminates when the forces tending to occlude the upper airway override the forces opposing it.

Lugaresi et al. (11,12) evaluated the mechanics of the passive pharynx using fiberoptic nasopharyngoscopy. They described the distribution of collapsible segments. They found that 75% of their patients had more than one site of narrowing. Primary nasopharyngeal narrowing was observed in 81% of these patients. They claimed that the soft palate is the most common site of narrowing in the pharynx of patients with OSA.

FACTORS INFLUENCING SNORING AND OSA

Poor Muscle Tone of the Pharyngeal Muscles

The first mechanism of hypopharyngeal narrowing is the delayed or absent contraction of dilator muscles during inspiration. This phenomenon was demonstrated in a study of upper airway closing pressure (13). The data showed that snorers tend to have pharyngeal collapse at a lesser degree of negative pharyngeal pressure, a finding indicative of the absence or insufficiency of dilator muscles' response to hypoxia. Hypotonia of the oropharyngeal muscles and abnormally high compliance of the velum palatinum and the pharyngeal walls are other proposed mechanisms (14).

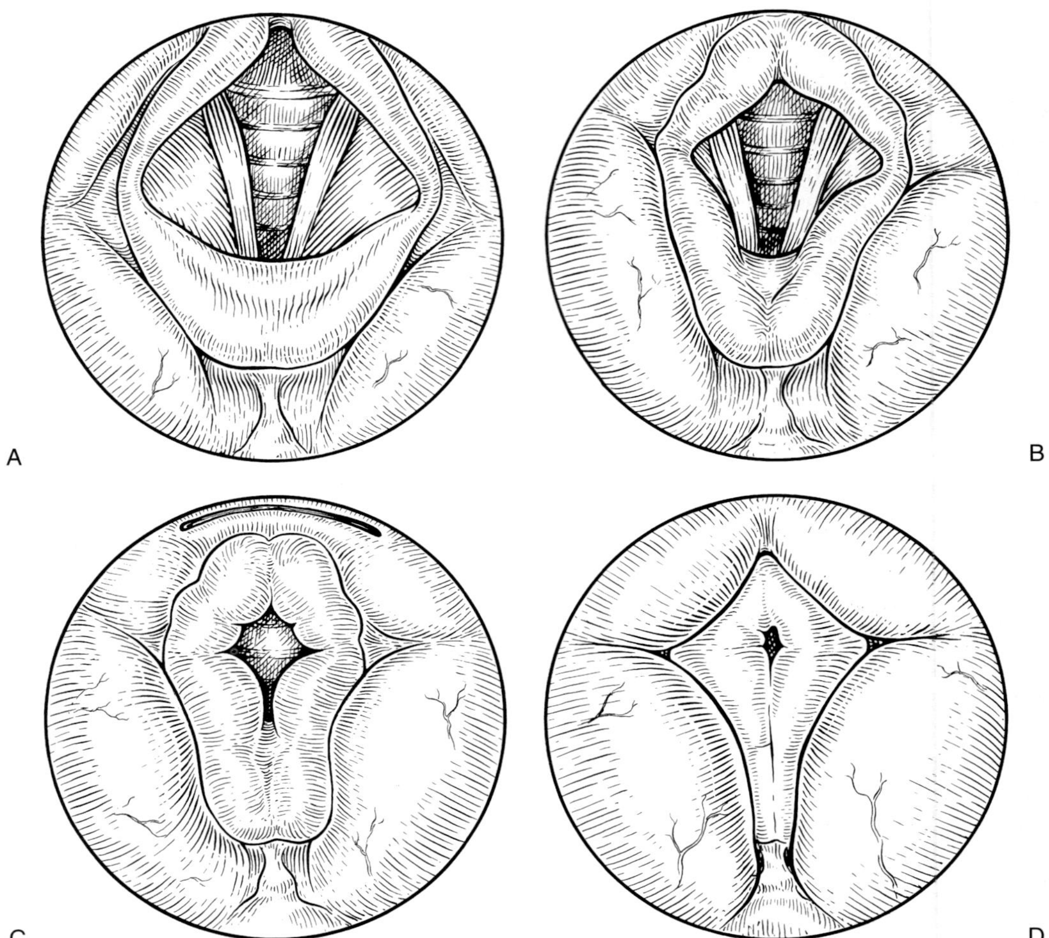

FIG. 2. (A) Hypopharyngeal airway during normal respiration. **(B)** Hypopharyngeal airway obstruction. **(C)** Moderate hypopharyngeal airway obstruction. **(D)** Severe hypopharyngeal obstruction (during Müller maneuver).

Maximal muscle relaxation occurs during rapid eye movement (REM) sleep, especially in the neck muscles. Therefore, snoring occurs predominantly during this sleep phase. A supine position aggravates this condition. Thereupon, the tongue tends to retract into the upper airway because of muscle relaxation, augmented by the pull of gravity and the Venturi effect.

Snoring and Obesity

The exact mechanisms by which obesity causes or aggravates snoring is unclear. How-

ever, it is known that thick and short cervical structures frequently seen in overweight people tend to narrow the air passages. Moreover, these individuals often have flabby tissues with poor muscle tone. Fat may actually infiltrate muscle fibers. Obese patients may have an abnormal submental electromyogram that becomes normal with weight loss.

Familial Predisposition

Familial occurrence of snoring is a common clinical finding, and familial forms of

OSA are also prevalent manifestations. It is not known whether this predisposition is primarily anatomic (ie, congenitally narrowed fauces), functional (defective coordination between diaphragmatic and pharyngeal dilator muscles), or constitutional (ie, plethoric habitus, with a short neck and a tendency toward the negative influence of obesity).

Drugs, Fatigue, and Smoking

Immoderate intake of tranquilizers, antihistamines, or alcohol prior to bedtime can aggravate snoring by deepening a person's sleep and causing excessive upper airway flaccidity. The negative influence of alcohol is twofold: peripherally, it induces vasodilation and consequent edema of the pharyngeal mucosa and, centrally, it depresses the respiratory centers in the medulla and selectively increases the hypotonia of the dilating muscles (15).

Overeating or overworking can also exaggerate the conditions that lead to snoring by increasing exhaustion and abetting over-relaxation of the upper airway. Smoking may exacerbate snoring by increasing upper airway resistance following changes in mucociliary clearance (16). Smoking causes increased production of mucus in the nose and throat and irritation and swelling of the upper air passage mucous membranes.

The role of progesterone in OSA is suggested by the increase in snoring in women during menopause and by the efficacy of medroxyprogesterone in some patients with sleep apnea. Progesterone is known to be a powerful respiratory stimulant; it may increase the tone of the muscles that stabilize the upper airways. Hormonal diseases favoring snoring and obstructive apneas include hypothyroidism, which induces structural (myxedematous) changes and altered muscular contractile properties, and acromegaly, which is associated with macroglossia, thickening of the pharyngeal mucosa, and facial skeletal changes (17).

UPPER AIRWAY RESISTANCE SYNDROME

Patients with isolated complaints of chronic sleepiness are usually classified as "idiopathic hypersomniacs" and treated symptomatically. The abnormal breathing pattern does not lead to drops in oxygen saturation or to apnea or hypopnea, as classically defined. However, upper airway resistance syndrome (UARS) leads to repetitive transient arousals, defined as appearances of alpha electroencephalogram (EEG) or fast theta EEG. These transient arousals induce sleep fragmentation. Progressively, this sleep fragmentation leads to a complaint of daytime tiredness and sleepiness.

Guilleminault (17) studied 50 subjects during nocturnal sleep and daytime naps. Most of these patients had sleep fragmentations caused by very short alpha EEG arousals throughout the sleeping period. These arousals were directly related to an abnormal increase in the respiratory efforts and to a reduction in title volume during sleep.

EVALUATION OF UARS SHOULD INCLUDE:

1. Monitoring of esophageal pressure (Pes) and its evolution during sleep.
2. Usage of nasal CPAP on a trial basis and observance of improvement in symptoms.
3. Usage of the multiple sleep latency test (MSLT) to indicate the degree of daytime sleepiness and status of daytime somnolence with nasal CPAP.

Subjects who presented with an abnormal increase in transient arousals were frequently, but not always, snorers. Nonsnorers with UARS are always women. Unfortunately, the only method currently available to recognize abnormal upper airway resistance reliably is systematic monitoring of Pes and flow limitation and demonstration of consistent reversal in daytime sleepiness with CPAP use.

Because chronic daytime somnolence is a major social, economic, and medical problem, accurate diagnosis of the syndrome and its cause is extremely important. The treatment for UARS is CPAP or surgical correction of the narrow air passages in either the nasal cavity or the oropharynx. Improved polysomnographic profiles and MSLT scores support the use of nasal CPAP to minimize or eliminate daytime sleepiness in patients with UARS. Certainly, laser-assisted uvulopalatoplasty (LAUP), submucous resection of the septum, and turbinectomy prove to be viable treatment options when long-standing relief from this syndrome is sought (17).

TREATMENT OF OSA AND UARS

The physical examination includes a complete evaluation of the nose, nasopharynx, oral cavity, oropharynx, hypopharynx, and larynx. Flexible fiberoptic nasolaryngoscopy is routinely used in this examination. Of particular importance is visual imaging while the patient performs the Müller maneuver (ie, when inhaling against a closed nose and mouth to create maximal negative pressure) (4). Polysomnography is performed to determine the presence and severity of OSA.

Treatment of snoring, UARS, and OSA begins by eliminating or reducing causative or exacerbating factors. The traditional plan involves weight loss, alteration of sleeping position, and avoidance of sedatives, smoking, and alcohol. Prosthetic and tongue-retaining devices are reportedly effective in 60% of patients with OSA and snoring (18), but patients have a poor compliance rate. The pharmacologic management of snoring with progesterone, mazindol, protriptyline, and other drugs is ineffective or provokes negative side effects that outweigh the benefits. In the management of all patients with UARS and OSA, weight loss and CPAP or surgery must be considered.

CPAP Management of OSA

Since the first report by Sullivan et al. (19), nasal CPAP has been the mainstream therapy for OSA patients. CPAP requires patients to wear a bulky nasal device attached to a bedside positive pressure generating machine. These machines help maintain upper airway patency in the treatment of OSA (19) (Fig. 3).This is

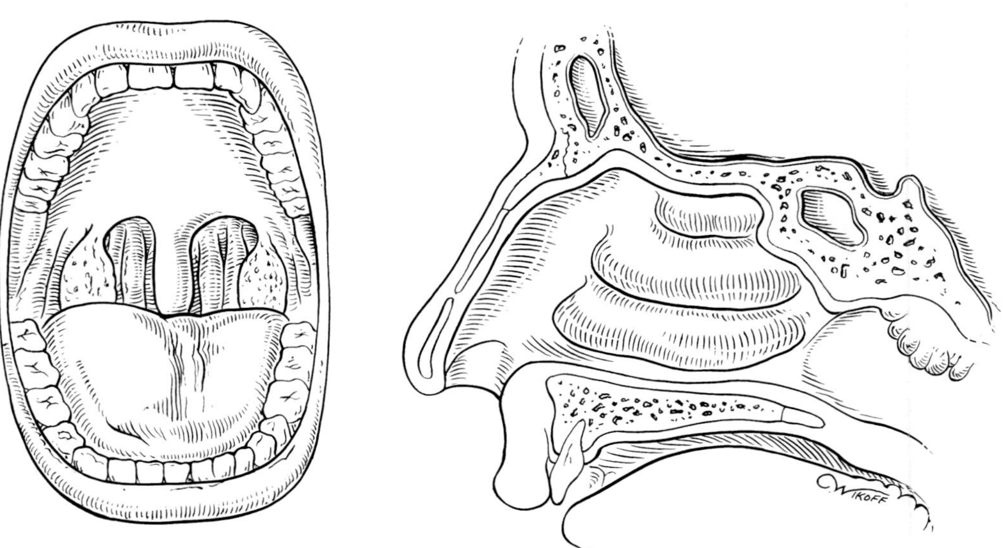

FIG. 3. Resolution of the hypopharyngeal obstruction using nasal continuous positive airway pressure.

the first treatment choice for OSA because it is noninvasive.

Compliance rates with CPAP range from 50% to 80% and vary among institutions (16,19,20). The implementation of a self-sealing, lightweight mask brought about a noteworthy improvement in compliance. A primary reason for the continuation of CPAP use is the immediate improvement in daytime performance, which apparently provides patients with a powerful source of motivation.

A question that is often asked is whether long-term CPAP use can cure sleep apnea. Clinical experience shows that, although it can greatly reduce the severity of the disorder, on its own, CPAP does not lead to a permanent cure (21). Despite a temporary reduction in apneas in patients who withdraw from CPAP treatment, there is a return of daytime sleepiness over a few days and a gradual progression toward the previous level of severity. The results suggest that improvement as a function of CPAP treatment occurs over the first 3–12 months and then stabilizes (21). There are a number of likely mechanisms for this early improvement. The soft palate is often elongated, swollen, and erythematous. This change in the soft palate, which is caused by the mechanical trauma of snoring, typically shows improvement after CPAP therapy, and has been confirmed via magnetic resonance imaging (21). Other reasons for early improvement include elimination of pretreatment chronic sleep fragmentation and improvement of the respiratory drive. Some patients who undergo long-term treatment with nasal CPAP do experience a marked improvement of their underlying sleep apnea to an extent that they can cease therapy entirely. However, this improvement tends to occur in obese patients who lose weight during CPAP therapy. Weight loss in isolation can cure sleep apnea (22). Hence, such improvement in a patient receiving CPAP therapy is not surprising. What is of great interest is that many of these patients appear to find weight loss much easier after they begin CPAP treatment. Restoration of normal daytime alertness, enhancement of

daytime physical activity, and motivation to lose weight may be crucial contributors.

By using CPAP therapy, the AHI and nocturnal oxygen desaturation improved appreciably. The percentage of slow wave and REM sleep were also significantly increased.

Surgical Treatment of UARS and OSA

When nasal symptoms are the primary complaint, success of nasal surgery may be predicted preoperatively by the nightly use of a long-acting decongestant spray or external nasal dilator. Nasal surgery, including septoplasty, turbinectomy, or repair of alar collapse, may be necessary in patients with nasal airway obstruction. The surgical treatment of choice for snoring and OSA, prior to the introduction of LAUP, was UPPP, which was also the most common procedure for treating OSA (5–7). UPPP is a single-stage procedure that provides maximal removal of the soft palate, tonsils, and uvula with conventional surgical equipment.

UPPP was first introduced by Ikematsu in 1964 as a surgical treatment for snoring (23). In 1981, UPPP was applied to OSA by Fujita (1). Since then, much effort has been devoted to improving and fine-tuning surgical intervention for OSA. Katsantonis et al. recommended UPPP to treat snoring as well as OSA, but, at the same time, recognized a number of serious surgical morbidities (5).

Potential complications of UPPP may also lead to reluctance on both patients' and surgeons' parts to undertake this procedure for the treatment of snoring alone. For traditional UPPP, general anesthesia and hospitalization are required. Induction of anesthesia and intubation is often difficult in this patient population, owing to the prevalence of short, full necks and relatively thick tongues (24). Postoperative complications (6) reported in the literature include hemorrhage in 2% of patients, temporary postoperative nasal regurgitation in 20%–60% of patients, permanent velopharyngeal insufficiency in 0.5% of patients, and nasopharyngeal stenosis, which is rare. Long-term complications include voice or resonance changes in a minority of patients and a foreign body sensation of "increased thick mucus." The latter may be attributed to loss of the uvula, which acts as a drip spout for pharyngeal mucus, and sweeps the posterior pharyngeal wall clear of secretions during swallowing.

Laser-Assisted Uvulopalatoplasty

Indications and Contraindications

Patient selection is critical when considering LAUP. Patients with grade II and grade III, persistent, position-independent, obnoxious, loud snoring that disrupts households are candidates for LAUP. LAUP in an office setting must be restricted to patients with loud snoring, UARS, and mild sleep apnea. Patients with severe OSA (AHI >40), mean oxygen desaturation of ≤80%, morbid obesity, and uncontrolled hypertension should be operated on in a hospital setting under general anesthesia. In patients with severe OSA, we still recommend the use of lasers to resect or ablate the palate and the tonsils over conventional UPPP performed with cold instruments. The incidence of bleeding, velopharyngeal insufficiency, stenosis, and postoperative edema is lower when lasers are used.

Anesthesia and Surgery

LAUP and laser-assisted serial tonsillectomy (LAST) in the office setting are performed in an upright sitting position. Topical anesthetic of benzocaine 20% (Hurricaine, Beutlich, Niles, IL) is used followed by the injection of a mixture of 1 mL lidocaine (Xylocaine, Astra, Westboro, MA) 2% with 1:100,000 epinephrine, and 0.5 mL of 0.5% bupivacaine hydrochloride (Marcaine, Winthrop Pharmaceuticals, New York, NY) into the junction of the soft palate and uvula bilaterally and into the base of the uvula. If laser ablation of the tonsils and tonsillar pillars is to be performed, the superior and mid portion of the anterior pillars are also injected bilaterally. Surgery using the carbon dioxide (CO_2)

laser is commenced after waiting 10 minutes. A special pharyngeal handpiece with backstop is used to incise the soft palate at a power setting of 20 W. Full-thickness vertical trenches measuring 1–2 cm are performed on the free edge of the soft palate on either side of the uvula. The overall surgical goal is to reduce the length and reshape the soft palate and uvula. Shortening and thinning of the uvula is carried out with the SwiftLase (Sharplan Lasers, Inc., Allendale, NJ) scanner attached to the CO_2 laser using 20 W (25). The uvula is reduced to 80%–90% of its original dimensions by removing its core from the bottom up, and by ablating the muscle from within, creating a "fishmouth" appearance, while preserving the mucosa of the base of the uvula. Excision of the uvula at its base using the CO_2 laser with a focus beam may cause undesired bleeding. The advantages of using the SwiftLase flashscanner are absence of char, precise layer-by-layer surface ablation, and the ability to seal small blood vessels. Redundant pharyngeal folds and enlarged tonsils can also be reduced using the SwiftLase scanner. The velopharyngeal dimensions are further enlarged by this method (Fig. 4).

LAUP for simple snoring typically requires two to three sessions. However, extended LAUP (LAUP-LAST) for UARS and mild OSA may require several treatments. At least 5 weeks should elapse between consecutive sessions to allow time for proper healing of the velopharyngeal mucosa. The endpoint of LAUP treatments for UARS and snoring is when snoring is significantly reduced and daytime sleepiness is reversed. This is confirmed by postoperative questionnaires and endoscopic evaluations. Postoperative polysomnography may be indicated to confirm the degree of success in patients with moderate or severe OSA, whether they are using CPAP or not.

COMPLICATIONS

A moderate to severe sore throat is the major side effect following LAUP. Pain intensity reaches its peak 4–5 days postoperatively with

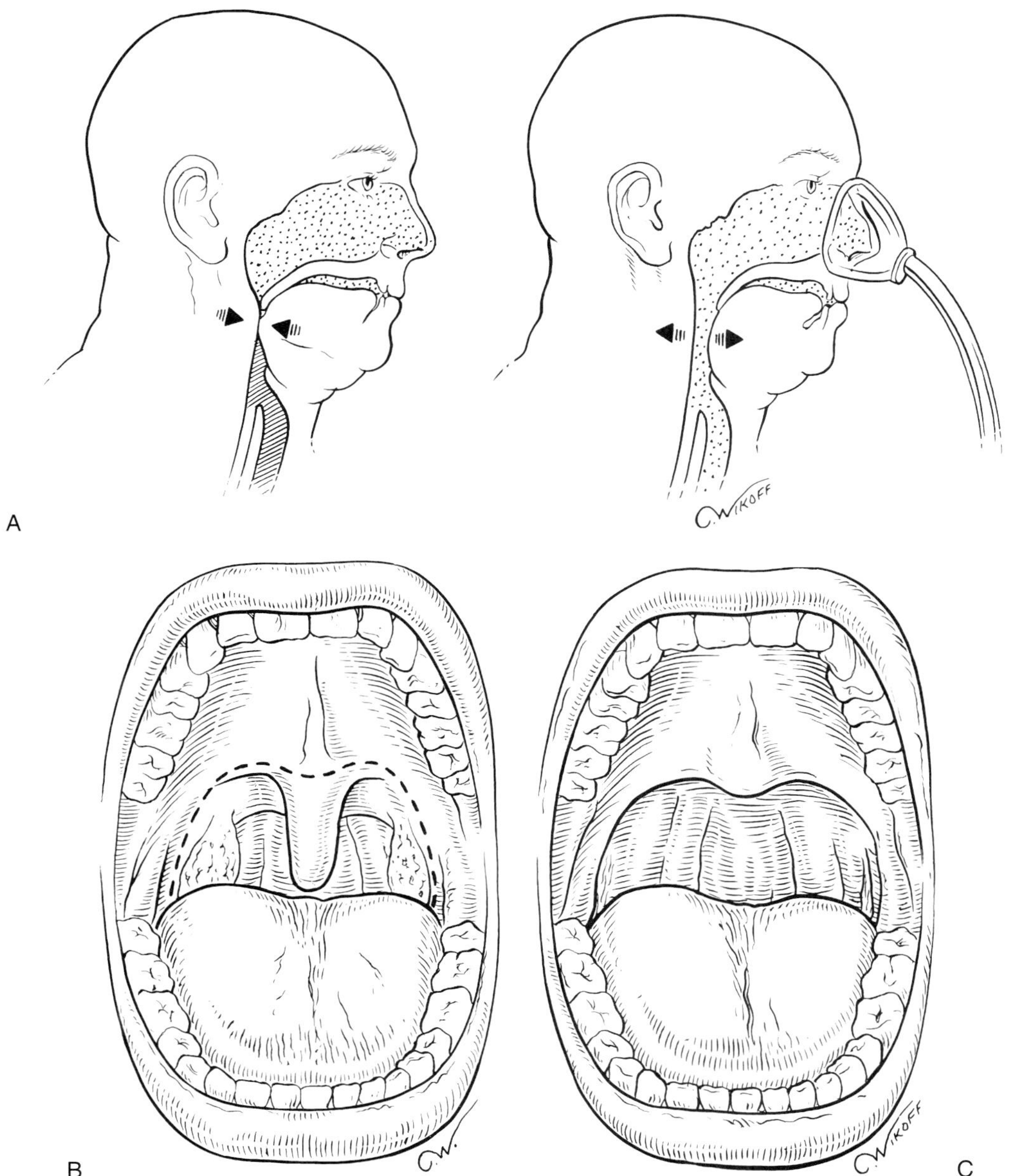

FIG. 4. (A) Tongue base collapse in a patient with OSA. Nasal CPAP stenting of the upper airway to improve OSA. **(B)** Extended laser-assisted uvulopalatoplasty involving resection of the soft palate, uvula, and palatine arches and laser ablation of the palatine tonsils. **(C)** Note significant enlargement of the velopharyngeal airway.

considerable relief of symptoms approximately 8–10 days after surgery. Mild bleeding, which was encountered during surgery in approximately 2% of the patients, was quickly controlled with silver nitrate cauterization. There was no need for electrocautery in any of the above cases. Delayed bleeding and infection was never encountered in our series. Vasovagal episodes occurred in four patients following injection of the local anesthetic.

In approximately 30% of our patients, LAUP was combined with other upper airway procedures. Such procedures included submucous resection of the septum, laser turbinectomy, LAST, or laser lingual tonsillectomy.

MATERIALS AND METHODS

From January 1993 to December 1996, 1100 patients were evaluated for snoring and sleep-related disorders. There were 940 men (85%) and 160 women (15%). Ages varied from 21 to 76 years with a median age of 49 years. Seven hundred ninety-four (73%) were married and 306 (27%) were not married. On the physical examination, 25% of these patients reported normal weight, 27% reported being overweight, and 48% reported being obese (body mass index >27). Among the group, 957 (87%) were white, 88 (8%) were black, 33 (3%) were Hispanic, and 19 (2%) were Asian. Of 1100 patients, 189 (18%) were hypertensive and 911 (82%) were normotensive; however, of this group, 20% were on antihypertensive medications. Of 1100 patients seen in consultation, 858 (78%) were found suitable for in-office LAUP. Of these, 177 (16%) were admitted to the hospital for extended LAUP and 65 (6%) were not surgical candidates.

Preoperative polysomnography was performed in 1068 of 1100 patients (97%) who had LAUP. Several patients operated on in the hospital who did not have polysomnography were simple snorers with strong gag reflexes. All patients with severe sleep apnea (AHI >40) were initially treated with CPAP as an adjunct to surgical intervention in the hospital. The efficacy of LAUP was evaluated with extensive analysis of pre- and postoperative patient questionnaires specifically designed for LAUP and OSA. In addition, patients with OSA completed Health Status Questionnaire (HSQ) version 2.0. The HSQ utilizes a collection of 40 brief items to develop 8 separate indices of functional health status and has been demonstrated to be both valid and reliable. The postoperative questionnaire was completed by 320 patients with UARS or OSA. Only 103 patients with moderate to severe sleep apnea underwent postoperative polysomnography.

Of the 1100 patients who had LAUP, 1068 underwent polysomnography, 317 were simple snorers, 96 had UARS, 419 had mild OSA, 163 had moderate OSA, and 73 had severe OSA.

RESULTS

Following the completion of single extensive LAUP or staged conventional LAUP procedures performed either in the office or in the hospital for UARS or OSA, the quality of sleep was significantly improved in 28%, slightly improved in 46%, and there was no change in 26% of patients. Daytime somnolence was significantly improved in 24%, slightly improved in 39%, and no change was noted in 37%. The overall energy level of the patients treated by LAUP was significantly improved in 42%, unchanged in 49%, and had evidence of deterioration in 9%. Deterioration of the energy level was attributed to significant weight gain. Following laser surgery, 28% of the patients had decreased weight, 4% had increased weight, and in 68% there was no change.

Further analysis of pre- and postoperative questionnaires in UARS and OSA patients revealed significant improvement following surgery in the following reported symptoms: sleep maintenance, fatigability, arising difficulties, daytime alertness, irritability, frustration, anxiety, worry, restlessness, sleeptime nasal obstruction, and sleeptime choking and gasping. The subjective ratings of sleep-related symptoms revealed significant reduction in their overall number (p <0.03).

A comparison of 43 pre- and postoperative polysomnograms in patients having moderate to severe OSA failed to reveal any statistically significant changes in sleep parameters. Although 60% of these patients had improved AHI and desaturation levels, this was attributed to significant weight loss and surgery combination rather than to LAUP alone.

CONCLUSION

LAUP is an effective method for treating patients with loud, habitual snoring. It is a safe, reliable method for the treatment of this sociomedical problem. LAUP is reserved for patients with either simple snoring or mild sleep apnea. The procedure is performed in an ambulatory setting using a CO_2 laser with a specialized handpiece under local anesthesia in several stages. Few patients were incapacitated by the postoperative pain, and all patients were able to immediately return to work. Another advantage of LAUP over UPPP is the ability to "titrate" tissue removal without the risk of over-resection. We have achieved an 85% success rate for reduction or elimination of snoring in 1100 patients.

Among our patients evaluated for snoring, 71% had polysomnography prior to surgical treatment. Various degrees of OSA or UARS were found in most of these patients. The initial treatment of choice for moderate to severe OSA is CPAP. CPAP and weight control in conjunction with extended LAUP (LAUP and LAST) is recommended for long-term management. The primary reason for the failure of LAUP in the management of OSA is usually lingual tonsil hypertrophy. Laser surgery directed to the tongue base is our preferred method to treat these failures. Skeletal advancement procedures are rarely necessary and should succeed lingual tonsil ablation.

UARS can be managed by CPAP or surgery directed at the site creating the maximal resistance. Most commonly these treatments are LAUP or intranasal surgery. Application of lasers to the treatment of OSA and UARS allows these diseases to be treated efficiently on an outpatient basis. These procedures are also safe, cost-effective, and compatible with the managed care concept.

OSA and snoring are ongoing disease processes. Snoring, once thought to be only a "social disease," may actually be a precursor to subsequent OSA, a concept we are now prospectively studying. Patients with the diagnosis of OSA and snoring, therefore, must be followed throughout their lifetime. Preliminary data from this study reveal a significant association between weight loss and the AHI regardless of the treatment modality used.

REFERENCES

1. Fujita S: Method of Fujita. In: Fairbanks DNF, Fujita S, Ikematsu T, Simmons FB, eds. *Snoring and obstructive sleep apnea.* New York: Raven Press, 1987:134–153.
2. Koskenvuo M, Kaprio J, Partinen M et al: Snoring as a risk factor for hypertension and angina pectoris. *Lancet* 1:893–896, 1965.
3. Partinen M, Palomaki H: Snoring and cerebral infarction. *Lancet* 2:1325–1326, 1985.
4. Sher AE: Obstructive sleep apnea syndrome: A complex disorder of the upper airway. *Otolaryngol Clin North Am* 23:593–608, 1990.
5. Katsantonis GP, Schweitzer PK, Branham GH et al: Management of obstructive sleep apnea: Comparison of various treatment modalities. *Laryngoscope* 98:304–309, 1988.
6. Maniglia AJ: Sleep apnea and snoring, an overview. *ENT J* 72:16–19, 1993.
7. Fujita S, Woodson R, Clark J et al: Laser midline glossectomy as a treatment for obstructive sleep apnea. *Laryngoscope* 101:805–809, 1991.
8. Riley RW, Powell NB, Guilleminault C: Maxillofacial surgery and obstructive sleep apnea: A review of 80 patients. *Otolaryngol Head Neck Surg* 101:353–361, 1989.
9. Riley RW, Powell NB: Maxillofacial surgery and obstructive sleep apnea syndrome. *Otolaryngol Clin North Am* 23:809–826, 1990.
10. Krespi YP, Har-El G, Levine TM et al: Laser lingual tonsillectomy. *Laryngoscope* 99:131–135, 1989.
11. Lugaresi E, Cirgnotta F, Cirignotta G, Piana D: Some epidemiological data on snoring and cardiocirculatory disturbances. *Sleep* 3:221–224, 1980.
12. Lugaresi E, Mondini S, Zucconi M et al: Staging of heavy snorers disease: A proposal. *Bull Eur Physiopathol Respir* 19:590–594, 1983.
13. Issa FG, Sullivan CE: Upper airway closing pressure in snorers. *J Appl Physiol* 57:528–535, 1984.
14. Smirne S, Iannoccone S, Ferini-Strambi L et al: Muscle fibre type and habitual snoring. *Lancet* 337:597–599, 1991.
15. Issa FG, Sullivan CE: Alcohol, snoring and sleep apnea. *J Neurol Neurosurg Psychiatry* 45:353–359, 1982.
16. Nino-Murdcia G, McCann CC, Bliwise DL et al: Compliance and side effects in sleep apnea patients treated with nasal continuous positive airway pressure. *West J Med* 150:165–169, 1989.
17. Guilleminault C, Stoohs R, Clerk A et al: A cause of excessive daytime sleepiness: The upper airway resistance syndrome. *Chest* 104:781–787, 1993
18. Miyazaki S: Prosthetic devices in the treatment of obstructive sleep apnea. *Oper Tech in Otolaryngol-Head and Neck Surg* 2:96–99, 1991.

19. Sullivan CE, Issa FG, Berthon-Jones M, Eves L: Reversal of obstructive sleep apnea with continuous positive airway pressure applied through the nares. *Lancet* 1: 862–865, 1981.
20. Sanders MH, Gruendl CA, Rogers RM: Patient compliance with nasal CPAP therapy for sleep apnea. *Chest* 90:330–333, 1986.
21. Lehrhaft B, Grunstein RR, Sullivan CE: Effects of long term treatment with nasal CPAP on severity of sleep apnea (OSA) and respiratory function. *Eur Respir J* 4:585S, 1991.
22. Harman E, Wynne JW, Block AJ: The effect of weight loss on sleep disordered breathing and oxygen desaturation in morbidly obese men. *Chest* 82:291–293, 1982.
23. Ikematsu T: Study of snoring, 4th report: Therapy. *J Jpn Otol Rhinol Laryngol* 64:434–435, 1964.
24. Norton ML, Brown ACD: Evaluating the patient with a difficult airway for anesthesia. *Otolaryngol Clin North Am* 4:771–785, 1990.
25. Krespi YP, Ling E: Tonsil cryptolysis utilizing CO_2 Swift-Lase [abstract]. *Lasers Med Surg* 197(suppl 5):40–41, 1993.

Office-Based Surgery of the Head and Neck
Edited by Yosef P. Krespi, MD
Lippincott–Raven Publishers, Philadelphia © 1998

11

Laser-Assisted Tonsil Ablation

Yosef P. Krespi and M. Morad Khosh

Chronic tonsillitis is the most common indication for tonsillectomy in adults. The dilated cryptic pockets in palatine tonsils can become obstructed with impacted debris or can simply harbor bacteria. Palatine tonsillectomy has long been the accepted surgical modality for the treatment of chronic tonsillitis. Although newer instrumentation and safer anesthesia techniques have reduced the morbidity associated with tonsillectomy, the need for general anesthesia and the risk of hemorrhage remain significant drawbacks to this procedure. The postoperative pain associated with tonsillectomy can be significant, resulting in loss of significant work time. In the adult population, some of these drawbacks can be avoided through carbon dioxide (CO_2) laser ablation of the surface of the palatine tonsils under local anesthesia in an office setting. The indications, technique, and efficacy of this novel procedure are discussed in this chapter.

CLINICAL INDICATIONS

Recurrent infections of the palatine tonsils remain a common affliction in the general population, particularly in pediatric patients. Chronic tonsillitis is the most common indication for tonsillectomy, a procedure that numbered 74,000 cases in 1990 (1). Tonsillar crypts have been shown to represent an important site for antigen presentation and processing in the tonsillar lymphoid tissue (2,3). In the adult population, persistent bacterial colonization or inflammation secondary to trapped debris within the tonsillar crypts may be important causes of recurrent tonsillitis,

halitosis, and dysgeusia. The morbidity associated with palatine tonsillectomy has been extensively studied (4–12). The most common risks include bleeding, which can be classified as intraoperative, early postoperative, and late postoperative. Intraoperative bleeding is technique-dependent and can be negligible to massive. Both early and late postoperative bleeding have a similar incidence of approximately 3% (4–12). Postoperative pain represents the most common morbidity due to this operation. Pain tends to subside in about 10–14 days, once the tonsillar fossa has remucosalized and the exposed pharyngeal muscle is covered.

In the adult population, the CO_2 laser can be used in the office setting to ablate the surface of the palatine tonsils in treating chronic cryptic tonsillitis. This procedure can also be performed in conjunction with laser-assisted uvulopalatoplasty to improve the pharyngeal airway affected by tonsillar hypertrophy in patients with mild obstructive sleep apnea.

TECHNIQUE

The procedure is carried out in the semisitting position without the use of a mouth gag. The patient and the office staff are equipped with safety eye goggles, and laser safety standards are carefully followed. The oropharynx is anesthetized by spraying a topical anesthetic such as benzocaine 20%. After several minutes, a 1 mL mixture of 2% lidocaine with 1:100,000 epinephrine, and 0.5 mL of 0.5% bupivicaine is injected into the superior junction of the anterior and posterior pillars, and the mid portion of the anterior pillar. Occasionally, in large tonsils the base of the tonsil is also injected. Glossopharyngeal nerve block is rarely indicated. The patient is instructed to inhale deeply prior to insertion of the laser handpiece into the oral cavity and to exhale slowly over 10–15 seconds while laser energy is being applied over the tonsil tissue. Inspiratory replenishment is cued by the surgeon only on deactivation and withdrawal of the laser handpiece from the oral cavity. This coordination is important for several reasons: It allows relative relaxation and stabilization of the soft palate and tongue, helps keep these structures away from the path of the laser, and minimizes laser plume inhalation. Inhalation of laser smoke can cause a coughing and choking sensation, and sometimes also initiate nausea, resulting in a vasovagal reaction. Therefore, effective and rapid smoke evacuation is mandatory for full patient comfort. In addition, we have found that the use of a large standing fan next to the patient provides great comfort for both the patient and the surgical staff.

We employ the CO_2 laser with SwiftLase or SurgiTouch scanner attachment (Sharplan Lasers, Inc., Allendale, NJ). The scanning device is a battery-powered accessory attached to the conventional CO_2 laser that distributes focused laser energy over a 3–4-mm treatment area in milliseconds, through the use of rotating mirrors. The laser energy is set at 15–18 W in the continuous mode. While the patient is exhaling, the pharyngeal handpiece is used to serially ablate the tonsil in a painting pattern. In small- to medium-sized tonsils, five to six passes (10–15 seconds each pass) may be necessary to complete the treatment on each side. The tonsils are ablated to the level of the pillars. By avoiding injury to the pillars, postoperative pain is reduced significantly. In some patients with deep, hidden, and dilated cryptic pockets, it may be necessary to incise or excise portions of the anterior pillar to gain access and marsupialize the pocket. Any repeated treatment can be done in 6-week intervals (Figs. 1–3).

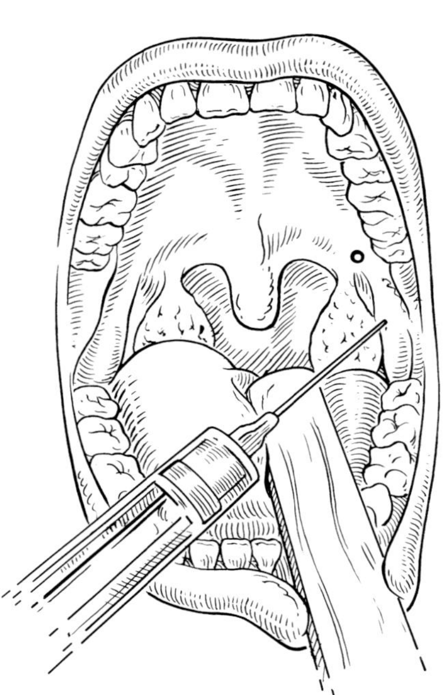

FIG. 1. Injection of local anesthetic to anterior pillar.

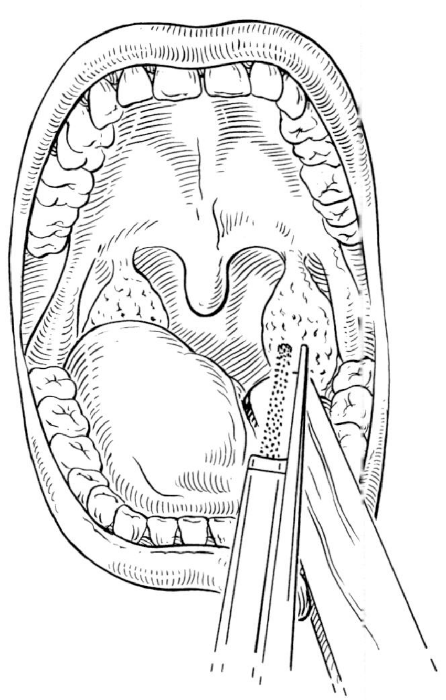

FIG. 2. Carbon dioxide (CO_2) laser ablation of palatine tonsils. Tongue blade positioned laterally to expose the tonsil.

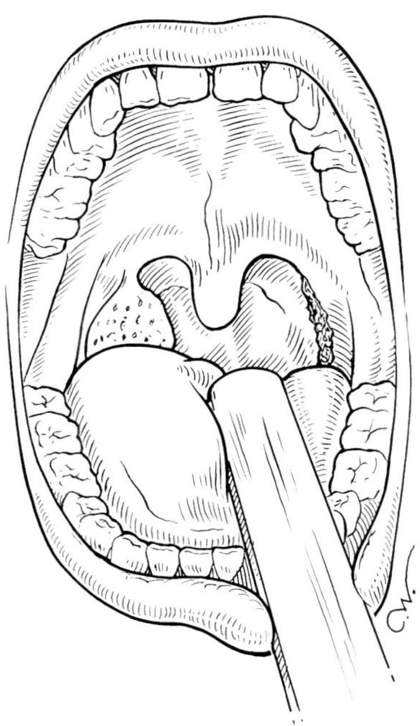

FIG. 3. Completion of tonsil ablation. Lymphoid tissue is ablated to the level of the pillars. Postoperative discomfort is minimal owing to preservation of the pillars.

Postoperatively, diluted peroxide rinses (three times a day) and throat lozenges are suggested for 5 days to promote the removal of debris and laser coagulum. Postoperative antibiotics are used for 1 week. Postoperative analgesics are prescribed on an individual basis. Steroids are not routinely used. Most patients tolerate a soft diet on discharge and are quickly advanced to a regular diet at home. The patient often returns to work or school the same day.

EFFICACY

Krespi and Ling (13), in a study of 120 adult patients, reviewed the results of laser-assisted serial tonsillectomy. In this study, 92% of the patients were treated in the office under local anesthesia; 8% of the patients were treated in the operating room under general anesthesia; and 96% of the patients experienced complete relief from recurrent tonsillar inflammation, during a 2–48-month follow-up. Twenty patients (17%) required more than one treatment. Only five patients (4%) reported insufficient improvement and underwent complete tonsillectomy using traditional methods.

There were no immediate postoperative complications in this study. The postoperative level of discomfort was described as minimal, and was well tolerated with oral analgesics (acetaminophen with codeine and viscous lidocaine). The degree of inconvenience was likened to a typical dental office visit. There were no reports of bleeding, rhinolalia, velopalatine insufficiency, or dysphagia beyond the initial postoperative period (Fig. 4).

ANATOMIC BASIS

Recurrent cryptogenic tonsillitis and recurrent tonsillolith formation are frequently treated with conventional tonsillectomy. Our understanding of tonsil anatomy and its histopathology, on the one hand, and innovations of the emerging laser technology, on the other hand, provide the link between theoretical framework and practical application of laser-assisted tonsil ablation. Whereas traditional tonsillectomy relied on extirpation, laser tonsil ablation offers an efficacious alternative treatment for these common tonsil problems.

Tonsillar crypts have been identified as an important site of primary immune antigen processing and response, which can lead to palatine tonsil inflammation. In addition, tonsillitis may also result from secondary infection related to the unique tonsil architecture. This inflammation may be the principal underlying cause of sore throats, halitosis, and dysgeusia.

The three-dimensional structure of tonsillar crypts has been elucidated, noting simple nonbranched crypts at the periphery and complicated branched units centrally (14). Just beneath the crypt epithelium are capillary vessels and lymphoid tissue (15). Changes in these capillary vessels correspond to the initiation of tonsillar inflammation (16). Although

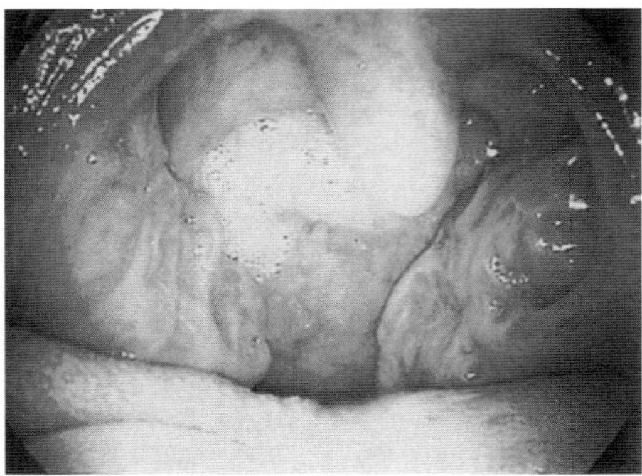 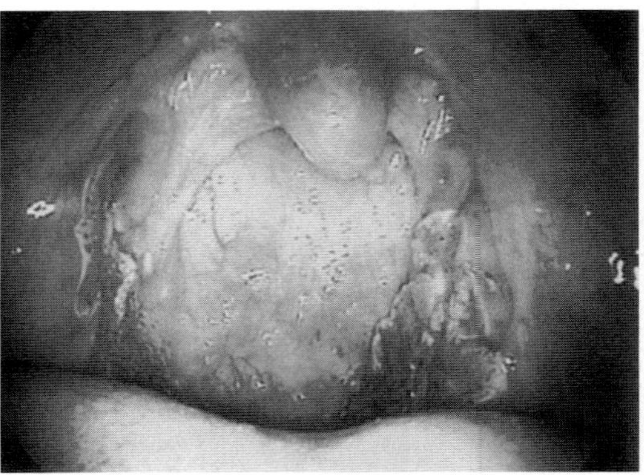

A   B

FIG. 4. (A) Preoperative and **(B)** postoperative view of the tonsils following laser-assisted tonsil ablation. Note the absence of bleeding and char in the surgical site.

this crypt architecture increases the surface area available for the microscopic capturing and processing of antigenic material (17), debris can be trapped and become the reservoir for recurrent secondary infection or the foci for tonsillolith formation (18). The ablation of tonsillar crypts, through the use of the CO_2 laser, eliminates this reservoir or focus (Fig. 5).

Although laser treatment, as described, is a surface-ablating procedure, tissue beyond the superficial openings of the tonsillar crypts is affected by the thermal results of laser energy. After healing, some cryptic pockets may undergo fibrosis and become obliterated. These closed crypts no longer collect antigenic or pathologic debris that may initiate inflammation. Other crypts maintain an epithelial lining and become marsupialized with a persistent opening analogous to a fistula. Crypts scarred open in this manner may trap less debris or permit discharge in spite of surrounding inflammatory swelling. Moreover, laser ablation of subepithelial capillaries limits their role in the development of potential inflammation. The diminished ability of antigen entrapment, and reduced subepithelial vascularity may account for the clinical improvement noted in the treated patients.

Patients or practitioners who have reservations about tonsillectomy may consider laser-assisted tonsil ablation as a tissue-conserving procedure. Tissue preservation is important for individuals in whom voice alteration is undesired, such as the professional speaker or singer. Laser-assisted tonsil ablation avoids significant changes of the tonsil bulk or scarring of the faucial arches and, therefore, maintains the position of the soft palate and leaves the voice intact.

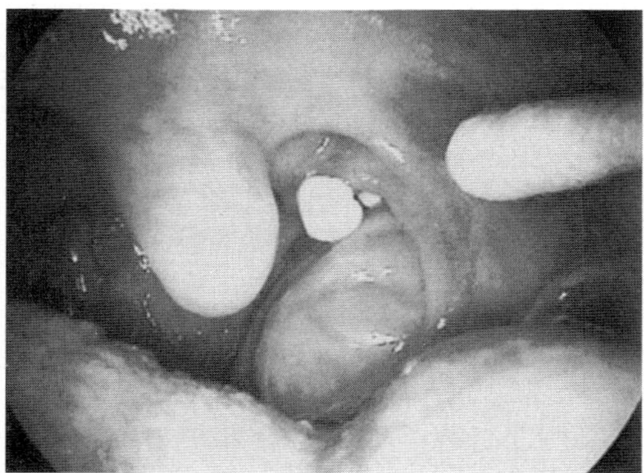

FIG. 5. Enlarged tonsil with a dilated cryptic pocket and tonsillolith. Note the removal of the tonsillolith using a cotton tip applicator.

CONCLUSION

Chronic inflammation of the tonsils has been treated by many therapies, from the application of iodine and massage in the preantibiotic era to today's common tonsillectomy. Although traditional tonsillectomy has proved to be an effective surgical treatment for chronic tonsillitis, the associated morbidity and cost has inspired other therapeutic modalities. In appropriately selected adult patients, laser-assisted tonsil ablation may provide the efficacy of traditional tonsillectomy with reduced cost and morbidity. Large, controlled, prospective studies are necessary to compare these two surgical modalities.

According to our experience, laser-assisted tonsil ablation offers some clear advantages, particularly when performed with the CO_2 laser with the SwiftLase/SurgiTouch scanning apparatus. The procedure can be performed safely in an ambulatory surgical or office setting under local or topical anesthesia. The ideal adult patient who is cooperative and has a low gag reflex can avoid the cost and risk of general anesthesia and total tonsillectomy. Limited tissue destruction significantly reduces operative and postoperative complication, discomfort, and recovery time (13,19, 20). To conclude, laser-assisted tonsil ablation is a safe and cost-effective method of treating tonsil pathology without unnecessary sacrifice of the organ and undue risks to the patient. We have demonstrated the long-term efficacy of this procedure with an equivalent cure rate as compared with conventional tonsillectomy.

REFERENCES

1. National Center for Health Statistics: *Health, United States, 1991*. Hyattsville, MD, Public Health Service, 1991:131.
2. Perry ME, Slipka J: Formation of the tonsillar corpuscle. *Funct Dev Morphol* 3:165–168, 1993.
3. Reibel J, Sorenson CH: Association between keratin staining patterns and the structural and functional aspects of palatine tonsil epithelium. *APMIS* 99:905–915, 1991.
4. Handler SD, Miller L, Richmond KH et al: Post-tonsillectomy hemorrhage: Incidence, prevention, and management. *Laryngoscope* 96:1243–1247, 1986.
5. Capper JWR, Randal C: Post-operative hemorrhage in tonsillectomy and adenoidectomy in children. *J Laryngol Otol* 98:365–368, 1984.
6. Tami TA, Parker GS, Taylor RE: Post-tonsillectomy bleeding: An evaluation of risk factors. *Laryngoscope* 97:11307–11311, 1987.
7. Colclasure JB, Graham SS: Complications of outpatient tonsillectomy and adenoidectomy: A review of 33,340 cases. *Ear Nose Throat J* 69:155–160, 1990.
8. Kristensen S, Tvetares K: Post-tonsillectomy hemorrhage. A retrospective study of 1150 operations. *Clin Otolaryngol* 9:347–350, 1984.
9. Crysdale WS, Russell D: Complications of T&A in 9409 children observed overnight. *Can Med Assoc J* 135:1139–1143, 1986.
10. Tan AK, Rothstein J, Tewfik TL: Ambulatory tonsillectomy and adenoidectomy: Complications and associated factors. *J Otolaryngol* 22:442–446, 1993.
11. Tay HL: Post-operative morbidity in electrodissection tonsillectomy. *J Laryngol Otol* 109:209–211, 1995.
12. Nicklaus PJ, Herzon FS, Steinle EW 4th: Short-stay outpatient tonsillectomy. *Arch Otolaryngol Head Neck Surg* 121:521–524, 1995.
13. Krespi YP, Ling EH: Tonsil cryptolysis using CO_2 SwiftLase. *Operative Techniques in Otolaryngology Head and Neck Surgery* 5:294–297, 1994.
14. Abbey K, Kawabata I: Computerized three-dimensional reconstruction of the crypt system of the palatine tonsil. *Acta Otolaryngol Suppl (Stockh)* 454:39–42, 1988.
15. Higashikawa R, Ohtani O, Masuda Y: Ultrastructures of the epithelial capillaries in rabbit palatine tonsils. *Arch Histol Cytol* 53:31–39, 1990.
16. Fujihara K: A study on the tonsil with focal infections: With special reference to the newly devised tonsillar cryptoscope and the architecture of the vessels in crypts. *Nippon Jibiinkoka Gakki Kaiho* 94:1304–1314, 1991.
17. Brandtzaeg P: Immune functions of human nasal mucosa and tonsils in health and disease. In: Beinestock J, ed. *Immunology of the lungs and upper respiratory tract*. Ontario, Canada: McGraw Hill, 1984;28–96.
18. Cooper MM, Steinberg JJ, Lasstra et al: Tonsillar calculi. *Oral Surg* 55:239–243, 1983.
19. Krespi YP, Ling EH: Laser assisted lingual tonsillectomy. *J Otolaryngol* 23:325–327, 1994.
20. Krespi YP: Tonsil cryptolysis utilizing CO_2 SwiftLase [abstract 197]. *Lasers Surg Med* (suppl 5):40–41,1993.

Office-Based Surgery of the Head and Neck
Edited by Yosef P. Krespi, MD
Lippincott–Raven Publishers, Philadelphia © 1998

12

Laser-Assisted Uvulopalatoplasty

Results and Complications in 1000 Patients

Yosef P. Krespi

Laser-assisted uvulopalatoplasty (LAUP) is an effective surgical procedure for the elimination of loud, habitual snoring. LAUP is performed under local anesthesia in either the physician's office or in an ambulatory surgery center. LAUP enlarges the oropharyngeal and nasopharyngeal air space by shortening and reshaping the uvula, velum, and pharyngeal pillars using the CO_2 laser. Our experience to date includes 1000 patients surgically treated within the past 3 years. We have evaluated more than 1500 patients for snoring or sleep-related breathing disorders over the same time period. Two thirds of these patients were determined to be appropriate candidates for surgery. By following strict selection criteria, we achieved 84% elimination of snoring. Of the remaining patients, 7% demonstrated improvement in the loudness of their snoring. Nine percent of our patients did not have any improvement in their snoring. It is important to note that the cure rate dropped to 76% when the follow-up was extended beyond 2 years. Similar rates of recurrent snoring were reported after conventional uvulopalatopharyngoplasty (UPPP). In summary, LAUP has proved to be a safe, simple, reliable procedure that can be performed in an ambulatory setting.

Habitual, loud snoring affects approximately 25% of the adult population, the incidence increasing with age. The incidence in men is higher than in women. Snoring is also a common finding in overweight or obese individuals (1,2). The sound of snoring originates in the collapsing portion of the pharyngeal airway, primarily from the vibration of the soft palate, uvula, tonsillar pillars, and pharyngeal folds. Reduced tone of the oropharyngeal and palatal muscles increases the loudness of these vibrations. It is postulated that the rhythmic vibrations of the uvula are produced by negative inspiratory forces pulling the uvula posteriorly against the posterior pharyngeal wall and the tensor veli palatini muscles drawing the uvula anteriorly against the tongue. These counteracting forces are thought to be responsible for the rumbling sound of snoring. Anatomic changes of the soft palate including a long uvula, low-lying velum, horizontal palate arch, and large tonsils can all contribute to the loudness of the snoring (3,4).

CLINICAL SIGNIFICANCE

Chronic snorers often report restless sleep, morning headaches, and excessive fatigue in the morning. Loud snoring can be associated with sleep fragmentation and daytime sleepiness. Memory difficulties, concentration deficits, behavioral and affective changes, impotence, and loss of alertness can be common findings in patients with loud, habitual snoring (5).

The following simple objective classification system is designed to rate snoring severity:

Grade I snorer: Occasional snoring usually occurring while the snorer is lying on the back or overtired or may have had too much alcohol prior to retiring.

Grade II snorer: Loud, frequent snoring that occurs in all body positions. Snoring continues through the night and may be associated with mild sleep apnea and upper airway resistance syndrome.

Grade III snorer: Extremely loud snoring that can be heard throughout the entire household and that is associated with obstructive sleep apnea.

A complete medical history is obtained from each patient, including completion of a comprehensive snoring evaluation questionnaire. A thorough head and neck examination is performed with visualization of the entire upper airway. Evaluation starts from the tip of the nose and extends down to the vocal cord region. Flexible fiberoptic nasolaryngoscopy provides an excellent tool in evaluation of the airway. During endoscopy, nasal and oral breathing, swallowing, "snorting," and Müller maneuver are performed to evaluate the anatomy and dynamic physiology of the palate, nasopharynx, and hypopharynx. A video recording of the fiberoptic examination provides an opportunity to review the airway with its dynamic changes pre- and postoperatively. The Müller maneuver (inhaling against a closed nose and mouth to create maximal negative pressure) allows an assessment of the upper airway and its response to maximal negative pressure. Excessive soft tissue can be detected as well as the amount of lateral and anteroposterior collapse of the pharynx that contributes to snoring and obstructive sleep apnea (OSA).

Polysomnography is recommended for all snoring patients to detect and measure OSA severity. Level I polysomnography includes electroencephalogram, electromyogram, electrocardiogram, airflow measurements, oxygen saturation, sleeping position, and manometry (5). Recently, the home polysomnography (level II) has become more popular in the diagnosis of OSA. An abbreviated study series that measures only one or two parameters is not considered valid (6). We recommend that all snoring patients undergo a sleep test prior to treatment to detect any underlying OSA.

PATIENT SELECTION FOR LAUP

Patients with grade II and grade III snoring that is habitual, obnoxious, and loud and that disturbs the household are candidates for LAUP. A detailed medical history, complete examination of the upper airway, and polysomnography must be performed in each candidate. Numerous nonsurgical measures may be successful in eliminating the snoring. When these behavioral measures fail, patients can be considered for LAUP. LAUP in an office setting must be restricted to patients with simple snoring, upper airway resistance, and mild sleep apnea. Patients with moderate to severe sleep apnea must be treated in a hospital setting under general anesthesia using conventional methods with or without laser. Ideally, these patients should be on continuous positive airway pressure (CPAP) for at least 4–6 weeks prior to surgery to normalize some of their sleep parameters and familiarize them with CPAP, which should be continued postoperatively until a repeat sleep study is obtained (7).

LAUP, ANESTHESIA, AND SURGICAL TECHNIQUE

LAUP is an office-based outpatient surgical procedure for the treatment of obnoxious, loud snoring, upper airway resistance syndrome, and mild sleep apnea (8). The CO_2 laser is used to sequentially vaporize the uvula and the free margin of the palate in a series of procedures. LAUP is performed in an upright, sitting position in a motorized otolaryngology examination chair. Prior to treatment, the patient is given instructions on relaxation of the tongue base, and on breathing, which, primarily, is to hold a deep breath during the lasing event followed by a forced exhalation on the termination of the laser pass. Forced exhalation blows any retained laser plume out of the oral cavity to avoid plume inhalation. Inhalation of the laser plume can be irritating, which may result in coughing, respiratory irritation, and nausea. Patients are also reminded that the back of the throat will become numb and that they may lose swallowing and breathing sensations (9).

Another helpful technique, particularly in a patient with a strong gag reflex, is to encourage vocalization during lasing. After careful instructions are given, 20% benzocaine (Hurricane, Beutlich, Inc., Niles, IL) topical anesthetic is sprayed on the posterior oral cavity over the soft palate, tonsil, and uvula. The nose is sprayed with a solution of equal parts 4% Xylocaine (Astra Merck Inc., Wayne, PA) and 0.5% neosynephrine, which also anesthetizes the posterior pharyngeal wall, facilitating the use of a backstop handpiece. The pharynx is then injected with a mixture of 1 mL, 2% lidocaine (Xylocaine) with 1:100,000 epinephrine and 0.5 mL 0.5% bupivacaine hydrochloride (Marcaine, Winthrop Pharmaceuticals, New York, NY) using a 3-mL syringe with a 27-gauge needle. Injections are performed bilaterally into the muscle at the junction of the soft palate and the uvula, and into the base of the uvula as well when it is long and thick. Adequate time is allowed for anesthesia and decongestion to take effect. During the infiltration of local anesthetic, it is important to avoid injecting superficially and creating a bleb or passing the needle through and through the velum beyond the muscle layer.

LAUP is performed using a CO_2 laser with specialized attachments. The attachments include a pharyngeal handpiece with a backstop, SwiftLase flashscanner (Sharplan Lasers, Inc., Allendale, NJ), and tongue depressor with a built-in smoke evacuator. The specially developed pharyngeal handpiece has a backstop that helps stabilize the soft palate and also protects the posterior pharyngeal wall. The tongue base is depressed inferiorly using an ebonized tongue blade with an integrated smoke evacuation channel. It is important to follow all laser safety parameters during the procedure for maximal safety of the patient and the personnel (10).

The CO_2 laser is used to make bilateral, vertical incisions in the palate on both sides of the uvula. These incisions are full-thickness through-and-through trenches approximately 1–2 cm in length from the free edge of the velum extending vertically and superiorly. These trenches are created using the SwiftLase scanner to create an inverted U-shaped defect. The laser is set at 18 W in a continuous mode. Without the SwiftLase scanner, the incision will appear like an inverted V, producing secondary webbing of this area during healing. To maintain an open velum and reduce possible future sessions, the SwiftLase is used at the same power settings, and the upper part of the trenches is further widened, thus creating the inverted U, keeping the palate arch wider and higher.

Once the palatal incisions have been made, the uvula is reduced. The length of the uvula is reduced by approximately 80%–90% using the same laser settings. The surgical goal is to shorten and reshape the soft palate in the uvula. Care must be taken not to excessively burn the mucosa, thereby exposing muscle and creating char. The uvula is shortened by ablating the muscle layer from within, creating a "fishmouth" appearance. This is accomplished by retracting the tip of the uvula anteriorly and vaporizing a central portion of the uvula muscle while preserving as much of the nasal and oral mucosa as possible. Minimizing denuded muscle results in less postoperative discomfort and facilitates healing. The advantages of using the SwiftLase are the absence of char, precise layer-by-layer surface ablation, and its ability to seal small blood vessels as the uvula is sequentially reduced (8,9).

LAUP usually requires two to three treatments, actually averaging 2.3 in our series, spaced 6–8 weeks apart. A minimum of 6 weeks is necessary between procedures to allow for proper healing of the soft palate mucosa. In subsequent procedures, the palate arches are lateralized and the uvula is shortened. The endpoint of LAUP is when the patient's snoring is totally eliminated; both the patient and the bed partner are happy, comfortable, and sleeping in the same bedroom; or if the patient is unable to generate a voluntary snorting sound (7,8).

POSTOPERATIVE CARE

Immediately following the procedure the patient gargles with a mixture of cold water and hydrogen peroxide. This will provide cooling of the soft tissues and clean off any char or debris that may collect during the procedure. Vigorous hydration, humidification, and steam inhalation are important to avoid drying of the oral mucosa. Oral analgesics, topical anesthetics, and antibiotics are prescribed for 7 days.

COMPLICATIONS

The overall complication rate for this procedure is extremely low. Moderate to severe sore throat is the major side effect following LAUP. The pain intensity reaches its peak 3–5 days postoperatively, with complete relief of symptoms usually occurring 8–10 days following surgery. Pain is usually controlled with topical lidocaine anesthetic gel and acetaminophen with codeine. Hydration, humidification, and intake of aloe vera juice usually facilitate healing.

The most common long-term complications are a sensation of a foreign body and increased mucus collection or thick mucus in the back of the throat, occurring in 46% of our patients. This is attributed to the absence of the mid portion of the velum and uvula, which acts as a pharyngeal sweeper, clearing the posterior pharyngeal wall of stagnant secretions during swallowing. In addition, the soft palate, which is rich in mucous and minor salivary glands, secretes large amounts of saliva and mucus, lubricating the pharynx (Fig. 1).

In our series, prolonged odynophagia (severe sore throat lasting ≥3 weeks) occurred in 1.4% of our patients. Weight loss, associated with postoperative odynophagia, averaged 5–12 pounds. Temporary taste alteration, lasting 1–3 months, occurred in 178 patients (18%). Decreased oropharyngeal transit time during swallowing, which manifested as a choking sensation, was reported by 9% of our patients. Changes in pharyngeal food transit

were directly related to the degree of the pharyngeal airway opening that resulted in poor control of the food bolus. These symptoms were temporary, and all patients eventually adjusted to their new palatal anatomy.

In our series of 1000 patients, we had no cases of severe bleeding; 3.8% of the patients had minor early bleeding or bleeding during the procedure that was controlled by silver nitrate application. Early bleeding is defined as that which occurs while the patient is still in the office. The incidence of late bleeding, patients needing to return to the office requiring cauterization or suture, was 0.3% We did not have any major bleeding requiring hospitalization, general anesthesia, or blood transfusion (Fig. 2).

Vasovagal reaction was encountered in several patients following the injection of local anesthetic into the soft palate (0.4%). The incidence of voice and resonance changes was 0.3%. An inability to roll a palatal "R" sound was reported by 121 patients (12%).

Infections were rare, occurring in only 14 patients. There were several patients (0.9%) who developed oral candidiasis following surgery, which was treated with an oral antifungal agent. Fungal infections were found solely in heavy smokers and alcohol drinkers (Fig. 3). Several patients (0.4%) also reported herpetic or aphthous ulcerations 7–10 days following the surgery. The use of prophylactic acyclovir (Zovirax, Glaxo Wellcome Inc., Research Triangle Park, NC) (400 mg twice daily) may be indicated in patients with a history of recurrent oral herpes. Laser-related complications were also uncommon. They can occur during the use of a straight handpiece as a direct burn of the palate and tongue or indirect burn with the use of a backstop handpiece (Fig. 4).

The incidence of occasional velopharyngeal incompetence was 0.7%, which was described as occasional nasal regurgitation. Permanent velopharyngeal insufficiency was not found. Severe nasopharyngeal stenosis did not occur in our series. However, we have evaluated and treated several cases of mild to moderate stenosis after LAUP referred to us

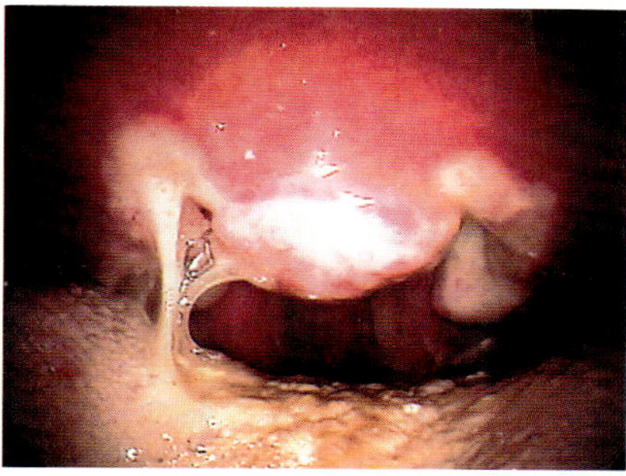

FIG. 1. Thick mucus over the healing palate, 10 days following extended laser-assisted uvulo-palatoplasty.

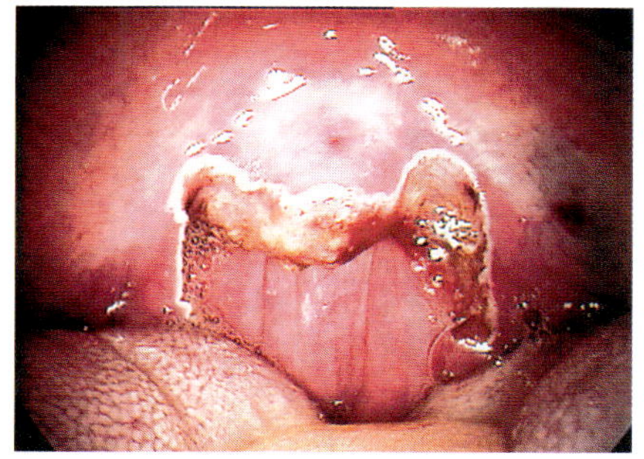

A

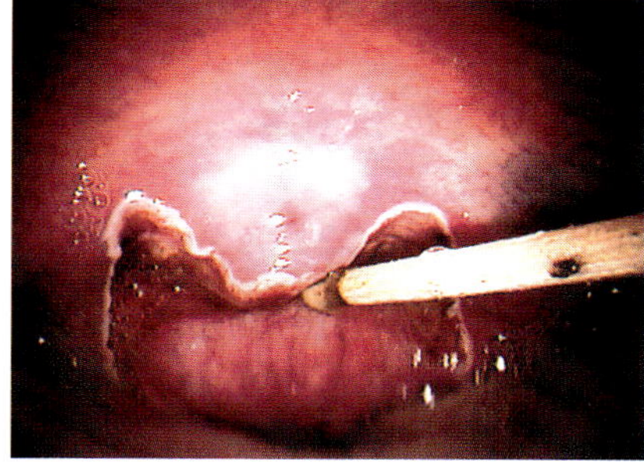

B

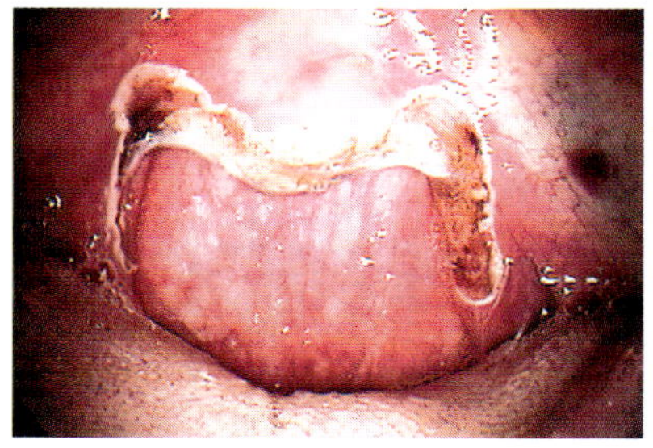

C

FIG. 2. (A) Minor bleeding from the left trench during surgery. **(B)** Silver nitrate cauterization of the bleeding site. **(C)** Minor bleeding controlled following LAUP. Note dry surgical field and absence of charring.

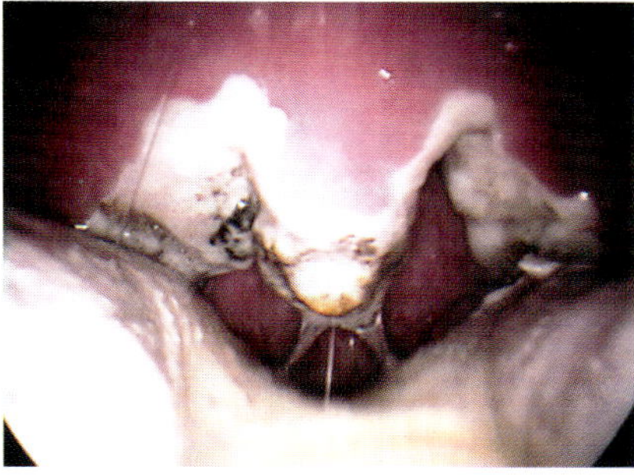

FIG. 3. Postoperative fungal infection of the palate, 7 days following laser-assisted uvulo-palatoplasty.

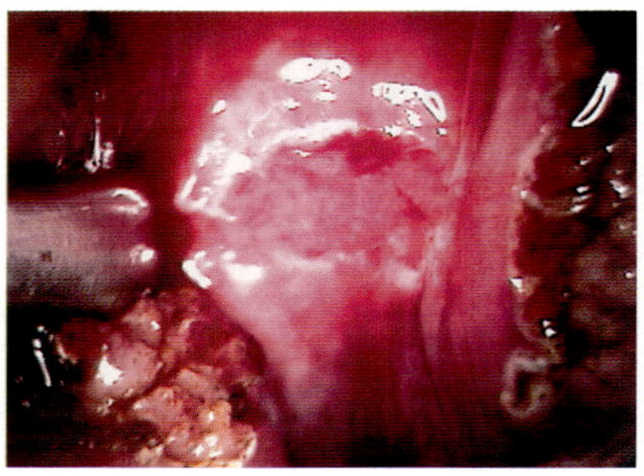

FIG. 4. Intraoperative indirect burn of the pharyngeal wall from overheated backstop handpiece.

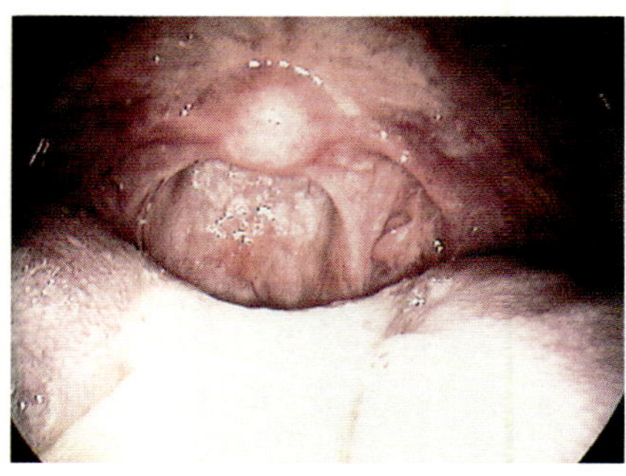

FIG. 5. Hypertrophic scar formation in the center soft palate following laser-assisted uvulopalatoplasty (British method).

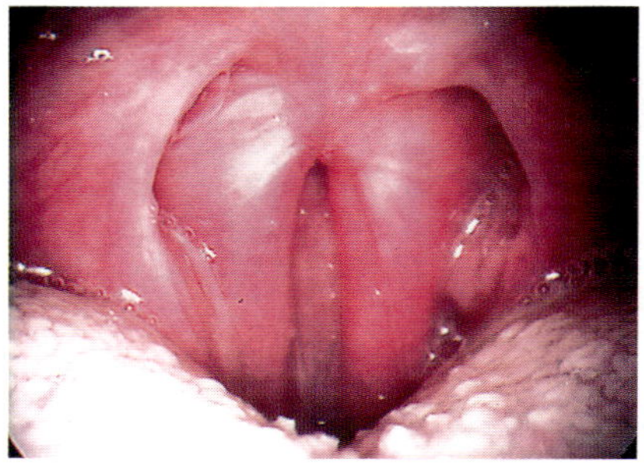

FIG. 6. Moderate nasopharyngeal stenosis.

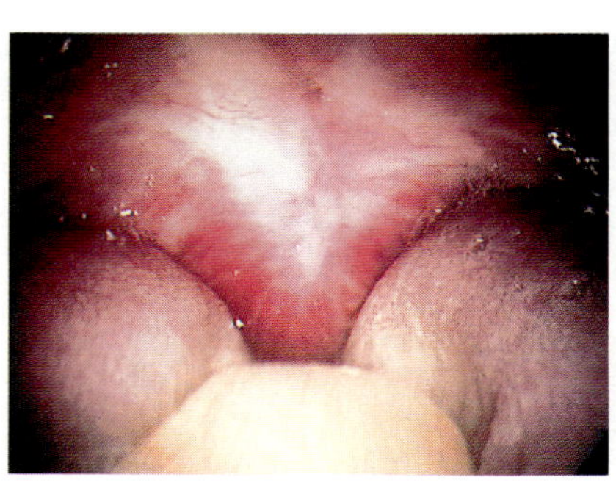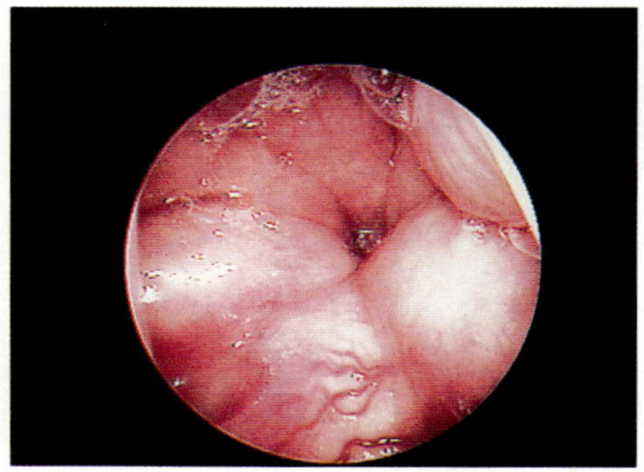

A

B

FIG. 7. Severe nasopharyngeal stenosis. Complete fusion of the lateral walls to the posterior pharyngeal walls. **(A)** Oral view; **(B)** Nasal view.

from other institutions. The incidence of mild stenosis, characterized as adherence of the lateral aspect of the palate to the posterior pharyngeal wall, was 0.5%. One patient developed a hypertrophic scar in the middle of the palate edge following the British LAUP method (Figs. 5–7).

The number of LAUP procedures required to achieve a cure ranged from one to five treatments, with an average of 2.3 sessions. Our experience in more than 1000 patients yielded an 84% cure and 7% improvement rate of snoring.

In conclusion, LAUP is an effective method in the treatment of loud, habitual snoring with a low incidence of complications. This procedure sequentially enlarges the airway at the level of the velum and uvula and reduces vibratory tissues. This procedure can be safely performed with the CO_2 laser in an office setting under local anesthesia. Other than the feeling of increased mucus, the incidence of long-term and severe complications is <1%. Therefore, LAUP has proved to be an effective, safe, simple, well-tolerated procedure and it is widely accepted by the otolaryngology community as the method of choice for the cure of habitual, loud snoring of palatal origin.

REFERENCES

1. Lugaresi E, Mondini S, Zucconi M et al: Staging of heavy snorers disease. A proposal. *Bull Eur Physiopathol Respir* 19:590–594, 1983.
2. Fujita S: Method of Fujita. In: Fairbanks DNF, Fujita S, Ikematsu T et al., eds. *Snoring and obstructive sleep apnea*. New York:Raven Press, 1987:134–153.
3. Ikematsu T: Study of snoring, 4th report: Therapy. *Nippon Jibiinkoka Gakkai Kaiho (Journal of the Oto-Rhino-Laryngological Society of Japan)* 64:434–435, 1964.
4. Kamami YV: Laser CO_2 for snoring—Preliminary results 1990. *Acta Otorhinolaryngol Belg* 44:451–456, 1990.
5. American Sleep Disorders Association, Standards of Practice Committee: Practice parameters for the use of portable recording in the assessment of obstructive sleep apnea. *Sleep* 17:372–377, 1994.
6. Zammit G, Lund S, Ghassibi J: Clinical polysomnography in the evaluation of snoring and sleep-related breathing disorders. *Operative Techniques in Otolaryngology-Head and Neck Surgery* 54:221–227, 1994.
7. Krespi YP, Pearlman SJ, Keider A et al: Laser assisted uvulopalatoplasty for snoring. *Insights in Otolaryngology* 9:1–8, 1994.
8. Krespi YP, Pearlman SJ, Keidar A: Laser assisted uvulapalatoplasty for snoring. *J Otolaryngol* October, 1994.
9. Krespi YP, Keidar A, Khosh M et al: The efficacy of laser-assisted uvulopalatoplasty in the management of obstructive sleep apnea and upper airway resistance syndrome. *Operative Techniques in Otolaryngology-Head and Neck Surgery* 54:235–243, 1994.
10. Krespi YP, Keidar A: Laser-assisted uvulopalatoplasty for the treatment of snoring. *Operative Techniques in Otolaryngology-Head and Neck Surgery* 54:228–234, 1994.

Office-Based Surgery of the Head and Neck
Edited by Yosef P. Krespi, MD
Lippincott–Raven Publishers, Philadelphia © 1998

13

Laser Treatment of the Lingual Tonsils

Yosef P. Krespi and Matthew E. Karen

The most common abnormality of the lingual tonsils is papillary hyperplasia. Although Waldeyer's ring tends to atrophy with age, the lingual tonsils can enlarge with allergy or chronic infections. Lingual tonsil hyperplasia is also encountered in patients with obstructive sleep apnea (OSA). Symptoms of lingual tonsil disease range from mild throat irritation to the feeling of choking and respiratory obstruction. The mainstay of therapy remains nonsurgical.

When conservative therapy fails, patients often benefit from surgical intervention. Laser tonsillectomy has undergone tremendous change with the advent of new instrumentation and technology. Patient selection is critical in facilitating laser use for this surgery.

CLINICAL SETTING

The lingual tonsil consists of lymphoid tissue incorporated within Waldeyer's ring, and sits at the base of the tongue between the circumvallate papilla and vallecula. It comprises two large laterally placed clumps of lymphoid tissue divided by the median glossoepiglottic fold. The size and deposition of this tissue are quite variable. Unlike the other lymphoid organs that compose Waldeyer's ring, the lingual tonsil does not involute with age, but can actually increase in size in response to environmental allergens or irritants. Speculation exists that this hyperplasia is a compensatory mechanism following pallatine tonsillectomy and adenoidectomy (1,2).

Diseases of the lingual tonsils and their treatment have long been ignored in both clinical practice and the medical literature. Physicians tend to overlook this anatomic area in their physical examination, differential diagnosis, therapeutic planning, and intervention. The rich vascular supply from the dorsal lingual artery that arises from the external carotid artery often makes transoral surgical excision of the lingual tonsils hazardous, particularly without proper equipment and experience. The lymphatic vessels drain into the suprahyoid, submaxillary, and deep cervical nodes. Sensory innervation is by way of the ninth and the superior laryngeal branches of the tenth cranial nerves (3,4).

Lingual tonsil hyperplasia is by far the most common pathologic state. Most often the hyperplasia is in response to allergens and irritants, such as smoke and dust, or is a result of chronic gastroesophageal reflux. Hormonal and immune mechanisms may also play a role in this enlargement. The incidence of lingual tonsil hyperplasia is greater in women than in men (5–6).

Clinically, lingual tonsil hyperplasia may manifest in a myriad of symptoms. These include constant throat irritation and globus to more serious complaints of choking and dysphagia. In obese individuals, lingual tonsil hypertrophy can contribute greatly to OSA (7–9). Conservative treatment includes avoiding the irritants or eliminating the inciting causes. This is often successful in obviating the need for surgical intervention.

Lingual tonsil hyperplasia can also result from infectious causes. Patients with acute lingual tonsillitis or chronic irritative tonsillitis usually respond to medical therapy. Antibiotics are the mainstay of therapy. Surgery is rarely indicated. However, in patients with chronic lingual tonsillitis refractory to antibiotics or those with excessive enlargement of the lingual tonsils, surgical intervention often brings relief and provides satisfactory resolution (10,11).

The traditional surgical armamentarium for lingual tonsillectomy includes scalpel, scissors, the special "lingual tonsillectomy snare," electrocautery, and cryoprobe (12–14). Excision by sharp dissection is uncommon, and remains an unpopular choice for surgeons owing to uncontrolled hemorrhage. Other surgical complications, such as postoperative edemas with resultant airway compromise, have dissuaded surgeons from performing lingual tonsillectomy. Cryosurgery has its advocates, but poor control of tissue damage with the cryoprobe has led to its demise as a surgical tool (15,16).

The carbon dioxide (CO_2) laser has proved superior to other surgical techniques in treating lingual tonsils. It is the ideal method for base of tongue surgery because of its precision and excellent hemostatic capability (17–19). Furthermore, it seals lymphatic vessels and nerve endings, thereby decreasing postoperative edema and discomfort. Avoidance of trauma to adjacent normal tissue is achieved, thus allowing more rapid healing.

INDICATIONS AND PATIENT SELECTION

Indications and patient selection for laser lingual tonsillectomy are important components of patient care. A diagnosis of lingual tonsil hyperplasia needs to be made prior full assessment. The medical evaluation includes a careful history and physical examination with the inclusion of fiberoptic visualization of the upper aerodigestive tract and an allergy assessment, if indicated. Patients with symptoms and findings consistent with lingual tonsil hyperplasia are placed on a 2-week course of antibiotic therapy. Owing to concomitant symptoms of gastroesophageal reflux or symptoms suggesting silent reflux, most patients should be treated with an anti-

reflux regimen as well. This consists of a combination of H2 blockers and antacids or proton pump inhibitors. Medical therapy must be rigorously reinforced and closely monitored through regular office visits. Flexible laryngoscopy is used to follow and document the clinical course after therapy has been instituted. If after 4 weeks of aggressive medical therapy the patient's symptoms persist and are considered intractable and intolerable, surgical intervention should be considered.

For patients who have mild to moderate disease of the lingual tonsil and can tolerate intraoral manipulation (minimal gag reflex), initial surgical therapy consists of CO_2 laser ablation using a pharyngeal handpiece with mirror tip. More advanced hypertrophy can be ablated with a CO_2 laser fiber (waveguide) passed through a flexible bronchoscope and coupled to a CO_2 laser. These procedures can be performed in the office setting in one or more sessions depending on the severity of the disease. They can be carried out under topical and local anesthesia.

In patients who have severe lingual tonsillar hyperplasia with associated OSA or in those with low tolerance to intraoral manipulation, laser surgery is carried out in the operating room under general endotracheal anesthesia. Suspension microlaryngoscopy with the newly developed lingoscope (Supraglottoscope, Richard Wolf Medical Instruments, Vernon Hills, IL) provides superior exposure and hemostatic control in cases requiring extensive resection at the tongue base.

PROCEDURES

Endoscopic Ablation of the Lingual Tonsil With CO_2 Laser Fibers (Waveguides)

The procedure is performed in an office or ambulatory setting using local or topical anesthesia. An operative adult flexible bronchoscope (4.2 mm) with a 2.2-mm working channel is employed for this procedure. After the nasal cavity is topically anesthetized and decongested, the bronchoscope is carefully passed through the nasal passage to the level of the tongue base. When the lingual tonsil is visualized, the CO_2 laser fiber (waveguide) is passed through the working channel until it is seen at the tip of the bronchoscope. A video camera or TV monitor aids in better visualization of the surgery. Anesthesia of the tongue base is achieved with topical 4% Xylocaine (Astra Merck Inc., Wayne, PA) spray followed by local infiltration of the lingual tonsils with 1–2 mL of 1% Xylocaine with epinephrine (1:100,000). The injection is performed either with a curved indirect laryngeal needle or a modified sclerotherapy needle introduced through the working channel of the flexible bronchoscope. The CO_2 laser is set at 10–15 W and in the super pulse continuous mode. Only 70%–80% of the actual laser energy is transmitted through the laser fiber. The remainder dissipates to the fiber wall as thermal energy. A constant stream of air flows through the fiber to keep it cool and clean.

Lingual tonsil ablation primarily involves contouring the cobblestone tonsil surface to achieve a smooth and level configuration, which effectively reduces the size of the lingual tonsil. In chronic tonsillitis, crypts are often present on the tonsillar surface and serve as a nidus for infection. Surgery is aimed at lysing these crypts. Care is taken to resect only the lymphoid tissue and to spare the underlying muscle layers, thus minimizing hemorrhage. Surgical exposure is enhanced by retracting the tongue forward. This is accomplished with the aid of a surgical assistant or with the help of the patient. The patient is asked to exhale slowly during the lasing to expel the laser plume. The procedure lasts 10–15 minutes and is well tolerated by the patient. At the end of the procedure, an oral rinse of H_2O/H_2O_2 mixture is given to the patient. Postoperatively the patient is observed for 1–2 hours before being discharged. Postoperative care includes hydration, humidification, analgesia, and antibiotics for 5 days.

Endoscopic Ablation of the Lingual Tonsil with Diode Laser

Similar endoscopic laser ablation of the lingual tonsils can be performed with the diode laser using 600–800-μm fibers. Fiber is inserted into the operating channel of the flexible nasolaryngoscope passed into the hypopharynx to ablate the lingual tonsils under direct vision.

Transoral Ablation of Lingual Tonsils Using CO_2 Laser Coupled to an Operating Microscope

This procedure is performed under general anesthesia with the use of a laser-safe endotracheal tube. A wide-mouth laryngoscope designed for laser surgery is best suited to provide adequate exposure of the tongue base and vallecula. The Supraglottoscope or lingoscope is ideal for this purpose. This scope has a much shorter blade when compared with the conventional laryngoscope; it can be adjusted independently for greater control and exposure. The lingoscope is positioned and stabilized by the Lewy suspension holder. Only one side of the tongue base can be exposed at any one time. Once the ablation is completed, the lingoscope has to be repositioned to treat the contralateral side. The newly developed SwiftLase or SurgiTouch flashscanner (Sharplan Laser Inc., Allendale, NJ) is ideal in ablating the lingual tonsil (20–23). It is of extreme importance to ablate only the lymphoid tissue, sparing the underlying muscle layers to avoid the risk of uncontrolled hemorrhage. The central portion of the tongue base (median glossoepiglottic fold) is best left intact. The laser power setting used for ablation is 12–15 W in continuous focused mode when using the SwiftLase flashscanner. In the absence of the SwiftLase, the power can be increased to 15–20 W in continuous defocused mode to cut and coagulate tissues simultaneously. The lingoscope has a built-in smoke evacuation port that is attached to a smoke evacuator for proper discharge of plume. In the rare incidence of bleeding, the laser beam in the same power setting can be changed to a defocused mode to coagulate small vessels. Persistent bleeding from larger vessels may require electrocauterization using the conventional suction cautery device.

Patients are often observed overnight in the hospital setting on continuous pulse oximetry. If limited surgery is performed, patients can be discharged later that same day. Postoperative care includes analgesics, humidification, hydration, and antibiotics.

CONCLUSION

Diseases of the lingual tonsils can present with a variety of signs and symptoms. They can be broadly categorized into chronic lingual tonsillitis or tonsillar hyperplasia. The pathogenesis of these diseases has been well described by many authors. The mainstay of treatment remains nonsurgical and includes oral antibiotics, anti-reflux treatment, or allergy therapy. Only when optimal medical therapy fails to alleviate the symptoms should surgical intervention be sought. The reluctance to pursue surgical therapy prior to the advent of the CO_2 laser is due to the morbid complications associated with sharp surgical dissection. These include massive hemorrhage, damage to surrounding tissues, and potential airway compromise as a result of postoperative edema. The CO_2 laser has revived the waning interest in performing lingual tonsillectomy. The CO_2 laser beam directed through a laser-safe laryngoscope, under microscopic control, provides an effective operative alternative to traditional methods. More recently, the CO_2 laser fiber (waveguide) has further expanded the role of the laser to treat the lingual tonsil in the office setting under local anesthesia. Careful patient selection is critical in ensuring success with these surgical techniques. The CO_2 laser seems to be a safe and effective surgical tool to eradicate disease within the lingual tonsil.

REFERENCES

1. Goeringer GC, Vidic B: The embryogenesis and anatomy of Waldeyer's ring. *Otolaryngol Clin North Am* 20(2): 207–217, 1987.
2. Wood DG, Whittet HB: The lingual tonsil: A neglected symptomatic structure? *J Laryngol Otol* 103:922–925, 1989.
3. Elfman LK: Lingual tonsils. *Laryngoscope* 59:1016–1025, 1949.
4. Elise CJ: Lingual tonsillitis. *Ann NY Acad Sci* 82:52–56, 1959.
5. Guarisco JL, Littlewood SC, Butcher RB: Severe upper airway obstruction in children secondary to lingual tonsil hypertrophy. *Ann Otol Rhinol Laryngol* 99:621–624, 1990.
6. Johnson MA, Mehdiabadi AJ, Ruff A: Infection and hypertrophy of the lingual tonsil as a cause of airway obstruction. *Tex Med* 82:29–31, 1980.
7. Jesberg N: Chronic hypertrophic lingual tonsillitis. *Arch Otolaryngol* 64:3–13, 1956.
8. Olsen KD, Suh KW, Staats BA: Surgically correctable causes of sleep apnea. *Otolaryngol Head Neck Surg* 89:726–731, 1981.
9. Wilson JF, Coutras S, Tami TA: Recurrent adult acute epiglottitis: The role of lingual tonsillectomy. *Ann Otol Rhinol Laryngol* 98:602–604, 1989.
10. Joseph M, Reardon E, Goodman M: Lingual tonsillectomy: A treatment for inflammatory lesions of the lingual tonsil. *Laryngoscope* 94:170–184, 1984.
11. Newman RK, Johnson JT: Abscess of the lingual tonsil. *Arch Otolaryngol* 105:277–278, 1979.
12. Cohen HB: The lingual tonsil: General consideration and its neglect. *Laryngoscope* 27:691–700, 1917.
13. Sluder G: Some clinical observations on the lingual tonsils. *Ann Otol Rhinol Laryngol* 26:1148–1153, 1917.
14. Hoover WB: The treatment of the lingual tonsils and lateral pharyngeal bands of lymphoid tissues. *Surg Clin North Am* 14:1257–1269, 1934.
15. Principato JJ: Cryosurgical treatment of the lymphoid tissue of Waldeyer's ring. *Otolaryngol Clin North Am* 20:365–370, 1987.
16. Von Leden H, Rand RW: Cryosurgery of the head and neck. *Arch Otolaryngol* 85:115, 1967.
17. Mihashi S, Jako GJ, Strong MS: Laser surgery in otolaryngology: Interaction of the CO_2 laser and soft tissue. *Ann NY Acad Sci* 267:263–294, 1976.
18. Strong MS, Jako GJ, Polanyi T et al: Laser surgery in the aerodigestive tract. *Am J Surg* 126:529–533, 1973.
19. Wouters B, van Overbeek JJM, Buiter CT, Hoeksema PE: Laser surgery in lingual tonsil hyperplasia. *Clin Otolaryngol* 14:291–296, 1989.
20. Krespi YP, Har-El G, Levine TM et al: Laser lingual tonsillectomy. *Laryngoscope* 99:131–135, 1989.
21. Krespi YP: Tonsil cryptolysis utilizing CO_2 Swiftlase [abstract 197]. *Lasers Surg Med* (Suppl 5):40–41, 1993.
22. Slatkine M, Krespi YP: Instrumentation for office laser surgery. *Operative Techniques in Otolaryngology Head and Neck Surgery* 5(4):211–217, 1994.
23. Krespi YP, Ling E: Tonsil cryptolysis using CO_2 Swiftlase. *Operative Techniques in Otolaryngology Head and Neck Surgery* 5(4):294–297, 1994.

Office-Based Surgery of the Head and Neck
Edited by Yosef P. Krespi, MD
Lippincott–Raven Publishers, Philadelphia © 1998

14

Laser-Assisted Endoscopic Laryngeal Surgery

Andrew Blitzer and Yosef P. Krespi

Operative laryngology was a natural outgrowth of the ability to examine the larynx with the mirrors of Garcia, Turck, and Czermak (1). A number of surgeons, most notably Morell MacKenzie, used these mirrors for examination and then designed instruments for biopsy and other operative procedures of the larynx. Once general anesthesia was available, Brunnings, Jackson, and others popularized operative laryngeal surgery via a direct laryngoscope (1). Many instruments were designed to fit through the laryngoscope to operate on vocal folds. With the introduction of the operative microscope, the surgery became much more precise, and small vocal fold lesions could be removed with minimal tissue damage. The next change in operative laryngology occurred with the development of the carbon dioxide (CO_2) laser, which allowed precise ablation of epithelial lesions with no bleeding and minimal scarring. For some lesions, such as recurrent papillomas, granulomas, and hemangiomas, the CO_2 laser is the modality of choice. A number of patient issues may make multiple procedures difficult, and so we attempted to find a way to provide accurate viewing and CO_2 laser energy in an awake patient in an outpatient setting.

EQUIPMENT AND LASER SPECIFICS

To accomplish the goal of direct CO_2 laser surgery with excellent visualization of the larynx under local anesthesia in an outpatient setting, we developed the use of a flexible optical waveguide that can be manipulated via an operative channel in a flexible fiberoptic laryngoscope. We use a 4.9-mm flexible fiberoptic laryngoscope or bronchoscope with a 2.2-mm working channel. We attach this endoscope to a halogen or xenon light source and a video camera. The procedures are performed while viewing the monitor, much the way we do other nonlaser surgical laryngeal procedures. To accomplish the laser surgery, we use a 30–40-W laser with a superpulse mode. The laser needs to be able to supply air pressure for fiber cooling. The laser energy is delivered to the articulated arm, which then delivers the power to a coupler that focuses the energy into the center of the thin plastic tube (waveguide). The flexible tube is coated with a dielectric silver-iodine film covered by a second metallic silver film. The optical coating is highly reflective from the multilayer at 10.6 μm wavelength. Multiple reflections from the waveguide walls enable the trapped optical radiation to propagate along the fiber and produce a 1-mm spot size at a distance of 1 mm from the fiber's distal end. The optical beam divergence is 80°, thus enabling considerable defocusing by slightly pulling back the fiber. The airflow through the fiber is synchronized with laser activation. Constant airflow is mandatory to keep the fiber walls from warming up, and to keep the channel free of debris. Power density is lost at 50% per meter of fiber length. The superpulse mode is recommended for laryngeal surgery to minimize char formation, eliminate bleeding, and allow layer-by-layer vaporization of the lesion (Figs. 1 and 2).

PATIENT SELECTION

At the present time, the laser-assisted endoscopic laryngeal surgery (LAELS) technique

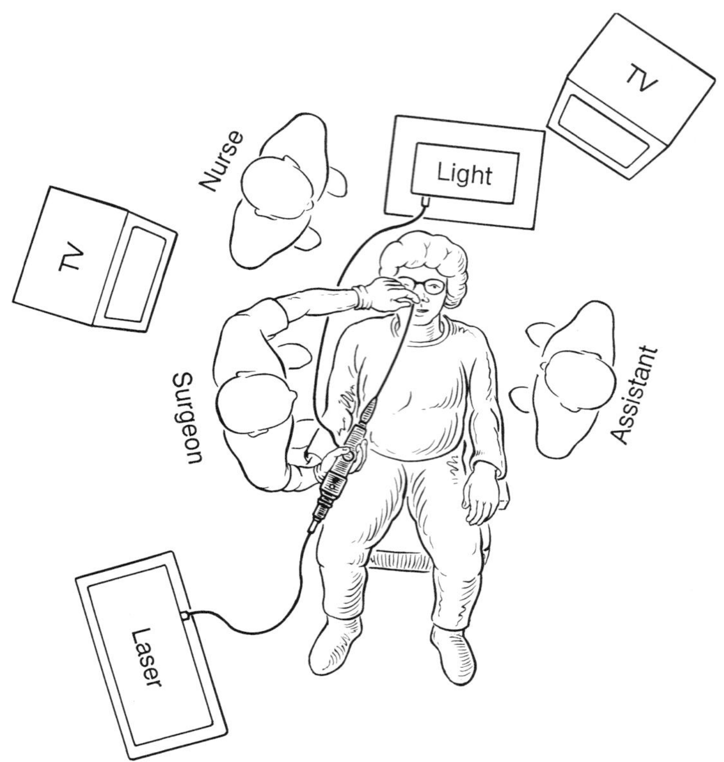

FIG. 1. Set-up of the endoscopic laser surgery suite. The procedure is performed via video control.

may be the only way to provide laryngeal surgery to patients with laryngeal lesions who are otherwise poor candidates for general anesthesia. The technique may also have a distinct advantage for patients who have a short neck and an anteriorly placed larynx, making rigid microendoscopy and laser surgery very difficult. Using a fiberoptic system with an awake patient, good visualization and vaporization of lesions are relatively easy. The LAELS technique is also advantageous for patients who have recurrent laryngeal papillomatosis, granulomas, or other recurrent lesions who may need multiple procedures. Often patients do not wish to have multiple general anesthetics; a procedure under local anesthesia is often better tolerated, and allows earlier intervention for a recurrent lesion. We have also found that patients who have small benign lesions are more likely to have a surgical intervention if they do not have to go to

the hospital and have a general anesthetic. Biopsies can be taken with a cup forceps passed through the operative channel, and then the rest of the lesion may be vaporized.

The lesions that seem well suited for the LAELS technique in the patients described above are of benign supraglottic pathology, such as vallecular cysts, aryepiglottic fold cysts, or hypertrophic lingual tonsillar tissue. At the level of the glottis, refractory vocal fold granulomas, vocal fold nodules or polyps, small webs and scars, small hemangiomas, and occasional vocal fold cysts exist in patients who cannot have more traditional surgery. Small areas of leukoplakia and even Tis lesions in patients who have contraindications to more traditional techniques can be treated effectively with the LAELS technique. We have even treated one patient effectively who had an extremely anteriorly placed larynx and a short neck who had an internal

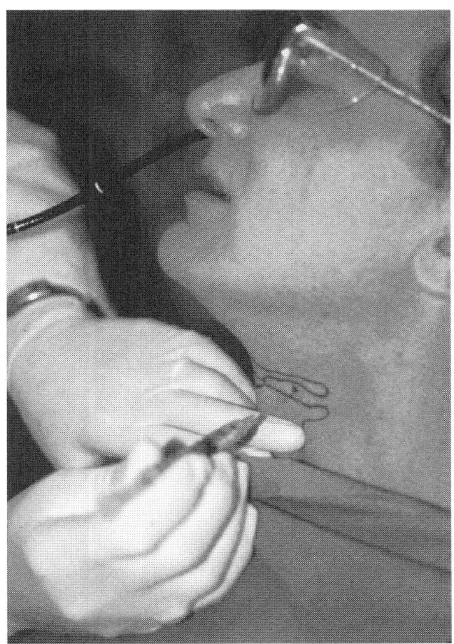

FIG. 2. Superior laryngeal nerve block. Note the site of injection between the hyoid and the thyroid cartilage at midpoint.

laryngocele that had failed to be corrected with three previous direct laryngoscopies and one external approach. With the LAELS technique, we were able to marsupialize the lesion, evacuate the mucoid contents, and then vaporize the lesion down to the saccule. One additional patient with bilateral vocal cord paralysis and a tracheostomy was treated with the LAELS technique because of her internist's concerns about general anesthesia. She had a Kashima type posterior cordotomy to allow for the possibility of decannulation.

The LAELS technique is not indicated in the uncooperative patient because it is performed under local anesthesia and may take 15–30 minutes of surgery with the endoscope in the nose. Most children would be poor choices for this procedure at present because they may not be able to sit quietly for the period of time necessary for this procedure. It is similarly not indicated in patients who have a very small nasal vestibule or severely deviated nasal septum because the endoscope is placed through the nose. Patients with extremely active gag reflexes may not be ideal because they may not be able to keep from swallowing or gagging. Patients with a tendency to bleed or with large vascular malformations would be poor choices for this procedure because it takes place in an unprotected airway. Until the spot size is made a little smaller and more experience is acquired, we would advise not using this procedure with a professional voice user. We do not know yet if the healing and vibratory characteristics will remain the same as with other more traditional techniques.

TECHNIQUE

The patient's nose is first sprayed with 2% lidocaine with 1:100,000 epinephrine. The throat is also sprayed with lidocaine. Following this, bilateral superior laryngeal nerve blocks are given to reduce the sensation and prevent laryngospasm and/or gagging. The superior laryngeal nerve can be found by injecting up against the thyrohyoid membrane midway between the greater cornua of the thyroid cartilage and the greater cornua of the hyoid bone, and halfway up the length of the greater cornua (Fig. 3). For patients with an excessive gag response, bilateral glossopharyngeal nerve blocks can also be employed.

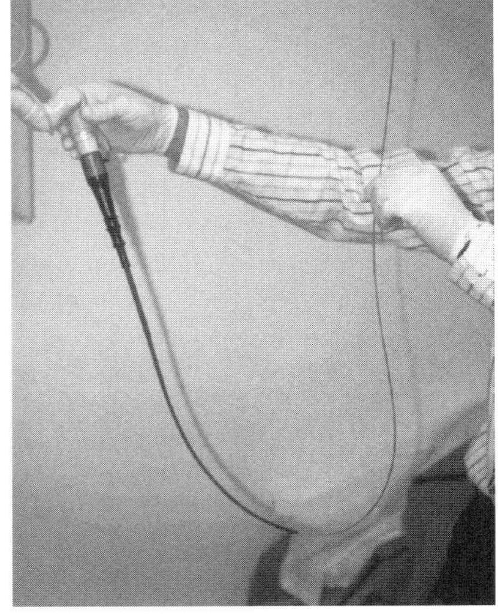

FIG. 3. The CO_2 laser waveguide and coupler.

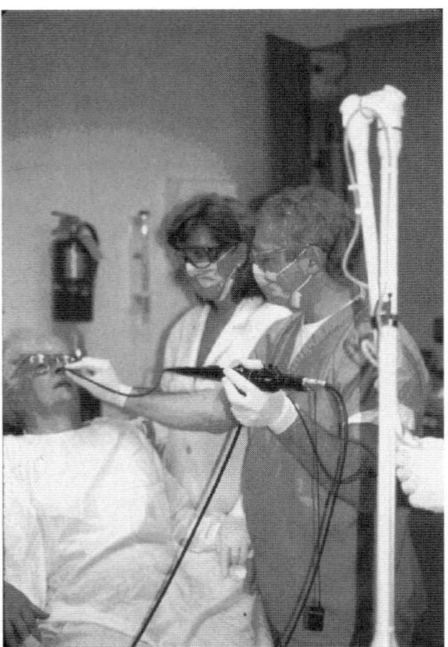

FIG. 4. Laser-assisted endoscopic laryngeal surgery in progress.

These injections are given at the midway point of the anterior tonsillar pillar. The endoscope is then placed through the patient's nasal chamber, and slowly advanced past the nasopharynx toward the larynx. When the endoscope is level with the tip of the epiglottis, lidocaine is injected via the endoscope aimed at the larynx to provide further topical anesthesia to the supraglottic larynx. The endoscope is then advanced toward the vocal cords, and some additional lidocaine is given to achieve topical anesthesia to the immediate subglottic larynx. When adequate anesthesia is achieved, the operative procedure may begin.

The endoscope is passed through the nose and down to the level of the lesion; a small cupped forceps can be passed down the operative channel to take a sample for biopsy. Once this is complete, the flexible waveguide is passed through the operative channel until it extends from the scope and is visualized on the monitor. The endoscope is advanced so that the waveguide is close to the lesion, and, on the superpulse mode, the laser energy is delivered in 200-ms bursts. Smoke evacuation is accomplished via another catheter placed in the oral cavity or opposite the nasal passage. Laser ablation continues as with any other laser surgical procedure until the lesion is completely vaporized. If some char is produced, the laser fiber can be removed, and a small spiral brush (such as used for bronchial brush cytology) is used to clean the area, and then the waveguide is replaced for further vaporization. In the case of inflammatory lesions (eg, granulomas), a flexible injection needle, such as the ones used for sclerotherapy, can be passed via the operative channel for steroid injection at the base of the lesion (Fig. 4). At the termination of the procedure, the endoscope is removed and the patient may go home.

COMPLICATIONS

No complications have been found in our series of patients. The potential complications, however, include those of any vocal fold surgical manipulation: bleeding, edema, and scarring. In addition, because of the significant local and topical anesthesia necessary, aspiration of vomitus is possible. The patient also has the theoretic possibility of aspirating a piece of

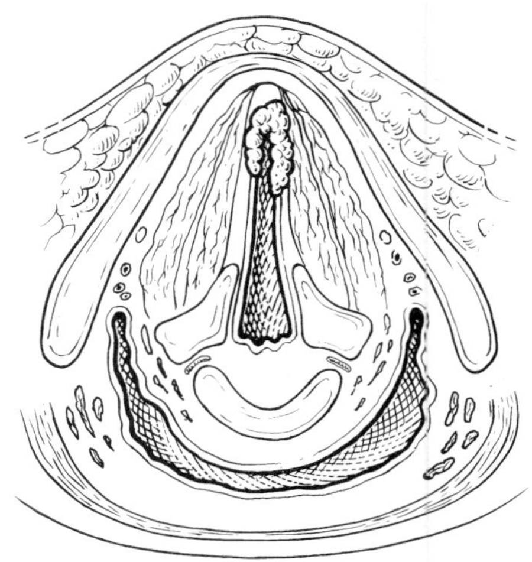

FIG. 5. Small anterior commissure lesion without cartilage invasion.

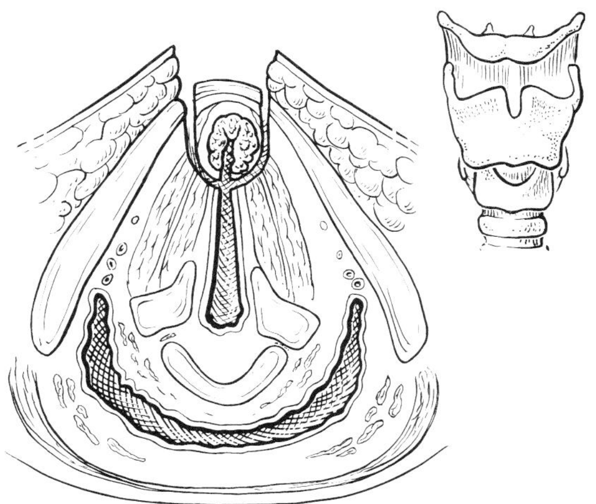

FIG. 6. Endoscopic laser incision of vocalis muscle with margins. External approach to the anterior commissure via small window to obtain margins.

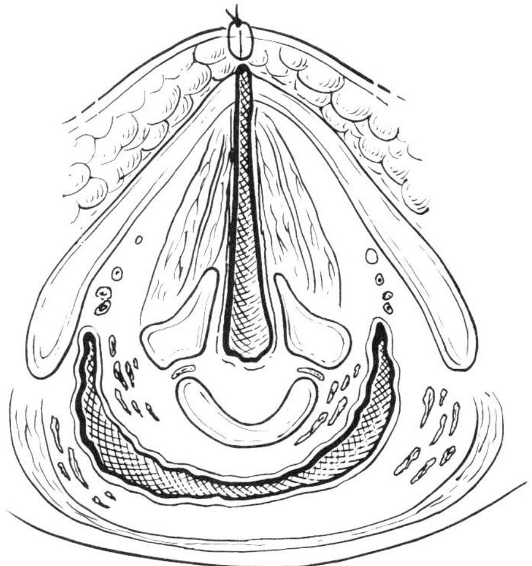

FIG. 7. Closure of the surgical defect.

the charred tissue produced by the laser vaporization. Laryngospasm due to the vocal cord manipulation is possible, but should be minimal if good anesthesia is achieved.

In cases where laryngeal cancer is suspected, initial biopsy can be obtained prior to lasing the tumor. Endoscopic laser ablation of vocal cord lesions is primarily reserved for benign lesions. Superficial malignant tumors can be treated with a CO_2 waveguide if the tumor is located at the mid-cord level. For suspicious lesions involving the anterior commissure, initial biopsy can be obtained and sent for frozen section. During the pathologic analysis, the remaining lesion can be ablated with the CO_2 waveguide. If the lesion proves to be benign, no further therapy is necessary. However, if the lesion is diagnosed as malignant, the patient is taken to the operating room for anterior commissure window laryn-

goplasty under local anesthesia with sedation, according to the method and surgical technique designed by Shapshay (2,3) (Figs. 5–7).

CONCLUSION

LAELS is possible with the advent of the flexible fiberoptic direct laryngoscope and a flexible waveguide. The procedure can be achieved in selected patients in an outpatient setting under local anesthesia. Small benign lesions are easily vaporized with minimal risk.

REFERENCES

1. Karmody CS: The history of laryngology. In Freid MP, ed. *The larynx*. St. Louis: Mosby, 3–11, 1996.
2. Shapshay SM, Wang Z, Reibez EE et al: Window laryngoplasty: A new combined laser endoscopic and open technique for conservation surgery. *Ann Otol Rhinol Laryngol* 103:679–685, 1994.
3. Wang Z, Pankratov MM, Reibez EE et al: Endoscopic diode laser welding of mucosal grafts on the larynx: A new technique. *Laryngoscope* 105:49–52, 1995.

PART 4

The Nose

Office-Based Surgery of the Head and Neck
Edited by Yosef P. Krespi, MD
Lippincott–Raven Publishers, Philadelphia © 1998

15

Conventional Turbinate Surgery

William Lawson and Anthony J. Reino

Excision of obstructing inferior turbinates was first described by Jones (1,2), who believed that their removal would relieve deafness and tinnitus. Holmes (3), in 1900, was the first to accurately describe stages of hypertrophic rhinitis and report his experience with the turbinectomy procedure in 1500 patients. Freer (4) criticized the procedure because of bleeding and prolonged crusting, but admitted that neither permanent chronic infection nor atrophic rhinitis was noted in his patients following complete inferior turbinectomy. In 1924, Strandberg (5) presented 1000 cases of submucous resection of the turbinate, and in 1931 Hurd (6) recommended electrocoagulation of the inferior turbinate mucosa to treat nasal obstruction.

Septal deviation is often associated with contralateral inferior turbinate hypertrophy. This association may be congenital, as in the cleft nose, the product of growth asymmetry, or the result of trauma (7). Unilateral hypertrophy in this setting often involves mucosa and bone. Turbinate enlargement in patients with allergic or vasomotor rhinitis is usually bilateral and due to mucosal thickening without hypertrophy of the underlying bone (7).

TURBINATE EVALUATION

Decisions about the effectiveness of surgery to relieve nasal obstruction can be made at the initial examination. For a thorough nasal examination, we prefer using a coaxial headlight along with a flexible fiberoptic scope. The nose is first inspected in its native state by anterior rhinoscopy without decongestion. The size, shape, and color of the turbinates are noted, as is the status of the septum. The color and character of the nasal mucosa and mucus are likewise assessed, along with the presence or absence of a string sign or nasal polyps. The string sign is the presence of tacky nasal secretions that bridge the nasal cavity; it has been closely associated with paranasal sinus infection.

Special consideration should be given to the anatomic differences of the platyrhine nose. The basic dissimilitude is the tubular shape of the nares, making the turbinates the primary cause of nasal obstruction. The shape of the nares is accompanied by a shortened pyramidal height, wider internal valve angle, and anteriomedially positioned turbinate; hence, turbinectomy is of prime importance in these patients when considering surgery for nasal obstruction.

Following topical vasoconstriction and anesthesia by atomizer with Neo-Synephrine (Sanofi Winthrop Pharmaceuticals, New York, NY) (0.25%) and Pontocaine (Sanofi Winthrop Pharmaceuticals) (2%), the nasal cavity is re-examined. It is important to ask the patient if the obstruction is completely relieved after adequate decongestion. Complete relief confirms the diagnosis of obstruction from mucosal congestion, whereas partial relief signals anatomic problems, such as septal deviation or valvular collapse.

If the turbinates fail to shrink after topical vasoconstriction, consider bony hypertrophy of the inferior turbinate, a pneumatized middle turbinate (concha bullosa), or rhinitis medicamentosa. Palpation of the turbinates usually confirms the diagnosis.

When the septum appears to be straight and the airway patent and the patient still complains of obstruction, a low nasal dyspnea syndrome may exist (8). This syndrome is a functional disorder that may be a form of nasal neurosis. Patients feel obstructed at normal levels of nasal airflow; to relieve their symptoms they may require an airway so patent that mucosal drying and its complications occur (8).

TREATMENT OPTIONS FOR OBSTRUCTING TURBINATES

Medical Management

Medical management should be attempted before surgery is performed (Table 1). After the proper diagnosis is established, antihistamines and decongestants should be prescribed. Sympathomimetic drops or sprays must be withdrawn from patients who habitually use them. In addition, patients on antihypertensives, beta-blockers, or antidepressants, which often have the side effect of turbinate engorgement, should be switched to a different preparation if possible. Complicating factors such as infection or hormonal abnormalities (ie, hypothyroidism, pregnancy, or oral contraceptive use) should be excluded. Allergic rhinitis, if suspected, should be diagnosed and treated appropriately with pharmacotherapy or hyposensitization. Maximal temporary relief of turbinate engorgement may require corticosteroids, given systemically or intranasally by either injection or aerosol. Only after the cause of turbinate hypertrophy has been identified and suitable medical management has failed should surgical remedies be pursued.

Submucosal Corticosteroids

The submucosal injection of corticosteroids was popularized by Simmons (9) in 1964. This technique may offer relief from nasal obstruction and rhinorrhea in properly selected patients. Simmons (9) and Mabry (10) have used this technique more than 10,000 times and report good results.

TABLE 1. *Nonsurgical Management of Turbinate Dysfunction*

Generalized Treatment
  Antihistamine/Decongestant
  Corticosteroids
    Systemic
    Intranasal
    Intraturbinal
  Environmental Control
    Cigarette smoke
    Air filtration
    Humidification
  Mucolytics
Complicating Factors
  Rebound rhinitis/rhinitis medicamentosa
    Discontinue nasal sprays or drops
    Alter antihypertensive medication regimen
  Endocrine abnormalities
    Check thyroid function
    Alter or discontinue oral contraceptives
    Inquire about early pregnancy
  Infection
    Diagnose and treat with appropriate
      scans and antibiotics
Allergic Rhinitis
  Specific therapy
    Cromolyn
    Corticosteroids
    Avoidance
    Immunotherapy
    Antihistamines
  Nonspecific treatment
    Mucolytics
      Alkalol (bicarbonate irrigation)
      Guaifenesin
      N-acetylcysteine
      Iodides
      Saline spray
      Steam

Indications for submucosal injection of corticosteroids include nasal allergy, rhinitis medicamentosa, rhinitis of pregnancy, vasomotor rhinitis, and in some instances, postseptorhinoplasty patients. Beekhuis (11), who described persistent engorgement of the inferior turbinates in 10% of his patients following rhinoplasty, suggested this treatment. Anderson (12) advocated intraturbinal steroid injection at the time of septorhinoplasty, and Mabry (13) advocated injection at the conclusion of all intranasal procedures. Both reported successes in diminishing turbinate edema and improving nasal airway.

Advantages of submucosal corticosteroid injection are its rapid onset and lack of systemic effect. The primary disadvantage is the short duration of action, which lasts only weeks to months.

Surgical Resection

Many surgical procedures are available to treat obstructing inferior turbinates (Table 2). Our personal preference is partial or anterior resection. The procedure is performed by first infracturing the turbinate using a Freer elevator. A right angle scissors is placed above the anterior tip of the turbinate and angled posterior and inferior at approximately a 45° angle. The cut is through mucosa and bone, and the detached segment is removed with a large Wilde forceps. The posterior tip of the turbinate should be resected only if it has undergone mulberriform degeneration. Bleeding is controlled with suction cautery, and the nose is packed tightly with petroleum jelly gauze. The patient is placed on oral antibiotics, and the packing remains in place for 48 hours.

This surgical resection technique has been supported by a number of authors. Bridger (14), in 1970, identified the flow-limiting segment of the nasal cavity in normal subjects to be in the upper cartilaginous vault. Within this segment he identified a point at which a marked pressure drop occurred at maximal flow; in normal subjects, this point related to the anterior end of the inferior turbinate. With mucosal congestion and turbinate enlargement, encroachment into this flow-limiting segment occurs. Pollack and Rohrich (7), in a study of 408 patients, reported that removal of the anterior one third to one half of the inferior turbinate was sufficient to relieve nasal obstruction, provided the posterior remnant was outfractured.

Partial turbinectomy has the advantage of directly removing varying amounts of hypertrophic and obstructive tissue. Its disadvantage has been reported to be increased intraoperative and postoperative bleeding (7). We have not found this to be the case, which is probably owing to avoidance of the sphenopalatine artery branches in the posterior turbinate tip, and the judicious use of suction cautery. To prevent osteitis-induced granulation tissue, prolonged crusting, and bleeding, all exposed bony edges should be carefully resected.

A second method of partial turbinate surgery is the submucous resection. In this procedure, a curvilinear incision is made at the anterior-inferior edge of the inferior turbinate and carried down to the bone. The submucosa

TABLE 2. *Surgery of the Inferior Turbinates*

Procedure	Results	Healing/Complications
Partial resection	Excellent; care must be taken to resect the anterior flow limiting segment completely	Minimal crusting for 1–2 weeks; postoperative bleeding rare
Total resection	Initially good; patients may then complain of progressive increased nasal obstruction	Crusting may be more severe or prolonged
Turbinoplasty	Good results reported in long- and short-term follow-up	Uncomplicated, low incidence of bleeding
Submucous resection	Temporary relief	Minimal bleeding or oozing
Lateral outfracture	Short-term results only	
Surface cautery	Little effect; of limited use	Complicated by ciliary dysfunction, crusting, persistent edema, and low-grade infection
Laser turbinectomy	Excellent results reported with approximately 83% of patients satisfied with their airway at 1 year	Significant postoperative crusting, bleeding, osteitis
Cryosurgery	More than 80% satisfied at 6 months; only 30% satisfied at 5–6 years	Prolonged crusting, edema, and infection; bleeding also a problem with slough of crusts; osteitis rare

is elevated off the bone as far back as possible, and the bone is removed with a Gruenwald forceps. The turbinate is outfractured and the nose is packed with gauze for 2–3 days.

House (15) states that submucous resection is best suited for cases of turbinate enlargement caused by a hypertrophic turbinate bone, and other means should be used to treat soft tissue turbinate enlargement. Controversy exists in the literature over the long-term results of this procedure, as well as the indications, postoperative complications, and technical difficulty of the surgery. House (15) reported that the removal of the bony support of the inferior turbinate allowed it to fall into a more lateral position, thereby increasing the size of the airway; however, the relief achieved by this shift was not permanent. Although House indicates that this procedure should be used for hypertrophy of the turbinate bone, Pollack and Rohrich (7) had their best results in patients with enlargement of both bone and mucosa. Bleeding during the procedure was reported to be minimal in the House study, but significant in the Pollack and Rohrich experience (7).

Mabry (16) described a variation of the submucous resection of the turbinate called "inferior turbinoplasty." Here, mucosa is dissected off the conchal bone medially. Then the turbinate bone and lateral mucosal flap are removed and a smaller neoturbinate is formed. These patients, who were followed for 1–3 years, had no postoperative crusting and an improved airway.

The management of nasal obstruction with total inferior turbinectomy remains controversial. Supporters of the procedure claim a decrease in nasal airway resistance, a marked subjective improvement in nasal airflow, and minimal postoperative bleeding and care. Martinez et al. (17) advocated total inferior turbinectomy in the belief that this was the only assured means of reducing mechanical airway obstruction, especially after failed septoplasty. However, supporters of the partial procedures claim that their resections include the high resistance area located at the anterior end of the turbinate, hence making radical resection unnecessary (8,15,16).

Complete turbinectomy has been shown to increase laminar nasal airflow, thereby reducing the humidifying capabilities of the nasal mucosa and resulting in drying, cilia destruction, mucous membrane atrophy, and chronic nasal infection (15,18–20). Traditional thought was that total turbinectomy produced rhinitis sicca, atrophic rhinitis, or ozena. Recent studies of a large series of cases contradict this. Courtiss et al. (21), Morgenstein and Krieger (22), Mabry (16), Martinez et al. (17), and Pollock and Rohrich (7), in a total of 586 cases, did not report a single case of rhinitis sicca, atrophic rhinitis, or ozena. In our experience, ozena is uncommon in the general population. An increased incidence has been noted in the East Indian population, which suggests either an environmental or hereditary predisposition. A common complaint of patients having an overpatulous nasal cavity was a paradoxical sense of nasal obstruction, which was believed due to excessive nasal drying. Some patients have also complained of an altered resonance to their voice following total turbinate removal.

Laser Resection

The recent development of lasers with free-hand delivery systems or those used in conjunction with the operating microscope or sinus endoscopes have extended laser application to the treatment of common sinus and nasal pathologies.

The laser, particularly the carbon dioxide (CO_2) type, has been used successfully to remove hypertrophic turbinate mucosa (Table 3). Selkin (23) and Fukutake et al. (24) have reported excellent initial results with improvement noted by 100% and 94% of patients, respectively. However, after 1 year, only a small percentage (6%–17%) of patients remained satisfied. Moreover, reported complications include significant nasal crusting requiring frequent care, prolonged nasal packing to prevent bleeding, synechia formation, turbinate bone osteitis, and photodamage of adjacent tissues.

In 1990, Levine (25) described the potassium-titanyl phosphate (KTP) laser treatment of turbinate dysfunction. He reported that 78%

TABLE 3. *Comparison of Laser Methods for Turbinectomy*

Laser Technique	Author	Initial Results	Follow-Up
Argon	Lenz (36)	80% with good response	6% required repeat procedure
CO_2	Fukutake et al. (24)	94% improved	23% complained of significant nasal obstruction at 1 year
CO_2	Selkin (23)	100% improved	6% had recurrence of obstruction at 6 months to 1 year
KTP/532	Levine (26)	Unavailable	78% had good results at 1 year

of patients remained satisfied 1 year after surgery. The main advantage of the KTP and argon lasers is that they do not require an aiming beam, which permits incisions to be made with greater accuracy. The preferential absorption of hemoglobin for the KTP and argon lasers is 532 nm and between 488 nm and 514 nm, respectively, which provides excellent hemostasis while cutting through tissue. Another important advantage is that their beams can be transmitted by a flexible delivery system that can be passed through the sinus endoscopes without obstructing the surgeon's vision.

Many theories attempt to explain the effectiveness of laser turbinectomy, the simplest being thermal ablation of hypertrophic mucosa. Fukutake et al. (24) showed fibrous proliferation and scar formation in the superficial layer of the submucosa. This scar tissue may prevent the rapid changes in turbinate size that so often cause a patient's symptoms (25). Photocoagulation may somehow alter the autonomic nervous system control of the vasoactive turbinate response and thus lessen symptoms. Levine (25) has speculated that the surface mucus-secreting glands could be decreased in either number or function by laser photocoagulation; this, however, has been refuted by other authors (23,24).

Cryosurgery

Cryosurgical techniques in otolaryngology began with Cahan and Montesa-Cruz in 1965, when they reported experimental cryotonsillectomy in dogs (26). Principato (27), Ozenberger (28), and Moszynski (29), in separate studies, reported their results with cryosurgical treatment of chronic rhinitis. However, Ozenberger (30), in 1973, had the best results and few complications in several hundred patients by using nitrous oxide cryosurgery. Recent advancements in sinus surgery and probe technology has led to greater cryosurgical success in the treatment of both turbinate hypertrophy and vasomotor rhinitis (31–33).

Cryosurgery reduces turbinate bulk through the formation of intracellular ice crystals and, ultimately, protein denaturation in the nuclear and cell membranes (27). Crystallization leads to cellular membrane destruction; small blood vessel thrombosis, intracellular dehydration, and hypertoxicity; and local ischemia, all of which cause tissue destruction. Karja et al. (32) also reported an immunologic reaction whereby antibodies were formed against necrotic tissue, which helped in its removal. Lundblad et al. (34) and Terao et al. (35) noted destruction of the parasympathetic noradrenergic fibers by the cryogenic process, thereby helping decrease the vasomotor reaction.

Cryosurgery can be performed with either local or general anesthesia. The liquid nitrogen medium is introduced onto the turbinate by means of a cryoprobe. Care must be taken to protect the ala, columella, and septum from the probe, as severe damage of these structures may ensue from inadvertent contact.

Following the procedure, serous or serosanguinous drainage occurs for the first week. The patient should understand that nasal congestion will continue for approximately 3 weeks after surgery. The frozen turbinate edge sloughs off over several days, with gradual healing taking place over a 6-week period. Immediate postoperative bleeding occurs rarely. Principato (27) noted an 11% incidence of bleeding requiring treatment, whereas 14%

had minor complications including prolonged crusting and infection. In approximately 6–8 weeks, a smaller turbinate forms that is covered by normal appearing mucosa.

Principato (27) found that approximately 80% of 350 patients were relieved of their obstructive symptoms 6 months postoperatively, and 30% of patients remained satisfied after 5–6 years. Other studies have demonstrated the diminished clinical effectiveness of cryosurgery after 1 year, with many patients requiring repeat surgery.

Electrocautery

Electrocautery produces its effects by thermocoagulation, necrosis, and scarring of the cavernous sinusoids within the turbinates. The two methods employed are linear and submucosal.

Linear surface cautery is performed by streaking the turbinate with a hot Nichromewire electrode, or through a high-frequency coagulating current applied with a ball-tip or needle electrode. The submucosal technique can be performed either by unipolar or bipolar methods. The unipolar approach coagulates tissue in a circumferential manner around the tip of the electrode, whereas the bipolar technique produces coagulation necrosis between two needle electrodes.

These methods are a simple and rapid way to reduce soft tissue turbinate bulk in patients without bony hypertrophy. Relief of obstructive symptoms lasts an average of 6 months to 2 years.

Turbinate Outfracture

Lateral outfracture is the simplest method of treating enlarged inferior turbinates; however, it is of limited use and provides only minor and temporary airway improvement. It partially crushes the turbinate, does not prevent engorgement, and displaces turbinates with bony hypertrophy into spaces that are too small to accommodate them. Although simple to perform, this procedure fails to address the

causes of turbinate enlargement, and, hence, does not provide long-lasting relief from airway obstruction.

CONCLUSION

Nasal obstruction may have a mucosal (atopy, vasomotor rhinitis) or anatomic (nasal vault narrowing, septal deviation, inferior turbinate hypertrophy) basis. Preoperative assessment is of great importance. Pharmacotherapy or immunotherapy must be attempted before surgery because many patients can be managed quite effectively in this manner. In cases that fail conservative therapy some form of invasive procedure will be necessary.

REFERENCES

1. Jones TC: Turbinotomy. *Lancet* 2:496, 1895.
2. Jones M: Turbinal hypertrophy. *Lancet* 2:879, 1895.
3. Holmes CR: Hypertrophy of the turbinated bodies. *NY Med J* 72:529, 1900.
4. Freer OT: The inferior turbinate: Its longitudinal resection for chronic intumescence. *Laryngoscope* 21:1136, 1911.
5. Strandberg O: A method of total removal of the inferior turbinate bone. *J Laryngology Otol* 39:65, 1924.
6. Hurd LM: Bipolar electrode for electrocoagulation of the inferior turbinate. *Arch Otolaryngol* 13:442, 1931.
7. Pollack RA, Rohrich RJ: Inferior turbinate surgery: An adjunct to successful treatment of nasal obstruction in 408 patients. *Plast Reconstr Surg* 74:227–236, 1984.
8. Goode, RL: Surgery of the turbinates. In: Krause CJ, Mangat DS, Pastorek N, eds. *Aesthetic facial surgery*, 1st ed. Philadelphia: JB Lippincott, 161–173, 1991.
9. Simmons MW: Intranasal injection of corticosteroid in nasal disorders: Further observations. *Trans Pac Coast Otoophthalmol Soc Ann Meet* 45:95–103, 1964.
10. Mabry RL: Corticosteroids in otolaryngology: Intraturbinal injection. *Otolaryngol Head Neck Surg* 91:717–720, 1983.
11. Beekhuis GJ: Nasal obstruction after rhinoplasty: Etiology and techniques for correction. *Laryngoscope* 86:540, 1976.
12. Anderson J: Twenty-five helpful hints in rhinoplasty. *Trans Pac Coast Otoophthalmol Soc Ann Meet* 72:113–117, 1970.
13. Mabry RL: Intraturbinal steroid injection: Indications, results, and complications. *South Med J* 71:789–791, 1978.
14. Bridger GP: Physiology of the nasal valve. *Arch Otolaryngol* 92:543–553, 1970.
15. House HP: Submucous resection of the inferior turbinal bone. *Laryngoscope* 61:637–648, 1951.
16. Mabry RL: Inferior turbinoplasty: Patient selection, technique, and long-term consequences. *Otolaryngol Head Neck Surg* 98:60–66, 1988.
17. Martinez SA, Nissen CR, Stock CR et al: Nasal

turbinate resection for relief of nasal obstruction. *Laryngoscope* 93:871–875, 1983.

18. Tremble GE: Methods of shrinking the inferior turbinate to improve the airway. *Laryngoscope* 70:175, 1960.
19. Richardson JR: Turbinate treatment in vasomotor rhinitis. *Laryngoscope* 58:834–837, 1948.
20. Moore GF, Freeman TJ, Ogren FP et al: Extended follow-up of total inferior turbinate resection for relief of chronic nasal obstruction. *Laryngoscope* 95:1095–1099, 1985.
21. Courtiss EH, Goldwyn RM, O'Brien JJ: Resection of obstructing inferior nasal turbinates. *Plast Reconstr Surg* 62:249–251, 1978.
22. Morgenstein KM, Krieger MK: Experiences in middle turbinectomy. *Laryngoscope* 93:871, 1983.
23. Selkin SG: Laser turbinectomy as an adjunct to rhinoseptoplasty. *Arch Otolaryngol* 111:446–449, 1985.
24. Fukutake T, Yamashita T, Tomoda K et al: Laser surgery for allergic rhinitis. *Arch Otolaryngol* 112:1280–1282, 1986.
25. Levine HL: The potassium-titanyl phosphate laser for treatment of turbinate dysfunction. *Otolaryngol Head Neck Surg* 104:247–251, 1991.
26. Cahan WG, Montesa-Cruz AF: Cryotonsillectomy in dogs. *Arch Otolaryngol* 81:372–387, 1965.
27. Principato JJ: Chronic vasomotor rhinitis: Cryogenic and other surgical modes of treatment. *Laryngoscope* 89:619–638, 1979.
28. Ozenberger JM: Cryosurgery in chronic rhinitis. *Laryngoscope* 80:723–734, 1970.
29. Moszynski B: Use of cryosurgery in the treatment of chronic rhinitis. *Otolaryngol Pol* 28:559–561, 1974.
30. Ozenberger JM: Cryosurgery for the treatment of chronic rhinitis. *Laryngoscope* 83:508–516, 1973.
31. Holden HB: Cryosurgery in ENT practice. *J Laryngol Otol* 86:821–827. 1972.
32. Karja J, Jokinen K, Palva A: Experience with cryotherapy in otolaryngological practice. *J Laryngol Otol* 89:519–526, 1975.
33. Bumstead RM: Cryotherapy for chronic vasomotor rhinitis: Technique and patient selection for improved results. *Laryngoscope* 94:539–544, 1984.
34. Lundblad L, Brodin E, Lundberg JM, et al: Effects of nasal capsaicin pretreatment and cryosurgery on sneezing reflexes, neurogenic plasma extravasation, sensory and sympathetic neurons. *Acta Otolaryngol* 100: 117–127, 1985.
35. Terao A, Meshitsuka K, Suzaki H et al: Cryosurgery on postganglionic fibers (posterior nasal branches) of the pterygopalatine ganglion for vasomotor rhinitis. *Acta Otolaryngol* 96:139–148, 1983.
36. Lenz H, Eichler J, Knof J, Salk J, Schazfer G: Argon laser: Strahlführungssystem und erste Klinishe Anwendungen bei der Rhinopathia vasomotoria. *Laryngol Rhinol Otol (Stuttg)* 56:749–755, 1977.

Office-Based Surgery of the Head and Neck
Edited by Yosef P. Krespi, MD
Lippincott–Raven Publishers, Philadelphia © 1998

16

Laser Photocoagulation of the Inferior Turbinates

Yosef P. Krespi, Michael Mayer, and Michael Slatkine

Allergic rhinitis is a common disorder, affecting nearly 15% of the population. Nasal obstruction from inferior turbinate hypertrophy is a frequent symptom among many allergic patients as well as patients with vasomotor rhinitis and rhinitis medicamentous. Longstanding swelling may become irreversible, owing either to the submucosal venous sinuses becoming varicose and unresponsive to sympathetic nervous system stimulation or to medical treatment.

Therapy for these patients includes allergic desensitization, medications delivered orally or through nasal inhalers, and nasal procedures to reduce the size of the inferior turbinates. Patients who fail the previously mentioned modalities require a more aggressive approach to achieve an adequate nasal airway.

Many surgical procedures are available to treat these patients, including surgical trimming and linear and submucosal diathermy. Unfortunately, initial optimism for submucosal diathermy has been reduced by studies that demonstrate that the initial improvement in nasal airflow is lost at 15 months (1–4).

Surgical excision of the inferior turbinates is frequently the next step in management of these patients. This procedure carries the risk of bleeding; it requires packing that causes significant discomfort leading to nasal crusting for several weeks after the surgery.

Alternatively, using laser technology on the inferior turbinates delivers a predictable, reproducible, and precise dose of photocoagulation. It is well tolerated under local or topical anesthesia, causes minimal postoperative crusting or discomfort, and carries a negligible risk of bleeding.

BACKGROUND

The inferior turbinates are vascular, glandular structures with large venous lakes that have the potential to swell in response to certain medical or environmental conditions. In patients with an atopic state of sensitivity to an allergen who are exposed to this allergen, histamine is released by mast cells, resulting in copious nasal discharge and edematous nasal mucosa. These conditions lead to obstruction of the nasal cavity from inferior turbinate hypertrophy. The patient subsequently complains of inability to breathe through the nose, which results in the loss of some very important nasal functions (eg, humidification, warming, and filtering the air).

THERAPY

Immunotherapy

Avoidance of the allergen is the easiest and most sensible way to alleviate the congestion; however, this is often extremely difficult. Immunotherapy involves identifying the responsible allergen and exposing the patient to the allergen through parenteral administration. This allows formation of IgG antibodies to the allergen, which competes with the antibodies for target sites on mast cells and basophils, thus preventing mast cell degeneration and histamine release.

Pharmacotherapy

Antihistamines compete with histamine for receptor sites on their target organs. This competitive inhibition relieves the itchiness, sneezing, and rhinorrhea, but will not usually relieve nasal obstruction.

Decongestants are substances that cause vasoconstriction and thereby decrease the edema of the mucus membranes. Although effective, these drugs have untoward effects such as elevated blood pressure and central nervous system stimulation.

Topical nasal decongestants are highly effective initially, but soon cause rebound swelling of the nasal mucosa, leading to abuse of and addiction to these medications. They are frequently counterproductive in long-term management.

Cromolyn stabilizes the mast cell membrane, preventing degranulation and release of histamine. It is primarily effective in prevention and anticipation of allergen exposure, but has no role in the acute management of allergic rhinitis.

Corticosteroids are the most potent agents available to relieve symptoms of allergic rhinitis. Given orally for a long term, they may produce undesirable side effects. Given nasally, they are well tolerated and effective and have almost replaced the oral administration of steroids. Systemic absorption is minimal and therefore side effects are eliminated.

Injection of depot steroids into the inferior turbinate was popular for some time, but has fallen out of favor.

SURGICAL MANAGEMENT

Turbinate outfracture produces a green stick fracture of the turbinate but the turbinate often returns to its initial position.

Cryosurgery causes mucosal and submucosal necrosis. This procedure produces prolonged postoperative edema and an eschar, which takes a long time to separate.

Submucosal resection of the inferior turbinate results in a floppy remaining turbinate and, commonly, bleeding. Similarly, resection of the inferior turbinate requires nasal packing to provide hemostasis. Nasal packing is often poorly tolerated by patients and usually causes bleeding at removal.

Lasers have been introduced for the surgical management of turbinate hypertrophy, usually as a tool to resect the inferior turbinate. We introduce the technique by two different methods. First, using the neodymium: yttrium aluminum garnet (Nd:YAG) laser, we insert the laser fiber directly into the inferior turbinate, causing photocoagulation. Second, using the carbon dioxide (CO_2) waveguide, we directly ablate the turbinate mucosa using the superpulse mode.

The Nd:YAG laser can be delivered through a flexible fiber. The beam is invisible and requires a second beam in the visible range to provide aiming capability. Energy, which is transmitted by scattering in all directions, usually penetrates 2–4 mm. The depth of penetration is thus predictable.

The Nd:YAG laser has a wavelength of 1.06 μ. Tissue absorption, which is dependent on color, is highly effective in vascular-rich tissue.

LASER TURBINECTOMY TECHNIQUE

Submucosal interstitial photocoagulation of the nasal turbinates is commenced initially to anesthetize the nasal mucosa with cocaine or 4% lidocaine. The Nd:YAG laser bare fiber is inserted under direct vision into the inferiomedial aspect of the turbinate and advanced about 3 cm posteriorly. The laser is set at an energy level of 8 W for 3 seconds, and a total of 24 J of energy is delivered. The laser is on while the fiber penetrates into the turbinate and is kept on while withdrawing, for a total exposure time of 3 seconds. Because there is no bleeding from the turbinate, no packing is required. The nasal cavity is filled with antibiotic ointment and the patient is discharged to regular activities.

The method of CO_2 laser ablation requires similar preparation and topical or local anesthesia. The CO_2 hollow waveguide can be easily attached to the articulated arm by an appropriate coupler. The superpulse mode is

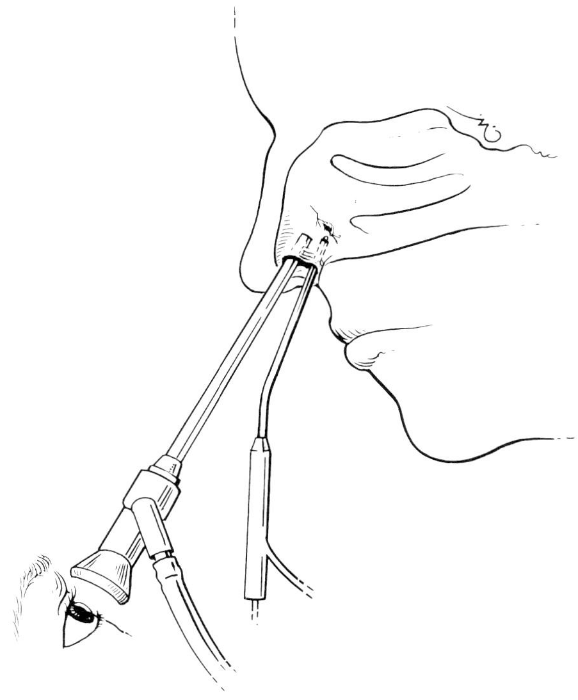

FIG. 1. Intranasal laser surgery under endoscopic control.

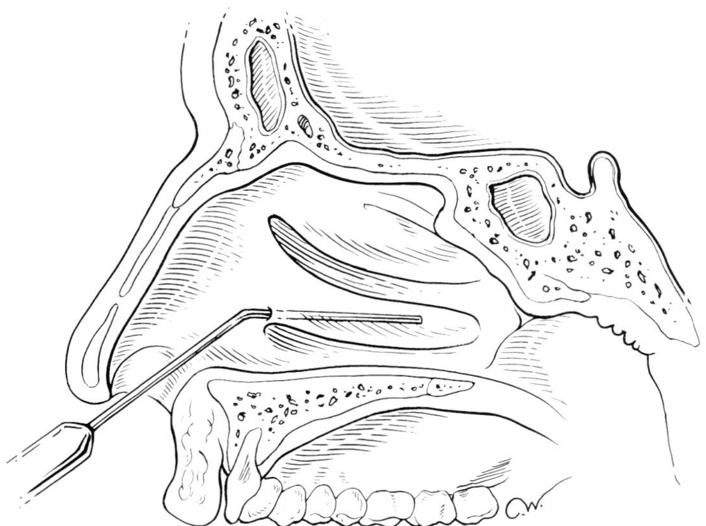

FIG. 2. Interstitial thermal therapy of inferior turbinate with Nd:YAG or diode laser fiber.

preferred to avoid excessive tissue damage, crusting, and charring. The laser is set to 6 W superpulse and the waveguide is introduced into the nasal cavity. The tip of the waveguide is kept 1 mm away from the turbinate mucosa during lasing. The inferior turbinate is ablated medially and inferiorly by about 30%. Only the anterior one half to two thirds of its length is ablated. It may be difficult to reach the posterior end of the turbinate with the currently existing waveguides. If the ablation of the posterior one third of the turbinate is indicated, we recommend the Nd:YAG laser (Figs. 1,2).

In general, we have not found any significant technical difference or long-term results between the Nd:YAG and the CO_2 lasers.

Safety Considerations

It is important to exercise safety precautions when using the laser. Eye protection should be worn by the doctors, patient, and nursing staff. Adequate smoke evacuation with the appropriate filters should be used. The appropriate nonreflecting nasal instruments should be available. And, finally, the operating suite should be equipped with room ventilation and adequate electrical supply.

Conclusion

Submucosal interstitial photocoagulation of the nasal turbinates using an Nd:YAG laser is an effective modality in combating the symptoms of allergic rhinitis. It is well tolerated under local anesthesia and can be performed in a doctor's office or other ambulatory setting. No packing is required, which is the usual source of discomfort in patients undergoing resection. There is minimal crusting postoperatively or risk of postoperative bleeding. The patient enjoys a rapid return to work.

Remaining unanswered is the question of duration of effectiveness using interstitial laser therapy. This question is currently under investigation.

DISCUSSION

Lenz et al. (5,6), in 1977, were the first to use a laser for hypertrophic turbinates. They successfully used the argon laser to create strips in the inferior turbinate for nasal obstruction secondary to vasomotor rhinitis. Eighty percent of their patients reported significant improvement in their nasal airway.

Mittleman (7) described the use of the CO_2 laser in 30 patients with chronic obstructive rhinitis refractory to medical therapy in whom the anterior one fourth of the inferior turbinate was vaporized. With a follow-up of 11–30 months, 27 of 30 reported an improved nasal airway.

Elwany and Harrison (8) compared four techniques in the treatment of chronic hypertrophic turbinates, including partial inferior turbinectomy, turbinoplasty, cryoturbinectomy, and laser turbinectomy (CO_2 laser). Outcome data included questionnaires, frequent examination, measures of mucociliary clearance, and olfactory assessment (follow-up at 1 year). Nasal obstruction was most frequently improved in the inferior turbinectomy and laser turbinectomy groups, although nasal discharge was not improved consistently in any of the groups. Benefits of laser turbinectomy were decreased bleeding, lack of postoperative pain, and faster healing.

Selkin (9) used a CO_2 laser to treat 102 patients concurrently with septorhinoplasty for chronic turbinate hypertrophy. The inferior turbinate was vaporized along its inferior aspect as far posteriorly as possible. Subjectively, all patients had improvement of their nasal airway postoperatively. Two patients experienced epistaxis 3 weeks postoperatively, one requiring cellulose to the affected area. Seven patients had recurrence of their nasal obstruction from 6 to 12 months after the surgery. No crusting or dryness was reported by any of the patients nor was pain an issue.

Fukutake et al. (10) performed a histologic study on lasered turbinates and found them to be replaced by scar tissue at 1 year, whereas the epithelium regenerated after 2 months.

Of the 58 patients treated by Levine (11) with a potassium-titanyl phosphate laser crosshatching the inferior turbinate, 85% reported improvement in their nasal airflow. Thick nasal discharge had stopped by 2 weeks and crusting had ceased by 6–8 weeks postoperatively. Of the patients who did not report improvement, 13 of 22 responded to medical treatment postoperatively while being refractory preoperatively.

The Nd:YAG laser was used by Krespi et al. (13) for allergic rhinitis by placing the fiber directly into the inferior turbinate, thereby coagulating its interior while preserving the epithelium. This provided improved nasal airflow without the sequlae of crusting and epistaxis postoperatively.

An animal study by Goldsher et al. (12) in which the Nd:YAG laser was inserted directly into the inferior turbinate demonstrated a reduction in turbinate size of 50% without bleeding or crusting at 9 months. Histologic examination confirmed that, although the epithelium remained intact, the stromal elements were replaced by scar tissue.

Lasers have become more commonplace in the otolaryngologist's office as prices have declined and as more office procedures are being refined with the use of the laser. Thus, laser turbinectomy will soon be the preferred method for treating the refractory hypertrophic turbinate. Managed care companies will no longer approve a turbinectomy performed in the hospital setting when an office procedure could suffice. The advantage of bloodless surgery when using the laser for turbinectomy or other surgery enables it to be used safely in the office setting.

The choice of laser will be determined by its cost, its ease of use, its versatility to perform varied procedures, and its ability to be inserted into fiberoptic endoscopes using laser fibers. It is apparent from the previous review that several lasers are adaptable to laser turbinectomy and that all can be safely used with the adherence to safety rules.

REFERENCES

1. Jones AS, Lancer JM: Does submucosal diathermy to the inferior turbinates reduce nasal resistance to air flow in the long term? *J Laryngol Otol* 101:448–450, 1987.
2. Wight RG, Jones AS, Beckingham E: Trimming of the inferior turbinates: A prospective long-term study. *Clin Otolaryngol* 15:347–350, 1990.
3. Dawes PJD: The early complications of inferior turbinectomy. *J Laryngol Otol* 101:1136–1139, 1987.
4. Williams HOL, Fisher EB, Golding-Wood DB: Two-stage turbinectomy: Sequestration of the inferior turbinate following submucosal diathermy. *J Laryngol Otol* 105:14–16, 1991.
5. Lenz H, Eichler J: Endonasal Ar+ laser beam guide system and first clinical application in vasomotor rhinitis. *Laryngol Rhinol Otol* 56:749–755, 1977.
6. Lenz H: Eight years experience of laser surgery of the inferior turbinate in vasomotor rhinitis using a laser-strip carbonization. *HNO* 33:422–425, 1985.
7. Mittleman H: CO_2 laser turbinectomies for chronic, obstructive rhinitis. *Lasers Surg Med* 2:29–36, 1982.
8. Elwany S, Harrison R: Inferior turbinectomy: Comparison of four techniques. *J Laryngol Otol* 104:206–209, 1990.
9. Selkin SG: Laser turbinectomy as an adjunct to rhinoseptoplasty. *Arch Otolaryngol Head Neck Surg* 111:446–450, 1985.
10. Fukutake T: Laser surgery for allergic rhinitis. *Arch Otolaryngol Head Neck Surg* 112:1280–1282, 1986.
11. Levine H: The potassium-titanyl phosphate laser for treatment of turbinate dysfunction. *Otolaryngol Head Neck Surg* 104:247–251, 1991.
12. Goldsher M, Joachims HZ, Gold A: Nd:YAG laser turbinate surgery animal experimental study: preliminary report. *Laryngoscope* 105:319–321, 1995.
13. Krespi YP, Mayer M, Slatkine M: Laser photocoagulation of the inferior turbinates. *Open Tech Otolaryngol Head Neck Surg* 5:287–291, 1994.

Office-Based Surgery of the Head and Neck
Edited by Yosef P. Krespi, MD
Lippincott–Raven Publishers, Philadelphia © 1998

17

Outpatient Endoscopic Sinus Surgery

Howard L. Levine and Cindi L. Davis

Modern treatment of paranasal sinus disease has undergone significant advancement over the past decade (1,2). Contemporary endoscopic sinus surgery (ESS) techniques with specially trained personnel and specialized instrumentation is ideally suited for the outpatient ambulatory surgery center because of the relatively short anesthesia and generally overall good health of the patients. Although some patients require an in-patient setting for their surgery because of significant medical problems, especially uncontrolled asthma, the rhinologist is generally comfortable operating in ambulatory facilities, which have become the mainstay site for this type of surgery.

Effective and safe outpatient ESS relies significantly on appropriate case selection, preoperative teaching by experienced personnel, and proper surgical instrumentation (3). In addition to the experienced surgeon, a well-trained ESS surgical team ideally includes the surgical nursing staff in charge of instrumentation and the patient in the operating room; the anesthesia team; pre- and postoperative nurses managing the patient before and after surgery; and the nurse clinician from the surgeon's office to coordinate outpatient office activity with the ambulatory surgical facility.

PREOPERATIVE EVALUATION

As with most other outpatient surgical procedures, patient selection and preparation take place during the initial surgical consultation (4). Patients with significant medical problems, especially cardiac or pulmonary

disease, may not be candidates for outpatient surgery or may require special preoperative assessment by primary care physicians, medical subspecialists, and anesthesiologists well in advance of the planned surgery. The results of this assessment may preclude surgery in an ambulatory facility.

Another group of patients that should not be treated in an ambulatory facility includes those with intracranial or intraorbital complications of sinusitis who will require monitoring their disease complications and sequelae by skilled nursing personnel, often in intensive care or step-down observation units.

Endoscopic biopsy should be done of endonasal and paranasal tumors in a surgical suite. Although biopsy of these tumors is usually carried out successfully in the outpatient setting, definitive excision is often reserved for an appropriate inpatient facility.

A history of previous surgery and intraoperative problems should be obtained. Past experiences of severe nausea and vomiting following anesthesia should be noted. A family history of bleeding problems and atypical anesthesia events should be obtained.

PREOPERATIVE TEACHING

Ideally, postsurgical instruction should begin during the preoperative office visit. Well in advance of the proposed surgery date, the patient should be given written information by the physician, nurse clinician, or surgery scheduling personnel that detail the operative recovery period. Such information should provide answers to many of the most commonly asked questions and concerns for postsurgical sinus patients. The patient will then have ample opportunity to review this material and to share it with others who will assist in providing care following surgery. Clinical staff are available to answer questions that may arise from this material. For selected patients, the process of informed consent is reinforced by use of videotape educational materials such as *Sinusitis and Sinus Surgery*, distributed by the American Academy of Otolaryngology–Head and Neck Surgery (5).

Specific instructions are provided to patients regarding the avoidance of aspirin, nonsteroidal anti-inflammatory drugs, and anti-coagulants for 2 weeks prior to surgery. An updated list of these medications is kept by physicians, nurse clinicians, and scheduling personnel to minimize the risk that they may be used by patients prior to surgery. This list should also be made available to each patient on request.

Successful preoperative teaching also necessitates instructing patients about the recovery period. Each patient is informed that several visits are required following surgery for removal of any intranasal dressings and debridement of eschar and exudate, which are nearly always present following surgery. This helps patients plan their postoperative work, school, home, or social schedules. Patients must understand that significant resolution of their sinus symptoms may not occur until 4–6 weeks following surgery. Patients are informed that "recovery is a process, not an event."

We generally use a nasal and sinus outpatient facility consisting of a freestanding ambulatory surgery center that is part of a larger group of independent office suites. This building also contains computed tomographic (CT) scanning equipment and laboratory facilities in association with a designated presurgical testing area. After patients have had the opportunity to schedule their procedure with the surgical scheduling staff, they are directed to the testing area for the requisite preadmission testing.

Preadmission test requirements vary from one facility to another. Some general preadmission guidelines include the following: Patients undergoing local anesthesia do not require any preoperative testing. Healthy pediatric patients aged 16 years or younger require no screening laboratory testing. African-Americans who have not previously been screened for sickle cell disease must have a sickle cell preparation performed. If a pediatric patient has a medical problem, appropriate tests may be done to clarify the extent or severity of that particular problem.

Adult patients are grouped into two categories:

1. Those aged 35 years or younger require complete blood count, glucose, potassium, blood urea nitrogen, and serum glutamic oxaloacetic transaminase. Electrocardiogram (ECG) is obtained if indicated by the patient's medical history.
2. Those aged 35 years or older require the same blood work, and the ECG is mandatory. A screening chest x-ray is required only if indicated by a patient's medical condition.

Because many patients undergoing endoscopic sinus surgery have chronic obstructive pulmonary disease, chronic bronchitis, or a recent pulmonary infection, a chest x-ray may need to be obtained in these individuals.

Adult patients are required by the Joint Commission on Accreditation of Hospitals to have a completed history and physical examination prior to a surgical or endoscopic procedure. This is accomplished through the preadmission testing center, where a nurse practitioner is responsible for completion of the history and physical. Children who do not undergo laboratory testing are examined by the nurse practitioner on the day of surgery, unless special arrangements have been made in advance with the patient's pediatrician or specialist.

There are exceptions to these guidelines, of course, which must be based on the patient's medical condition and the problem being treated.

Pediatric patients and their families often visit with a child life specialist to introduce them to the surgical procedures and facility.

As with any surgical procedure, it is of utmost importance to maintain an open dialogue with the anesthesia staff responsible for the patients at each facility to resolve potential conflicts before they have negative impact on the surgery schedule (6).

Patient care is of paramount importance; by following the guidelines outlined above, perioperative morbidity will be minimized in the outpatient surgical setting.

As a final step before surgery, the patient's office chart is completed and reviewed by the operating surgeon and/or nurse clinician. It is convenient and useful to place a copy of the patient's sinus CT scan in the permanent medical record. In this way, the CT scan can be easily located by the operating surgeon on the day of surgery. This also minimizes the risk that the CT scan will be inadvertently misplaced during a transfer from the radiologic facility to the physician's office and finally to the ambulatory surgical facility.

The clinical staff ensures that the history, physical examination, consultation forms, and supporting laboratory data are present on the chart. Standard nasal-sinus physician postoperative orders are completed by the clinical staff in advance of the surgery.

A key feature of the patient's office chart is the nasal-sinus surgery checklist devised by one of the authors (H.L.L.) (Fig. 1). This chart ensures that the appropriate procedures can be noted specifically at the time of surgery. Other information that can be noted on the chart includes the nature and extent of sinus disease and any adjunctive procedures, such as septoplasty and turbinate reduction; preoperative and intraoperative medications; unusual operative findings and events; and the patient's home-going medications, nasal dressings, splints, or other implants. The clinical office staff will find much of this information invaluable in providing follow-up care to the patient within the first 12–24 hours following the procedure. This document becomes a valuable reference for the

physician, scheduling personnel, supporting nursing staff, and clinicians in following the patient. Those who are responsible for interacting with third-party payers quickly realize the utility of such information in documentation of care. It becomes a permanent component of the patient's medical records.

PERIOPERATIVE PERIOD

A transition from the preoperative area to the operating room and finally to the postanesthesia room and postoperative recovery area must be arranged in a fashion that allows the patient to feel as comfortable as possible on the day of surgery. Minimal emphasis is placed on the actual preparation of the patient for surgery. Most of these issues have been addressed prior to the day of surgery. Instead, the patient is supported by the nursing staff, attending anesthesiologist and certified registered nurse anesthetist (CRNA), attending surgeon, nurse clinician, and other appropriate support personnel (eg, child life worker).

Preoperative sedation is generally not needed, but the anxious patient may be given intravenous midazolam (Versed, Roche Pharmaceuticals, Nutley, NJ). Oxymetaxoline or an appropriate topical decongestant may be placed in the nose during this time to begin the nasal decongestion. All eye makeup should be removed prior to entering the surgical suite so that the globes may be easily observed during surgery.

The anesthesia team may choose to use medications such as metoclopramide (Reglan, AH Robins, Richmond, VA) or ordansetron (Zofran, Glaxo Wellcome, Research Triangle, NC) for the patient who has had a previous experience with nausea or vomiting following surgery. This allows for more rapid anesthesia recovery and avoids the occasional hospital transfer for nausea, vomiting, or fluid management. Passage of an oral gastric tube prior to anesthesia emergence empties the stomach of blood and gastric secretions and also reduces nausea and vomiting (6).

OPERATIVE FINDINGS

NAME: _________________________ DATE: _____________ ANESTHESIA: <u>LOCAL</u>   <u>GEN</u>   <u>MAC</u>

SERVICE LOCATION: _________________________ PATIENT STATUS: <u>OUT-PT</u>   <u>OBSERVE</u>   <u>INPATIENT</u>

PRE-OP DIAGNOSIS: ____

POST-OP DIAGNOSIS: ____

PROCEDURE

31231	R L	Nasal Endoscopy, Diagnostic
31237	R L	ESS; with Biopsy, Polypectomy, Debridement
31238	R L	with Control Epistaxis
31240	R L	with Concha Bullosa Resection
31254	R L	ESS, with Ethmoidectomy (Partial)
31255	R L	with Ethmoidectomy, (Total)
31256	R L	ESS, with Maxillary Antrostomy
31267	R L	with Removal Tissue Maxillary Sinus
31276	R L	ESS, with Frontal Sinus Exploration,
31287	R L	ESS, with Sphenoidotomy
31288	R L	with Removal Tissue Sphenoid Sinus
69421	R L	Myringotomy
69436	R L	Tympanostomy (Insert Vent Tube)
*****		Excision lesion _____cm x _____ cm of_____________
*****		Tonsillectomy
*****		Adenoidectomy
42145.52		LAUP
42415		UPPP

21320	Closed Treatment Nasal Fracture
30410	Rhinoplasty, Complete
30420	including Septum Splints
30520	Septoplasty Splints
30140	SMR of turbinate
30802	Turbinate Ablation, Laser, Cautery
31600	Tracheostomy
31525	Laryngoscopy, Diagnostic
31541	Laryngoscopy / Micro, VC strip
31622	Bronchoscopy
43200	Esophagoscopy
42415	Parotidectomy, superficial
60220	Thyroidectomy
OTHER:	

LOCATION	SINUSITIS	POLYPOSIS	MEDICATIONS
NASAL			*INTRAOPERATIVE:*
MEDIAL MIDDLE TURBINATE			STEROIDS: __________ ANTIBIOTICS: __________
TURBINATE			OTHER: __________
ANT ETHMOID			*HOME GOING:* TYLENOL/ELIXER
POST ETHMOID			TYLENOL/CODEINE DARVOCET-N
SPHENOID			MEDROL/PREDNISONE:__________ ANTIBIOTIC:__________
FRONTAL RECESS			MUCOLYTIC:__________ OTHER: __________
FRONTAL SINUS			
MAXILLARY SINUS			

DRESSINGS	SURGICAL NOTES		
NONE	BLEEDING __________ cc.	R	L
TELFA	DIPLOPIA	R	L
MEROCEL	ORBITAL ECCHYMOSIS	R	L
AVETENE	ORBITAL HEMORRHAGE	R	L
OXYCEL	ORBITAL FAT	R	L
INSTAT	EXPOSED DURA	R	L
SURGICEL	CSF LEAK	R	L

OPERATIVE COMMENTS:__________

CULTURES

NURSING NOTES: ____

FIG. 1. Nasal-sinus surgery checklist.

The actual surgical procedure takes place much in the same way as it would in a standard inpatient facility. The technique generally utilizes propofol (Diprivan, Zeneca, Wilmington, DE) because of its short half-life. The patient experiences a shorter time in the postanesthesia recovery area and is able to return home in an expedient manner, which helps maintain the tempo of the ambulatory surgery facility, which is usually more rapid than that of its inpatient counterpart.

During surgery, blood pressure is maintained at the lowest possible level that is safe for each patient, which greatly facilitates the dissection, improves surgical visualization, and keeps the blood loss to a minimum.

Available instrumentation may vary among institutions and surgeons. Arrangements must be made in advance if special equipment is required, such as C-arm imaging fluoroscopy, surgical lasers, or drills. The attending surgeon must be familiar with the instrumentation that is available in each ambulatory surgery center. Ideally, all video equipment should be stored in single rolling cabinet to minimize setup time and reduce maintenance.

A special surgical nursing team designated and specifically trained to assist with endoscopic sinus surgery can greatly enhance the efficiency of performing multiple procedures on a given day. This personnel should be specifically trained to handle the video equipment, light sources, printers, and endoscopes. Departments (eg, biomedical engineering), which are normally found in larger inpatient settings, are usually not available in smaller freestanding ambulatory facilities.

During surgery, the use of video imaging maintains the appropriate level of interest by others in the operating room, such as the anesthesiologist, circulating nurse, and scrub technician. Video imaging may aid the anesthesiologist in lowering the blood pressure if excessive bleeding is seen and in predicting the conclusion of the procedure; it promotes operating room efficiency by not delaying the wake-up time of the patient; and it assists the skilled scrub technician in anticipating the instrumentation needs of the surgeon.

Video imaging can also document the patient's chart through the inclusion of photographs or videotape. This helps during postoperative office visits in recalling specifics of the operation and unique intraoperative findings.

POSTOPERATIVE PERIOD

Following surgery, the patient is transferred to the postanesthesia care unit. Preprinted written orders concerned with both general and specific aspects of the care of the patient who has undergone ESS are provided to the postanesthesia nursing staff. These order sheets have "fill in the blank" categories to customize the recovery orders for specific patient needs. These include vital signs, intravenous fluids, diet, analgesia, antibiotics (when applicable), antinausea medications, dressing changes, oxygen, and humidity. Special considerations are given to the surgical patient with pulmonary problems for the use of appropriate respiratory aerosol treatments.

Freestanding ambulatory surgical centers may limit the physician's access both to the patient and to medical resources. The operating physician who may have to leave the facility while the patient is still recovering must have some method of communicating with the ambulatory unit. Nursing staff personnel are often the ones to provide immediate assessment and attention to problems to ensure early intervention and prevent permanent postoperative morbidity. Therefore, the postoperative nursing team must become knowledgeable about nasal and, most importantly, sinus surgery. An understanding of what occurs intraoperatively and how this can affect the postoperative period is extremely helpful. This can best be accomplished through in-service training and observation of actual surgical procedures. In this way the anatomy of the region and the potential complications are better understood.

The postoperative nursing team should become familiar with how much nasal bleeding is expected following surgery, which is usually best assessed by dressing change frequency. Supplies and equipment to manage nasal hemorrhage must be available if needed by the nursing staff, nurse clinician, or operating surgeon. The nasal dressings are removed by the nursing staff or nurse clinician and any unusual drainage is noted and reported to the surgeon.

The presence of ophthalmologic problems requires careful assessment and often immediate management by the postoperative nurses. If a patient exhibits proptosis, orbital ecchymosis, or subconjunctival hemorrhage-associated visual impairment, the attending physician or nurse clinician is notified immediately. An ophthalmologic consultation may be needed to assess the patient. Because an ophthalmologist might not always be available in the ambulatory surgical facility, one should be contacted and notified of an impending problem. In the interim, the operating surgeon and nursing staff must be able to initiate care to avert further problems.

Most patients achieve adequate pain control with acetaminophen with codeine or an equivalent narcotic analgesic. Occasionally, patients require intramuscular pain medication, such as meperidine. Orders for these medications are included in the standard nasal and sinus physician's postoperative sheet. The nurse clinician or surgeon is notified of any pain that is not adequately controlled with these medications. Postural headache or severe ocular pain needs to be evaluated by the nurse clinician or surgeon prior to the patient's discharge from the center.

Family members of patients under the age of 16 are permitted in the postanesthesia recovery area. They provide a familiar face for the patient recovering from anesthesia and generally make the postoperative nurse's task easier.

At the time of discharge, the nurse clinician reviews with the patient and a responsible adult the postoperative home-going instruction booklet, which had been given to the patient at the time of the initial preoperative counseling. It includes avoidance of excessive exertion, bending, or lifting, refraining from sneezing and expectoration through the nose, and strict avoidance of aspirin and nonsteroidal anti-inflammatory drugs. If excessive headache, bleeding, or other unusual symptoms occur, patients are instructed to call the surgeon immediately.

Patients are given a home-going care supply bag that contains nasal cotton tip applicators to clean away any accumulated blood in the vestibule of the nose, 2 × 2-inch gauze dressings and one-half-inch nonallergic paper tape to absorb any nasal drainage, and a starter bottle of saline nasal spray to be used several times a day. The supply bag also includes the office telephone number for contacting staff regarding any problems. A written prescription for acetaminophen and codeine tablets or another appropriate analgesic is also included in this package. Antibiotics and steroids are prescribed selectively depending on the specific patient problem.

OUTPATIENT CARE

Patients may choose to be accompanied home by a friend or relative who is responsible for transportation should they feel the need. Patients are instructed to consider taking half to a full dose of their home-going pain medication 30 minutes before each of the several office visits following surgery. During the first visit, any nasal splints or middle meatus dressings are removed following topical application of an aerosol anesthetic and decongestant. During this and subsequent visits, crusts, clots, secretions, and absorbable dressing materials are removed endoscopically using specially designed postoperative suctions and forceps. Intraoperative culture results are reviewed and any necessary changes in the antibiotic regimen are undertaken at this time. Patients are counseled to expect continued expectoration and drainage of secretions and clot material and nasal congestion intermittently for several weeks following surgery (3,7).

CONCLUSION

Endoscopic sinus surgery represents a significant advance in the treatment of paranasal sinus disease and has allowed major sinus surgical procedures to be done in the ambulatory surgical setting. Compared with the days of Harris Mosher, when operating in the region of the paranasal sinuses was associated with significant risk and morbidity to the patient, ESS can be done with greater efficacy and safety. Perhaps no other procedure in the specialty of otolaryngology—head and neck surgery has evolved so closely with the transition of much of the surgical practice to outpatient-based facilities. Treatment of paranasal sinus disease is ideally suited for either the freestanding surgical center or an outpatient facility that exists as part of a larger inpatient center. Regardless of the facility available,

ESS requires considerable preoperative preparation, instrumentation, and personnel who are familiar with surgical techniques and perioperative care. Careful attention to coordination between office staff and personnel at the outpatient surgical facility will ensure a smooth and efficient flow that facilitates safe and successful surgery.

REFERENCES

1. Stammberger H: Endoscopic endonasal surgery—concepts in treatment of recurring rhinosinusitis. *Otolaryngol Head Neck Surg* 94(2):143–156, 1986.
2. Kennedy DW, Zinreich SJ, Rosenbaum AE, Johns ME: Functional endoscopic sinus surgery. *Arch Otolaryngol* 111:576–582, 1985.
3. May M, Levine HL, Mester SJ, Porta M: Endoscopic sinus surgery. In: Levine HL, May M, eds. *Endoscopic sinus surgery*. New York: Thieme Medical Publishing, 105–175, 1993.
4. May M, Levine HL, Mester SJ, Porta M: Office evaluation of nasaosinus disorders: Patient selection for endoscopic sinus surgery. In: Levine HL, May M, eds. *Endoscopic sinus surgery*. New York: Thieme Medical Publishing, 3:60–90, 1993.
5. American Academy of Otolaryngology—Head and Neck Surgery: *Sinusitis and sinus surgery* (videotape). Patient Education Video Series, distributed by Milner-Fenwick Timonium, MD.
6. Al Haddad S: Anesthesia for endoscopic sinus surgery. In: Levine HL, May M, eds. *Endoscopic sinus surgery*. New York: Thieme Medical Publishing, 91–104, 1993.
7. Gross CW, Gross WE: Post-operative care for functional endoscopic sinus surgery. *Ear Nose Throat J* 73:(7) 476–479, 1994.

PART 5

The Ear

Office-Based Surgery of the Head and Neck
Edited by Yosef P. Krespi, MD
Lippincott–Raven Publishers, Philadelphia © 1998

18

Laser-Assisted Tympanostomy

Herbert Silverstein, Jeffery J. Kuhn, Daniel I. Choo, and Seth I. Rosenberg

Continuous middle ear aeration is indicated when conservative measures fail to clear fluid from it. An accepted technique is to make an incision in the tympanic membrane, aspirate the fluid, and insert a pressure equalizing (PE) tube that will maintain ventilation and prevent recurrence of fluid. A myringotomy without PE tube insertion usually remains open for only 1–2 days and is no more effective than medical treatment for persistent serous otitis media (SOM) (1–4). The length of time a myringotomy must remain open to adequately treat persistent SOM has yet to be determined. Armstrong initially believed that 2–3 weeks was sufficient (5). To create a tympanostomy that will remain open for several weeks, the carbon dioxide (CO_2) laser can be used to vaporize an opening in the tympanic membrane without inserting a PE tube (6–11).

This chapter reports our experience using laser-assisted tympanostomy (LAT) to treat persistent SOM, conditions of abnormal eustachian tube patency, and other otologic conditions that require an opening in the tympanic membrane (1).

INDICATIONS FOR LASER-ASSISTED TYMPANOSTOMY

Indications for LAT include adult patients with persistent SOM who fail medical management, patients who wish to have immediate relief from symptoms of SOM, and patients with abnormal patency of the eustachian tube (ie, eustachian tube dysfunction and patulous eustachian tube). Older, cooperative children with persistent SOM who do not require long-term middle ear ventilation may also benefit from the procedure and also avoid the risk and cost of general anesthesia. LAT can be repeated in selected cases of recurrent otitis media that fail the initial procedure. A PE tube is inserted when long-term ventilation is determined necessary. LAT will prevent painful descent with air travel in patients susceptible to recurrent barotrauma. LAT is performed in patients with patulous eustachian tube prior to PE tube insertion to determine whether middle ear aeration will be successful in relieving symptoms. In performing middle ear exploration with the otoendoscope, LAT creates a bloodless opening that makes endoscopy easier.

METHOD

The Zeiss OPM1 microscope with a 300-mm objective lens is adapted for the Sharplan CO_2 laser (Model 1030, Sharplan Lasers, Inc., Allendale, NJ) using a microslad optical delivery system. The smallest spot size (0.65 mm at 0 setting) is obtained by aiming the beam perpendicular to a tongue blade. The eyepieces of the microscope are adjusted so that the surrounding area is in focus. Either a focused or a defocused beam technique can be used to vaporize an opening in the tympanic membrane. Because CO_2 laser energy is readily absorbed in water, either technique is suitable for treating persistent SOM.

Focused Beam Technique

An initial power setting of 1 W, 0.1-second pulse duration in the regular mode, was used for the focused beam technique. The energy may be increased from 1.5–3.0 W, if needed. A thicker tympanic membrane may require a higher power setting. Multiple hits are made in a circular fashion to create the desired size opening. Defocusing the microslad to two units and vaporizing the edges and bridges of the tympanic membrane enlarges the opening to the desired size. A defocused beam at low power settings will not cause laser injury to the promontory bone. Making the tympanostomy anterior to the malleus allows the laser beam to penetrate the tympanic membrane in a more perpendicular plane. Also, the promontory is at a greater distance from the tympanic membrane in this region (Fig. 1).

Defocused Beam Technique

When a shorter procedure with fewer laser bursts is desired (ie, LAT in children), a defocused beam technique is used. With the microslad beam defocused to three units at 15 W or four units at 20 W in the regular mode, an opening of 1.5–2.0 mm can be produced with one laser burst. Occasionally, two or three laser bursts may be necessary to achieve a larger opening.

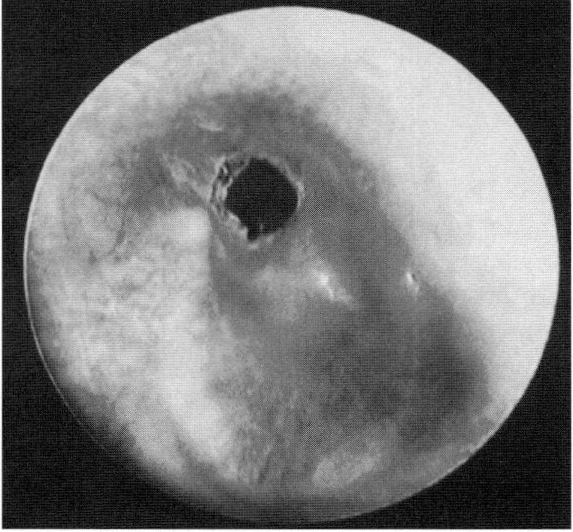

FIG. 1. Video print showing a 2-mm diameter laser-assisted tympanostomy (LAT).

Anesthesia

In 29 patients (40 ears), the tympanic membrane was anesthetized using topical tetracaine base (160 mg of powder dissolved in 0.2 mL of isopropyl alcohol) just prior to use (12,13). The solution is delivered into the external canal by dropper and allowed to remain in contact with the tympanic membrane for 5–8 minutes. The solution is then suctioned from the canal prior to beginning the procedure. This technique provides up to 2 hours of anesthesia.

LAT has been performed in eight patients (8 ears) without anesthesia using the focused, multiple burst technique. Usually, little pain is associated with this procedure; however, the psychological stability of the patient should be considered when performing LAT without anesthesia. Thus far, no patient has asked to stop the procedure because of pain.

Patient Evaluation and Treatment

Thirty-seven patients (48 ears) were included in our study. Thirty patients (39 ears) had persistent SOM, four patients (5 ears) had patulous eustachian tube, and three patients (4 ears) had eustachian tube dysfunction. The diagnosis of persistent SOM was based on several factors, including careful observation of the mobility of the tympanic membrane under the microscope with pneumatoscopy, the appearance of fluid behind an intact tympanic membrane, and audiometric evidence of a conductive loss with a type B tympanometry curve.

A diagnosis of patulous eustachian tube was made in four patients, all of whom presented with symptoms of echo sensation, tinnitus when breathing through the nose, and ear fullness or pressure that improved in the supine position. One of the patients with patulous eustachian tube demonstrated tympanic membrane movement with nasal respirations.

A diagnosis of eustachian tube dysfunction was made in three patients who presented with symptoms of fullness and pressure in the ears related to either an upper respiratory illness or recent air travel. On microscopic examination by pneumatoscopy, a normal or retracted tympanic membrane was seen without middle ear fluid and a type C tympanogram. Most patients in the study had symptoms for <1 month prior to presenting at the Florida Ear and Sinus Center. Initially, medical treatment was given, which usually included a systemic decongestant, antibiotics, and auto-inflation of the middle ear. If symptoms of persistent SOM and eustachian tube dysfunction persisted for 3 weeks despite medical management or if the patient requested immediate relief of symptoms, LAT was used. Patients with patulous eustachian tube were scheduled for LAT without any intervening treatment. Although the focus of this study was persistent SOM, there appeared to be applicability in patients with eustachian tube dysfunction and patulous eustachian tube. Patients with eustachian tube dysfunction and patulous eustachian tube whose symptoms resolved after LAT but then returned after the tympanic membrane healed, were treated with myringotomy and PE tube.

Audiometric testing with pure tone audiometry, tympanometry, and speech discrimination were performed on each patient prior to and at 1 week following LAT. Patients were subsequently examined weekly until closure of the tympanostomy. The healed tympanic membrane was examined under the microscope, photographs were taken, and audiometry was performed. Patients were followed for a minimum of 3 months after closure of the tympanostomy.

RESULTS

Forty patients (51 ears) underwent LAT. Data were completed on 37 patients for a total of 48 ears (24 left, 24 right). Three patients (3 ears) were lost to follow-up. Patient ages ranged from 8 to 87 years with a mean age of 67 years and a median age of 75 years. Patients tolerated the procedure well with only one patient having complained of slight pain at laser impact. There was one case of transient postoperative otorrhea, which was treated successfully with an antibiotic otic solution. When fluid was present in the middle ear, laser injury of the promontory did not occur. However, several patients without middle ear fluid had inadvertent laser burns of the promontory when a higher wattage with focused beam was used or when multiple bursts were used to enlarge a tympanostomy.

Twenty-nine adults and 1 child (39 ears) with persistent SOM were initially treated using LAT without PE tubes. Persistent SOM was cured in 24 patients (31 ears) after the first LAT and in 1 patient (1 ear) after a second treatment for an overall success rate of 78%. Four patients (5 ears) eventually required PE tubes. One of these patients had two LAT procedures performed in both ears prior to the insertion of PE tubes. While the tympanostomy remained open, four patients (5 ears) with patulous eustachian tube and three patients (4 ears) with eustachian tube dysfunction were symptom free (Table 1). One patient with patulous eustachian tube required PE tube insertion for recurrent symptoms following closure of the tympanostomy. Another patient with eustachian tube dysfunction had recurrent symptoms following clo-

TABLE 1. *Cures or Failures by Diagnosis*

Diagnosis/Ears (patients)	Ears (patients) Cured/Ears (patients) Fail	Cure/Fail Rate
SOM/39 (30)	32 (25)/7 (5)	78.1%/21.9%
PET/5 (4)	5 (4)/0 (0)	100%/0%
ETD/4 (3)	4 (3)/0 (0)	100%/0%

SOM, serous otitis media; PET, patulous eustachian tube; ETD, eustachian tube dysfunction.

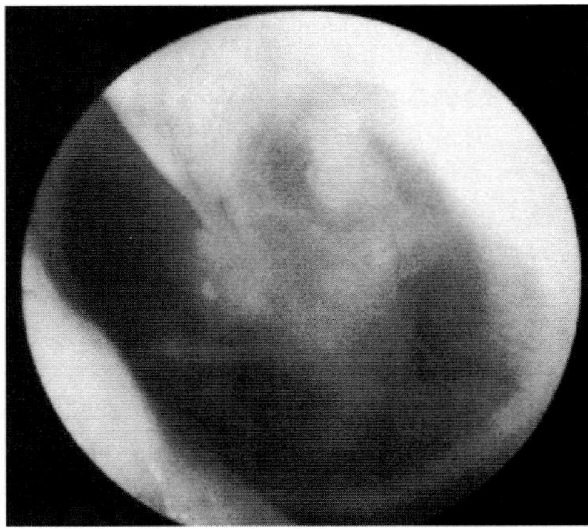

FIG. 2. Video print of healed, normal appearing tympanic membrane after laser-assisted tympanostomy (LAT).

sure of the tympanostomy, but did not want further treatment.

The tympanostomy size in 48 ears varied from 0.5 to 3.0 mm with an average of 1.6 mm. The patency time (ie, time for the tympanic membrane to heal) ranged from 1 to 7 weeks with an average of 3.17 weeks. All but one tympanostomy healed without evidence of scarring on microscopic examination (Fig. 2). The average patency time based on tympanostomy size was studied in all 48 ears. The results are summarized in Table 2. The average patency time per tympanostomy size was also studied for each diagnostic group and results are summarized in Tables 3 and 4. The average patency time for patients with a tympanostomy $\leq$1.0 mm (N = 17) was 2.12 weeks; 1.5 mm (N = 10) was 3.0 weeks; 2.0 mm (N = 12) was 4.04 weeks; and

TABLE 3. *Average Patency Time (weeks) per Tympanostomy Size (mm) for Each Diagnostic Group*

Size (mm)	SOM (ears)	Weeks	PET (ears)	Weeks	ETD (ears)	Weeks
$\leq$1.0	11	2.00	2	2.00	4	2.50
1.5	7	2.43	3	3.67		
2.0	12	4.04				
$\geq$2.5	9	4.17				

SOM, serous otitis media; PET, patulous eustachian tube; ETD, eustachian tube dysfunction.

$\geq$2.5 mm (N = 9) was 4.17 weeks. There was a definite trend toward increasing patency time with increasing tympanostomy size for openings <2.5 mm in diameter (Fig. 3). There appeared to be little advantage in creating an opening >2.0 mm, as patency time did not increase appreciably with openings $\geq$2.5 mm in diameter. A larger tympanostomy (ie, 3 mm) may increase the risk of a permanent perforation.

Ototopical agents were not used routinely in patients following LAT. Early in the study we noticed a prolonged patency time in patients receiving a combination of dexamethasone ophthalmic solution (0.1% Decadron, Merck, West Point, PA) and sulphacetamide sodium prednisolone (Vasocidin ophthalmic solution, IOLAB Pharmaceuticals, Claremont, CA). In an effort to delay healing and prolong patency time, seven patients (11 ears) were treated post-LAT with Decadron drops three times per day and Vasocidin drops at night until closure of the tympanostomy. The average tympanostomy size in this group of

TABLE 2. *Average Patency Time (weeks) per Tympanostomy Size (mm)*

Size (mm)	Ears	Average Weeks
$\leq$1.0	17	2.12
1.5	10	3.00
2.0	12	4.04
$\leq$2.5	9	4.17

TABLE 4. *Average Patency Time (weeks) for Each Diagnostic Group*

Diagnosis (ears)	Average Size Opening (mm)	Average Patency Time (weeks)
SOM (39)	1.74	3.21
PET (5)	1.15	3.00
ETD (4)	0.75	2.50

SOM, serous otitis media; PET, patulous eustachian tube; ETD, eustachian tube dysfunction.

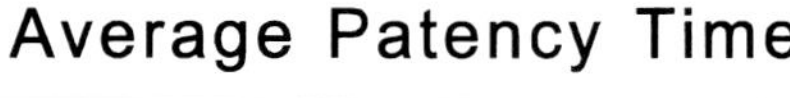

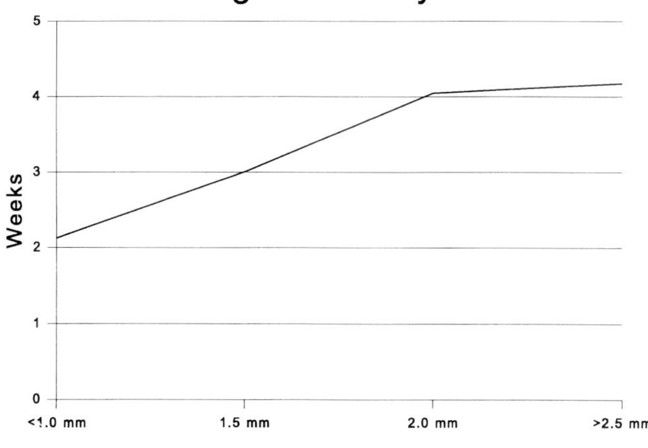

FIG. 3. Patency time related to tympanostomy opening.

patients was 1.86 mm and the average patency time was 3.36 weeks. This compared with an average tympanostomy size of 1.54 mm and an average patency time of 3.12 weeks in 30 patients (37 ears) not receiving post-LAT treatment (Table 5). The average patency time for each tympanostomy size was compared for the two groups and the results are summarized in Table 6. This comparison is illustrated in Figure 4. There was no statistical difference in average patency time between ears that received post-LAT treatment and those that did not.

In 30 patients (38 ears) with persistent SOM, the average pre-LAT speech reception threshold (SRT) was 44.1 dB and the average air-bone gap was 25 dB. The average post-LAT SRT improved to 28 dB and the average air-bone gap decreased to 8.0 dB (ie, 17 dB improvement). No patient had a sensorineural hearing loss following LAT (Table 7).

DISCUSSION

Myringotomy with PE tube insertion is a common procedure for treating chronic SOM and conditions related to abnormal patency of the eustachian tube. The use of PE tubes, however, is not without consequences. The incidence of early postoperative otorrhea ranges from 12% to 40% (4,14–16) and may occur in as high as 68% of patients during the time the tube is functional. Short-term PE tubes remain functional for a period of 6–12 months, with functional time varying slightly among the different types commercially available. While open, the PE tube may permit bacterial contamination of the middle ear from extrinsic causes and, as theorized by Bluestone et al., the presence of the tube may facilitate reflux of nasopharyngeal secretions into the

TABLE 5. *Average Patency Time (weeks) for Ears Receiving Ototopical Treatment versus No Treatment Post-Tympanostomy*

Ears (patients)	Average Tympanostomy Size (mm)	Average Patency Time (weeks)
Drops 11 (7)	1.86	3.36
No drops 37 (30)	1.54	3.12

TABLE 6. *Average Patency Time (weeks) per Tympanostomy Size (mm) for Ears Receiving Treatment versus No Treatment Post-Tympanostomy.*

Size (mm)	Drops (ears)	Weeks	No drops (no. of ears)	Weeks
≤1.0	2	2.00	15	2.14
1.5	3	2.67	7	3.14
2.0	2	4.5	10	3.95
≥2.5	4	4.00	5	4.31

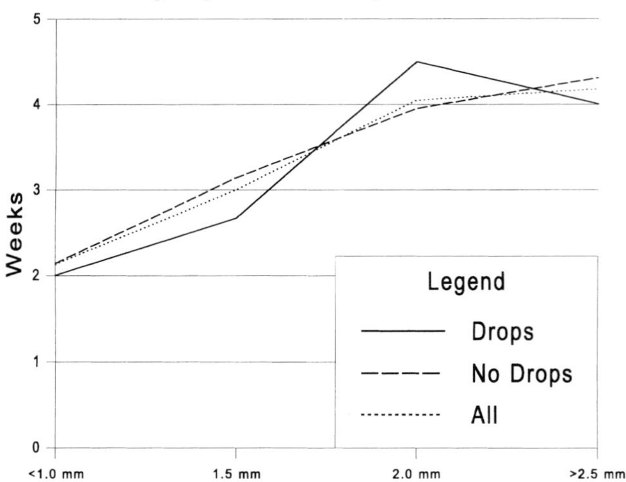

FIG. 4. Comparison of post-tympanostomy treatments.

middle ear (17). The anatomic sequelae of PE tubes, including tympanosclerosis, atrophy, and permanent perforation, have been reported to occur in 57%, 25%, and 18% of patients, respectively (2,4). The minimal length of time that a PE tube must remain functional to adequately treat chronic SOM is not known. In many cases, a shorter period of aeration may suffice. To create a tympanostomy that would remain open for several weeks and heal with minimal scarring, the CO_2 laser was used without a PE tube.

Wilpizeski was the first to use the microsurgical CO_2 laser for making perforations in the tympanic membrane of the squirrel monkey (7). He performed partial myringectomies by vaporizing the posterior quadrant of the tympanic membrane in 40 monkeys and found that all perforations "healed quickly." Lyons et al. used a modified CO_2 laser with an alternat-

ing current power supply that consistently caused damage to inner ear structures in the guinea pig (9). Even at low-power settings and short exposure times, the laser application was too unpredictable to warrant continued use. Saito et al. created myringotomies in 50 patients using a small electrocautery device that produced openings equaling one quarter of a quadrant of the tympanic membrane. This opening remained open for >6 months in eight of eight patients (18). Lau et al. used a battery-powered heating element with a Nichrome wire tip to create myringotomies in 10 pediatric and 15 adult patients with persistent SOM (19). They reported a patency time of 1–3 weeks. Fifty percent of their pediatric patients' ears were controlled and only 40% of their adult patients' ears were controlled with heat myringotomies. Soderberg et al. performed CO_2 laser myringotomies in 22 rats

TABLE 7. *Hearing Results (average dB) for Each Diagnostic Group*

Diagnosis/Ears (patients)	Pre-SRT	Post-SRT	Pre A-B Gap	Post A-B Gap
*SOM 38 (30)	44.1	28.4	25.0	8.1
PET 5 (4)	25	25	0	0
ETD 4 (3)	12.5	16.3	5	6.3

*One patient with no response in one ear. SRT, speech reception threshold; A-B gap, air-bone gap; SOM, serous otitis media; PET, patulous eustachian tube; ETD, eustachian tube dysfunction.

and found that most of the openings closed within 3 weeks. Histologic studies showed that the perforations began to close at day 9 when the proliferating squamous epithelium had reached the edge of the perforation. Further closure of the perforation was governed by the presence of a hyperplastic squamous epithelium with pronounced keratin production (11). Most recently, Derowe et al. performed CO_2 laser myringotomies in 30 guinea pig ears using a hand-held otoscope and fiberoptic delivery system (10). They noted a dose-dependent relationship between total energy used and the duration of the open myringotomy, with the most important variable being exposure time. Myringotomy size in their study varied from 1.5 to 2.0 mm. Although the surgeons did not consider a size difference of 0.5 mm a significant factor, our study shows an average of a 1-week difference in patency time for tympanostomies of 1.5 and 2.0 mm in diameter (see Table 1). Histologic studies failed to support a direct relationship between total energy and patency time. Goode used the CO_2 laser to create myringotomies in 4 fresh temporal bone specimens, 10 cat ears, and 11 human patient ears (8). Fifty percent of his patients redeveloped middle ear fluid within 1 month following the procedure. Six patients were treated without anesthesia, and pain was experienced only when multiple bursts of the laser were used to create a 2.0-mm opening. One 4.0-mm myringotomy and one opening in an atrophic area failed to heal; however, the remainder healed within 6 weeks. Our results were better than those reported by Goode, due in part to the fact that four of his patient failures had developed persistent SOM following radiation therapy to the head and neck. Dr. Juan Coma treated 168 ears with SOM using the CO_2 laser (personal communication, 1994). Seventy-four percent of his patients were children ranging in age from 4 to 9 years. Coma found that patency time correlated with myringotomy size. Openings of 1.5 mm remained open for 2–3 weeks, whereas those 2.0–2.5 mm in diameter remained open for 4–6 weeks. He reported that repeat myringotomy was "minimal" in his group of patients.

To apply the CO_2 laser efficiently in patients, a variety of power settings and exposure times were first tested on temporal bone specimens, temporalis fascia, and tongue blades. Laser spot size was also varied (ie, focused and defocused beam) while energy parameters remained constant. In patients, the usual laser settings were 0.1- or 0.2-second pulse duration, using a single burst of 15–20 W in regular mode with a defocused beam of three or four units, or multiple burst technique of 1–3 W with a focused beam. Defocusing the beam to two units of low wattage (ie, 1 W) allows the tympanostomy to be enlarged without injury to the promontory bone. Tympanostomies were generally made smaller in patients with patulous eustachian tube and eustachian tube dysfunction (ie, average size is 1.15 mm and 0.75 mm, respectively) as compared with patients with persistent SOM (ie, average size is 1.74 mm) (see Table 3). Average patency time was directly related to tympanostomy size for each diagnostic group (see Table 2). In patients without middle ear fluid, inadvertent laser injury to the promontory was prevented by inserting saline-soaked Gelfoam (The Upjohn Co., Kalamazoo, MI) through a 0.5-mm laser opening beneath the tympanic membrane. The tympanostomy was then enlarged with additional laser bursts until the desired size was achieved. In patients with persistent SOM, middle ear fluid prevents injury to the tympani promontorium, as CO_2 laser energy is readily absorbed by water. After middle ear fluid is removed, the tympanostomy can be enlarged by lowering the power setting to 1 W at 0.1-second pulse duration and defocusing the beam to two units. This technique will prevent injury to the promontory.

There has been some criticism regarding the use of the CO_2 laser to make an opening in the tympanic membrane to treat SOM (6). In the past, the main drawback to laser tympanostomy was the need for an office CO_2 laser. However, with the popularity of laser-assisted uvulopalatoplasty (LAUP), many otolaryngologists are now using the CO_2 laser for office-based surgery. The CO_2 laser used for office LAUP can easily be adapted for use in the ear.

At the Florida Ear and Sinus Center, LAT has been an effective method for performing rapid, painless middle ear aeration. This procedure is particularly suited for adult patients with persistent SOM (ie, 78% cure rate). The tympanostomies made with this procedure remain open for several weeks and heal without excessive scarring. The tympanic membrane appears to heal in three layers and functions normally on pneumatoscopy. Patency time is directly related to tympanostomy size (ie, larger opening equals longer healing time) (see Table 1). The average patency time for a tympanostomy that is 1.6 mm in diameter is approximately 3 weeks. Because of the risks of atrophic healing and permanent perforation, tympanostomies >3.0 mm in diameter have not been attempted. Other surgeons have also warned against making openings larger than 2.5–3.5 mm, in diameter (19,20). In our study, there appeared to be little advantage in making tympanostomies >2.0 mm, as patency time did not increase significantly for openings ≥2.5. Only one patient developed early postoperative otorrhea following LAT. While the tympanostomy is open, patients are advised to use cotton and petroleum jelly or a commercially available ear plug when showering or swimming.

In patients who fail to respond to short-term middle ear aeration, we generally recommend PE tubes. Two patients with recurrent SOM underwent a second LAT with one patient being cured and the other eventually requiring PE tube insertion. In older, cooperative children (ie, 8–10 years of age), aeration of the middle ear for several weeks may be sufficient to treat persistent SOM. The office procedure avoids the cost and risks of general anesthesia and the psychological trauma of an operating room procedure. Patients can swim after the tympanic membrane heals and water precautions are unnecessary beyond the 2–4 weeks needed for tympanostomy closure. However, in young children and in cases of persistent SOM that do not respond to LAT, PE tubes are indicated.

LAT can be used as both a diagnostic and a prognostic procedure in patients with patulous eustachian tube and eustachian tube dysfunction. A 0.5-mm tympanostomy is helpful in diagnosing patients with suspected eustachian tube dysfunction and it may relieve symptoms of fullness and pressure in the ears. LAT can help determine whether middle ear aeration with a PE tube will relieve symptoms associated with patulous eustachian tube. In these cases, LAT is usually performed with a focused beam at 1 W, 0.1-second pulse duration, without anesthesia. Four patients (5 ears) with patulous eustachian tube and three patients (4 ears) with eustachian tube dysfunction were successfully treated with LAT. One patient (1 ear) with patulous eustachian tube eventually required a PE tube for long-term symptomatic relief.

The length of time needed to aerate the middle ear to prevent the recurrence of SOM is not the same in all cases. In adults who develop SOM in conjunction with an upper respiratory illness or as a result of barotrauma during air travel, aeration of the middle ear for a 2- to 4-week period appears sufficient in most cases. Of the patients in our study with persistent SOM who were successfully treated with LAT (78%), most were noted to have thin, amber fluid in the middle ear space. Most of the patients were treated medically for at least 3 weeks prior to undergoing LAT for persistent SOM. Obviously, some of these cases would have resolved over a longer period of observation. However, an advantage of LAT is that symptoms are usually immediately relieved after the procedure without subjecting patients to the risks of longer term aeration with PE tubes. Surgical aeration of the middle ear is indicated when middle ear fluid fails to clear after 3 weeks of medical treatment or when the patient requests immediate relief of ear pressure and restoration of hearing. LAT appears to be a safe, cost-effective procedure that can easily be performed in an office setting when an opening in the tympanic membrane is needed for either treatment or diagnosis.

OTOENDOSCOPY TECHNIQUE

Otoendoscopes (Smith & Nephew Richards, Memphis, TN) (1.7 mm in diameter, 0°

and 30°, and 10 cm in length) are used to evaluate the middle ear anatomy. The most useful endoscope for middle ear otoendoscopy is the Smith & Nephew Richards 1.7-mm, 30° otoscope. The 30° lens allows visualization of the under surface of the tympanic membrane, a direct view of the round window, and a view directly down the eustachian tube. The middle ear is viewed by watching a TV monitor. Video and photo documentation of the procedure and middle ear anatomy are obtained by attaching the Olympus camera (OTV-S4, Deerfield Beach, FL) to the endoscope and observing a 13-in Olympus (OTV-141) color video monitor.

Video prints are taken with a Sony (Park Ridge, NJ) color video printer, (UP-1200) and the procedure is recorded with a 0.5-in Sony Super VHS recorder (SVO-9500MD-VR-1 B).

INDICATION FOR MIDDLE EAR EXPLORATION

Laser-assisted otoendoscopy can be used in the following situations (6,7):

1. Visualization of the oval and round windows in suspected perilymph fistulas.
2. Visualization of the middle ear before chronic ear surgery. This allows the surgeon to evaluate the ossicular chain, the extent of cholesteatoma, whether skin has grown onto the under surface of the tympanic membrane, and the status of the eustachian tube and middle ear mucosa. Small, benign perforations can be repaired at the same time with ear lobe adipose tissue.
3. Evaluation of a middle ear mass or unexplained conductive hearing loss.
4. Evaluation of the round window niche for the presence of obstructing mucosal bands prior to chemical perfusion of the inner ear with dexamethasone or gentamicin.
5. Evaluation of the eustachian tube in recurrent SOM prior to inserting a PE tube.
6. Visualization of the eustachian tube in cases of patulous eustachian tube prior to inserting a PE tube, or materials to decrease the patency of the eustachian tube.

Using the laser to perform the tympanostomy provides a bloodless opening for endoscopic middle ear exploration, which reduces the need for frequent cleaning of the endoscope lens. Office operating room procedures reduce the need for hospitalization and the cost of surgery for the patient. More procedures are being performed in the office and outpatient centers that, in the past, would have required expensive treatment in the hospital.

CONCLUSION

The office CO_2 laser, used mainly for LAUP, can easily be adapted for microsurgery using a microslad mounted on the Zeiss OPM1 microscope with a 300-mm lens. For cases of persistent SOM, LAT may obviate the need for a PE tube. Of the 38 adult patients' ears and 1 pediatric patient's ear with persistent SOM that underwent treatment using LAT, 78% were cured and 5 patients (7 ears) eventually required PE tubes. In addition, LAT can be used in patients with eustachian tube dysfunction or patulous eustachian tube, and for endoscopic evaluation of the middle ear.

In our study, we found a direct relationship between tympanostomy size and patency time. LAT appears to be a safe, cost-effective procedure that can easily be performed in an office setting when an opening in the tympanic membrane is needed for either treatment or diagnosis.

REFERENCES

1. Silverstein H, Kuhn J, Choo D: Laser assisted tympanostomy. *Laryngoscope* 106:1067–1074;1996.
2. Le CT, Freeman DW, Fireman BH: Evaluation of ventilation tubes and myringotomy in the treatment of recurrent or persistent otitis media. *Pediatr Infect Dis J* 10:2–11, 1991.
3. Mandel EM, Rockette HE, Bluestone CD et al: Myringotomy with and without tympanostomy tubes for chronic otitis media with effusion. *Arch Otolaryngol Head Neck Surg* 115:1217–1224, 1989.
4. Mandel EM, Rockette HE, Bluestone CD et al: Efficacy of myringotomy with and without tympanostomy tubes for chronic otitis media with effusion. *Pediatr Infect Dis J* 11:270–277, 1992.
5. Armstrong SW: A new treatment for chronic secretary otitis media. *Arch Otolaryngol* 59(6):653–654, 1954.

6. Parkin JL: Lasers in tympanomastoid surgery. *Otolaryngol Clin North Am* 23(1):1–5, 1990.

7. Wilpizeski C, Majorello RP, Reddy JB et al: Otological applications of lasers: Basic background. *Trans Pa Acad Ophthalmol Otolaryngol* 30:185–192, 1977.

8. Goode RL: CO_2 laser myringotomy. *Laryngoscope* 92:420–423, 1982.

9. Lyons GD, Webster DB, Mouney DF et al: Anatomical consequences of CO_2 laser surgery of the guinea pig ear. *Laryngoscope* 88:1749–1754, 1978.

10. Derowe A, Ophir D, Katzir A: Experimental study of CO_2 laser myringotomy with a hand-held otoscope and fiberoptic delivery system. *Lasers Surg Med* 15:248–253, 1994.

11. Sodenberg O, Hellstrom S, Stenfors LE: Myringotomy made by CO_2 laser. An alternative to the ventilation tube? An experimental study. *Acta Otolaryngologica* 97:335–346, 1984.

12. Silverstein H, Call DL: Tetracaine base: An effective surface anesthetic for the tympanic membrane. *Arch Otolaryngol* 90:150–151, 1969.

13. Silverstein H, Rosenberg S: *Middle ear aeration procedure. Part A: Tympanostomy and pressure-equalizing tubes.* Philadelphia, Lea & Febiger, 106–108, 1992.

14. Bulkley WJ, Bowes AK, Marlow JF: Complications following ventilation of the middle ear using Goode T tubes. *Arch Otolaryngol Head Neck Surg* 117:895–898, 1991.

15. Gates GA, Avery CA, Cooper JC Jr et al: Chronic secretory otitis media: Effects of surgical management. *Ann Otol Rhinol Laryngol* 98(suppl 138, part 2):1–32, 1989.

16. Bluestone CD: Pathogenesis of otitis media: Role of eustachian tube. *Pediatr Infect Dis J* 15(4):281–291, 1996.

17. Luxford WM, Sheey JL: Myringotomy and ventilation tubes: A report of 1,568 ears. *Laryngoscope* 92:1293–1299, 1982.

18. Gates GA, Avery C, Prihoda TJ et al: Delayed onset post-tympanostomy otorrhea. *Otolaryngol Head Neck Surg* 98:111–115, 1988.

19. Saito H, Miyamoto K, Kishimoto S et al: Burn perforation as a method of middle ear ventilation. *Arch Otolaryngol* 104:79–81, 1978.

20. Lau P, Shelton C, Goode RL: Heat myringotomy. *Laryngoscope* 95:38–42, 1985.

Office-Based Surgery of the Head and Neck
Edited by Yosef P. Krespi, MD
Lippincott–Raven Publishers, Philadelphia © 1998

19

Middle Ear Endoscopy

Seth I. Rosenberg and Herbert Silverstein

In many surgical fields, there has been a trend toward minimally invasive, "band-aid," or "key-hole" surgery. Procedures that traditionally have been performed through large openings are now being performed through very small surgical incisions. The actual procedure is typically guided by a thin, rigid or flexible endoscope. In these procedures, patients benefit from decreased operative time and postoperative morbidity, as well as from an improved cosmetic result. Also, these procedures often decrease hospital stay, and patient and insurance company cost. Sometimes, these procedures can be performed in an office-based setting, further reducing cost. A recent increase in literature describes how endoscopic techniques have either enhanced or have been used to replace standard otologic and neurotologic procedures (1–8). This chapter describes how minimally invasive endoscopic techniques can be used in an office-based setting.

Although middle ear endoscopy was first described by Mer et al. in 1967, only recently have the optics associated with small endoscopes approached microscopic quality (8). Takahashi et al. endoscopically studied the middle ears of patients with otitis media with effusion (7). Their study showed the usefulness of otoendoscopy as a research tool in elucidating the natural history and pathology associated with middle ear problems. Otoendoscopy can also be used as an adjunct in middle ear diagnosis, such as in the presence of a middle ear mass or unexplained conductive hearing loss. Endoscopic examination could reduce the need for open exploration in a hospital setting. Poe et al. demonstrated that a transtympanic endoscopic examination of

the middle ear avoided a traditional middle ear exploration for perilymph fistula (3–5). Intratympanic gentamicin instillation into the middle ear has been used to control vertigo associated with Meniere's disease (9). Exposing the round window membrane endoscopically helps assure that the medicine is applied to that area. Overall, middle ear exploration is done to check suspected perilymph fistula, evaluate a middle ear mass, check unexplained conductive hearing loss, rule out cholesteatoma, and apply a drug to the round window membrane. In recurrent serous otitis media the eustachian tube can be visualized for obstructive narrowing or swollen mucosa. In patulous eustachian tubes a wide open eustachian tube can be seen. The advantage of the 30° endoscope is that it allows visualization of areas that cannot be seen with the traditional operating microscope.

Laser-assisted tympanostomy (LAT) with middle ear otoendoscopy is an office-based technique devised to allow for direct inspection of the middle ear with a rigid endoscope. The tympanic membrane is first anesthetized with a topical solution of tetracaine base powder (160 mg) dissolved in 0.20 mL of isopropyl alcohol applied for 8 minutes (10). This anesthetic lasts for about 2 hours. The tetracaine solution is irrigated out of the external auditory canal with sterile water. If perilymph fistula is suspected, injectable local anesthesia is avoided because the solution could potentially enter the middle ear and confound the results. For more extensive endoscopic procedures, the external ear canal is injected with 1–2 mL of 1% Xylocaine (Astra Merck, Wayne, PA) and adrenaline 1:100,000,

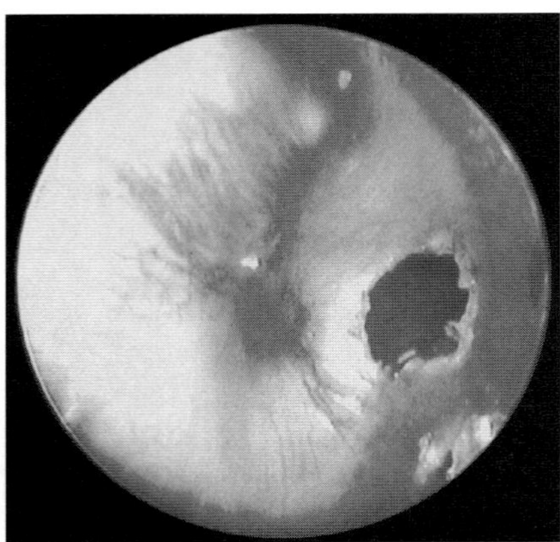

FIG. 1. Dry 2-mm tympanostomy using CO_2 laser.

similar to stapes surgery. A Sharplan CO_2 laser (Sharplan, Allendale, NJ; model 1030) with a microslad attached to a Zeiss Opmi I microscope (Zeiss, Thornwood, NY) is then used to create a tympanostomy 2 mm in diameter, posterior to the umbo and over the round window niche. If examination of the eustachian tube is the primary goal of otoendoscopy, the tympanostomy is made anterior to the umbo. For the past year, in our office, the LAT has been used to treat serous otitis media without pressure equalizing tubes (see Chapter 18). The main advantage of using the laser is that there is a bloodless opening through which the endoscope may be passed (Fig. 1). Also, there is little chance of a transudate forming as with a middle ear exploration with a tympanomeatal flap. A 2-mm opening can be made through a normal tympanic membrane using one burst of the laser at a setting of 15 W, for 0.1 second using a defocused beam at three units. Another method is using the laser to create a rosette using a setting of 1 or 2 W, for 0.1 second with a focused beam. The laser is then defocused to two units and the perforation enlarged to the desired diameter. Multiple laser bursts are used to vaporize the opening to 2 mm in diameter.

Otoendoscopes (Smith & Nephew Richards, Memphis, TN) (1.7 mm in diameter, 0° and 30°, and 10 cm in length) are used to evaluate the middle ear anatomy. The most useful endoscope for middle ear otoendoscopy is the Smith & Nephew Richards 1.7-mm, 30° otoscope. The 30° lens allows visualization of the under surface of the tympanic membrane, a direct view of the round window, and a view directly down the eustachian tube. The middle ear is viewed by watching a TV monitor. Any mucosal bands present are removed with small otologic picks. This is especially important if medication is being applied to the round window membrane. However, there is usually excellent visualization of both the round and oval windows (Figs. 2 and 3). Video and photo documentation of the procedure and middle ear anatomy are obtained by attaching the Olympus camera (OTV-S4) (Deerfield Beach, FL) to the endoscope and observing a 13-in Olympus (OTV-141) color video monitor. Video prints are taken with a Sony (Park Ridge, NJ) color video printer (UP-1200) and the procedure is recorded with a 0.5-in Sony Super VHS recorder (SVO-9500MD-VR-1B). After the procedure, patients are given Vasocidin ophthalmic solution (IOLAB Pharmaceuticals, Claremont, CA) to use before bedtime. The perforation closes in 2–4 weeks. There have been no complications associated with office middle ear endoscopy.

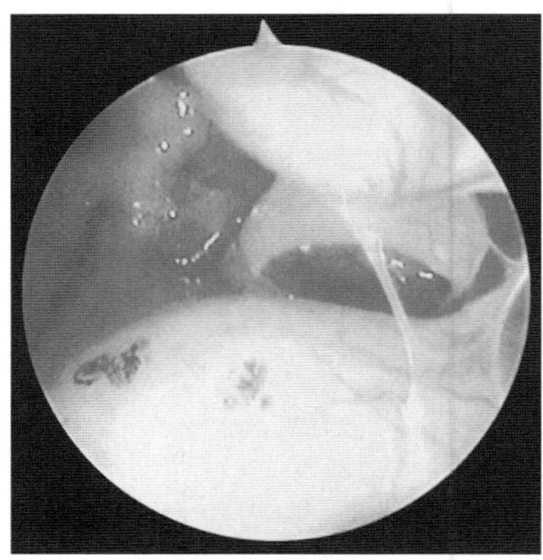

FIG. 2. View of anterior and posterior crus of the stapes using a 1.7-mm, 30° endoscope.

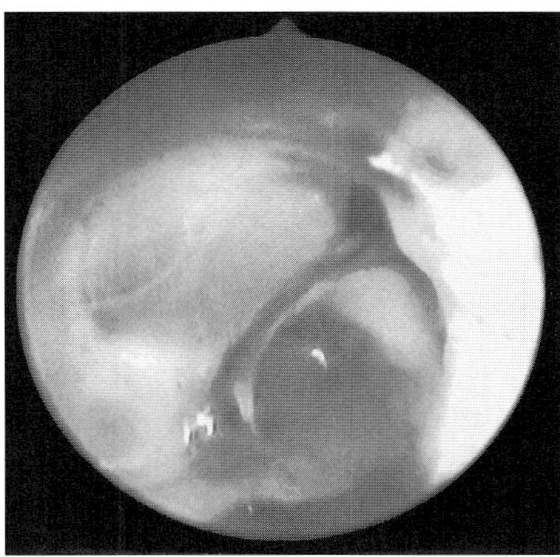

FIG. 3. Endoscopic picture of mucosa over the round window membrane (1.7-mm, 30° endoscope).

The following cases help illustrate how office otoendoscopy can be used.

CASE 1

A 42-year-old woman presented with hearing loss in the left ear after a recent plane flight. Prior to the flight, she was suffering from a viral upper respiratory infection. During the plane's descent, the patient suffered from severe otalgia and then noted a hearing loss in the left ear. She did not have any vestibular symptoms. A week later, the patient was found to have areas of hemorrhage on the left tympanic membrane as well as a tea-colored middle ear effusion. Audiologic assessment demonstrated a 30-dB low-frequency conductive hearing loss in the left ear with normal hearing in the right ear. LAT was performed and the tea-colored effusion was removed by suction. Otoendoscopy was performed using a 30°, 1.7-mm endoscope. The patient was found to have an intact ossicular chain, but had marked edema of the eustachian tube mucosa (Fig. 4). The patient was reassured and sent home with antibiotic ear drops. After 3 weeks, the perforation was completely healed and the patient had normal hearing.

CASE 2

A 73-year-old diabetic woman presented with a 5-month history of acute left facial paralysis that was slow to recover. Because of the patient's corneal problems, a local ophthalmologist had performed a lateral tarsorrhaphy 2 months after the onset of the facial paralysis. Magnetic resonance imaging was normal, but computed tomography demonstrated "increased soft tissue" in the vicinity of the horizontal facial nerve. When the patient was evaluated by us 5 months after the onset of her paralysis, she was found to have a House-Brackmann III/VI left facial paralysis. Audiologic assessment demonstrated a 10-dB low-frequency conductive hearing loss in the left ear with normal hearing in the right. Middle ear otoendoscopy demonstrated marked thickening of the chorda tympani that was not appreciated on otoscopic examination (Fig. 5). There was no evidence of a tumor in the middle ear. In light of the patient's age and medical status, no further medical or surgical intervention was recommended.

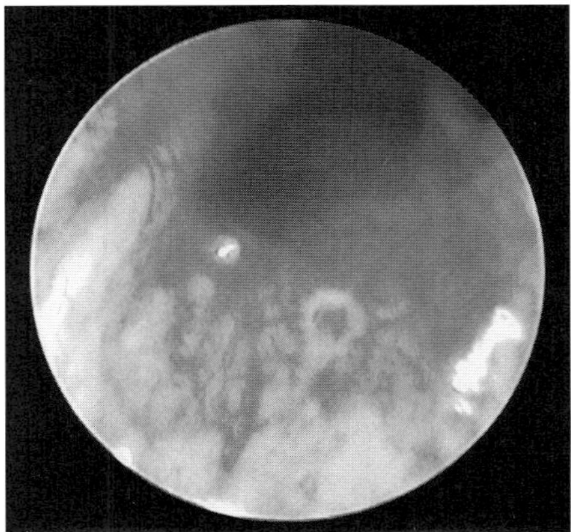

FIG. 4. Endoscopic view of the eustachian tube after LAT for serous otitis media (1.7-mm, 30° endoscope).

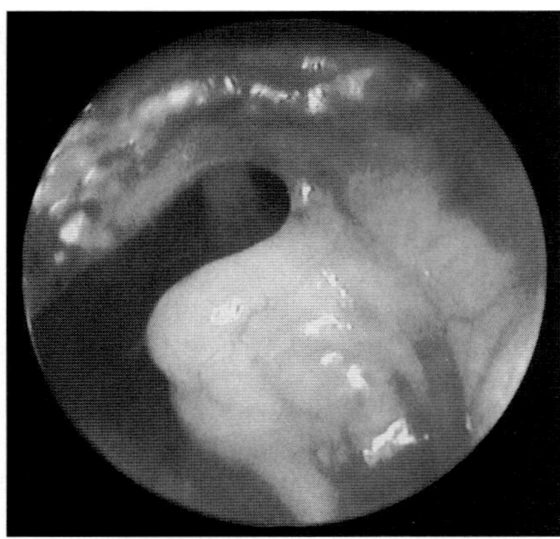

FIG. 5. View of enlarged chorda tympani after LAT (1.7-mm, 30° endoscope).

CASE 3

A 39-year-old woman presented 2 weeks after sudden and profound hearing loss in her right ear after scuba diving. Audiologic assessment showed a pure-tone average of 97 dB in the right ear with 0% discrimination score and normal hearing in her left ear. She also complained of tinnitus, but had no vestibular symptoms. Middle ear endoscopy demonstrated perilymph fluid coming from the round window niche area. This finding was confirmed by an exploratory tympanostomy, in which the round window was patched with lobular fat. Three weeks postoperatively, the patient's hearing in her right ear returned to a pure-tone average of 18 dB and 92% discrimination score. Prior to this case, our series of 14 patients who were suspected of having a perilymph fistula revealed no fistula, either endoscopically or with microscopic exploration.

CONCLUSION

Office otoendoscopy may alleviate the need for a formal middle ear exploration for perilymph fistulas. Office otoendoscopy can also be used to diagnose middle ear pathology and unexplained conductive hearing loss. Otoendoscopic techniques are an adjunct to the instillation of drugs in the round window niche.

PITFALLS IN OTOENDOSCOPY

Perilymph fistulas may heal intermittently with mucosal bands giving a false-negative endoscopic examination for a fistula. If there is a strong indication for a perilymph fistula and visualization of the oval and round windows is not perfect, the patient probably should have a formal exploration of the middle ear with palpation of the stapes and round window membrane. At present, no good endoscope holder exists that allows the surgeon to use both hands when operating in the middle ear. Mucosal bands may obstruct critical areas that cannot be removed in an office setting. The surgeon must learn how to evaluate depth because the endoscope gives a one-dimensional view. When using a traditional myringotomy, blood from the incision can be an annoying feature by clouding the endoscope lens. If the patient moves suddenly, the incus or stapes could potentially be dislocated by trauma from the endoscope.

REFERENCES

1. Rosenberg SI, Silverstein H, Willcox TO et al: Endoscopy in otology and neurotology. *Am J Otol* 15:168, 1994.
2. Rosenberg SI, Silverstein H, Hoffer M et al: Use of endoscopes for chronic ear surgery in children. *Arch Otolaryngol Head Neck Surg* 121:870,1995.
3. Poe DS, Bottrill ID: Comparison of endoscopic and surgical explorations for perilymphatic fistulas. *Am J Otol* 15:735, 1994.
4. Poe DS, Rebeiz EE, Pankratov MM: Evaluation of perilymphatic fistulas by middle ear endoscopy. *Am J Otol* 13:529, 1992.
5. Poe DS, Rebeiz EE, Pankratov MM et al: Transtympanic endoscopy of the middle ear. *Laryngoscope* 102:993, 1992.
6. Thomassin JM, Dorchia D, Doris JMD: Endoscopic-guided otosurgery in the prevention of residual cholesteatoma. *Laryngoscope* 103:939, 1993.
7. Takahashi H, Honjo I, Fujita A et al: Transtympanic endoscopic findings in patients with otitis media with effusion. *Arch Otolaryngol Head Neck Surg* 116:1186, 1990.
8. Mer SB, Derbyshire AJ, Berushenko A et al: Fiberoptic entoptoscopies for examining middle ear. *Arch Otolaryngol Head Neck Surg* 85:387, 1967.
9. Nedzelski JM, Chiong CM, Fradet G et al: Intratympanic gentamicin instillation as treatment of unilateral Meniere's disease: Update of an ongoing study. *Am J Otol* 14:278, 1993.
10. Silverstein H, Call DL: Tetracaine base: An effective surface anesthetic for the tympanic membrane. *Arch Otolaryngol* 90:150, 1969.

Office-Based Surgery of the Head and Neck
Edited by Yosef P. Krespi, MD
Lippincott–Raven Publishers, Philadelphia © 1998

20

Techniques of Office Myringoplasty

Anthony F. Jahn

The current trend in otolaryngology toward more office-based procedures also encompasses ear surgery. The main limitations to office-based otologic surgery have been threefold:

Sterility
Need for specific microinstrumentation
Postoperative recuperation

Although the middle ear is contiguous with the rest of the upper aerodigestive tract, it is generally sterile, and its mechanisms for coping with introduced contaminants or bacteria are more limited than those of the nose, sinuses, or pharynx. In procedures such as stapedectomy, opening the inner ear in a substerile environment introduces an even greater potential risk. Extensive surgery on a sterile middle ear, therefore, requires a degree of sterility that usually exists only in a conventional operating room.

The cost of microinstrumentation and the need for meticulous maintenance and replacement of these instruments are also limiting factors. Unless a practice has a large and constant volume of such procedures, it may not be cost-effective to invest in a full set of middle ear instruments. Office microsurgery may also require upgrading the microscope.

Postoperative recovery facilities may not be able to cope with an acutely vertiginous patient who requires observation and prolonged intravenous hydration.

Taking these limitations into account, myringoplasty is an ideal office-based procedure: it does not significantly invade the middle ear, it requires few instruments, and the immediate postoperative recovery is usually uneventful. Myringoplasty, in contrast to tympanoplasty, is defined here as a patch or graft applied to cover a tympanic membrane perforation, without opening the middle ear by means of a tympanomeatal flap. Several techniques for office myringoplasty are in current practice. The choice should be based on preoperative evaluation of the perforation, as well as physician preference.

PREOPERATIVE EVALUATION

The patient should be free of any active infection, and should not be suffering from a medical condition that contraindicates what is a minor but elective procedure. Preoperative assessment should also take into account perforation size, condition duration, remaining tympanic membrane state, middle ear state, degree of hearing loss, and eustachian tube (ET) function (1).

Perforation Size

Small perforations are more easily covered by office myringoplasty. Because any graft requires healing, either by vascularization of autograft tissue or by new growth from the edge of the membrane remnant, perforation size is critical. In an office setting, the edges of the perforation cannot normally be as thoroughly prepared as in the operating room.

Perforation Duration

Most acute perforations heal spontaneously, even if the opening is large. Acute perforations, in the absence of complicating factors, require minimal or no assistance to heal. Acute perforations that fail to heal usually have complicating factors, such as persistent middle ear disease or poor ET function.

Remaining Tympanic Membrane State

For a graft to take, or a perforation to heal by secondary intent, the surrounding drum remnant must be healthy and well vascularized. A graft will not take if the surrounding membrane remnant is tympanosclerotic, because tympanosclerosis is an avascular submucosal hyalinization. Neither will healing occur if the drum remnant is thinned ("monomeric") as a consequence of prolonged negative middle ear pressure.

Middle Ear State

Perforations occur commonly as a consequence of trauma or otitis media. Before considering myringoplasty, it is important that the middle ear mucosa be free of infection or inflammation. Even once purulent discharge has stopped, a graft is unlikely to take if there is persistent edema or mucorrhea. An atrophic or hyalinized middle ear mucosa is not a contraindication to myringoplasty, except insofar as what this implies about the health of the drum remnant.

Degree of Hearing Loss

Tympanic membrane perforations are normally associated with some conductive hearing loss. Because the degree of loss varies with the size and location of the perforation, there are no simple rules to correlate physical appearance and audiologic results. In the absence of a cholesteatoma, which can act as a sound-conducting structure, a conductive hearing loss of <20 dB usually indicates that the ossicular chain is intact (2). Greater degrees of hearing loss are more difficult to attribute. Certainly, if the patient has a large conductive hearing loss with a small pars tensa perforation, ossicular dysfunction should be suspected. This is especially the case in chronic perforations, where ossicular resorption, ankylosis, or ligamentous fibrosis may cause additional hearing loss. If the presence of ossicular disease cannot be easily inferred from an audiogram, a simple office patch can be applied prior to audiologic testing. This not only gives an estimate of the hearing gain that may be expected, but also helps in deciding whether the patient will require a formal tympanotomy and middle ear exploration.

ET Function

Poor ET function is a major cause for persistent or recurrent perforations. Although the literature has not agreed on what constitutes a physiologic test of ET function (3), nor has it shown a predictable correlation between ET function and surgical outcome, my preference is to test ET function in some fashion before any attempt to close a perforation. The simplest technique is to listen over the ear with the bell of the stethoscope while the patient performs a modified Valsalva maneuver. Classically, a Toynbee tube can also be used, placing one end in the patient's ear, and the other end into the examiner's ear, or into a glass of water. The appearance of air bubbles implies an open ET. More physiologic, and quantifiable, is the use of a tympanometer-monitored swallow to clear positive or negative pressure generated by the impedance bridge.

The best candidate for an office myringoplasty is the patient with an acute small pars tensa perforation who has a healthy drum remnant, normal middle ear mucosa, and good ET function. In many cases, patients meeting all these criteria will heal spontaneously. Patients failing to meet all these criteria are still potential candidates for office myringoplasty, but the surgeon should weigh the implications, because outcome may be adversely affected.

ANESTHESIA

Office myringoplasty should be done with local anesthesia. My method is to layer the area with EMLA (Astra Merck, Wayne, PA) cream. This can be introduced with a 3-mL syringe and a 22-gauge needle. The cream is expressed over the edges of the perforation under direct microscopic vision. The area is normally anesthetized after 15 minutes. At this time, the cream is suctioned away. Care is taken not to introduce any EMLA cream into the middle ear.

If more extensive manipulation is anticipated, the external auditory canal is coated with EMLA cream, left for 60 minutes, and suctioned out; the canal is then injected with 2% Xylocaine (Astra Merck) with epinephrine 1:10,000. The injection is prepared by mixing 9 mL of 2% Xylocaine plain with 1 mL of epinephrine 1:1000. A 30-gauge needle is used, and no more than 1 mL should be slowly injected. Rapid or excessive injection can produce extavasation into the middle ear and cause vertigo, tinnitus, and even hearing loss owing to absorption through the round window. I infiltrate the deep canal in three quadrants, and also anesthetize the lateral rim of the canal where the speculum sits. Patients under local anesthesia often complain more of discomfort from the speculum than from the surgery. Hypertension and drug allergies are contraindications to the injection described above.

Anxious patients can be premedicated with 10 mg of Valium (Roche Pharmaceuticals, Nutley, NJ) 1 hour before the procedure.

Simple patching does not require antimicrobial cleansing; however, techniques involving a tissue graft do. The auricle and ear canal should be prepared in the customary fashion. Some surgeons feel that Betadyne (Purdue Frederick, Norwalk, CT) is irritating to the middle ear, and prefer aqueous Zephiran (Winthrop Pharmaceuticals, New York, NY). I usually use Betadyne, taking care, however, to wash it completely out of the ear with copious amounts of lukewarm saline.

SURGICAL TECHNIQUE

Onlay "Paper Patch" Technique

After anesthesia, the edges of the perforation are freshened with a 1-mm stapes hook.

The hook is used to evert the edges circumferentially. Instead of the traditional cigarette paper, I currently use a Steristrip patch. This is trimmed to the appropriate size, grasped at one corner with alligator forceps, and pressed over the perforation. The patch is flattened and pressed against the drum remnant with the elbow of the stapes hook or with a small ring wax curette.

The above method is a good first attempt at patching, and is especially useful in cases where a postoperative patient returns with a small perforation. It can also be used with marginal dehiscences, such as when a short tympanomeatal flap has pulled away from the bony annulus. The Steristrip should be made large enough to provide good adherence to the drum remnant or adjacent canal. Over the following 2 months, the Steristrip falls away from the drum and migrates laterally (Fig. 1).

Fat Myringoplasty

Fat myringoplasty is a technique suitable for small perforations. After adequate anesthesia, the edges of the perforation are freshened, using the 1-mm stapes hook. The edges are everted, and the hook is swept around the medial aspect of the perforation to roughen up the recipient surface. Through a small earlobe incision, fat is harvested. The incision is closed with a single nylon suture. The fat is trimmed, making sure that no epidermis or dermis remains, and then plugged into the opening. Fat should protrude on either side of the perforation, like a dumbbell. Over time, the graft dries and thins and closes the perforation (Fig. 2). This technique is only useful for small perforations, because the new membrane formed is quite thin and not of good acoustic quality. Care is also taken in harvesting the fat to avoid earring tracts, to prevent accidental implantation of epidermis.

Tragal Perichondrium Underlay Graft

Although most surgeons prefer formal exploration of the ear, it is possible to insert a

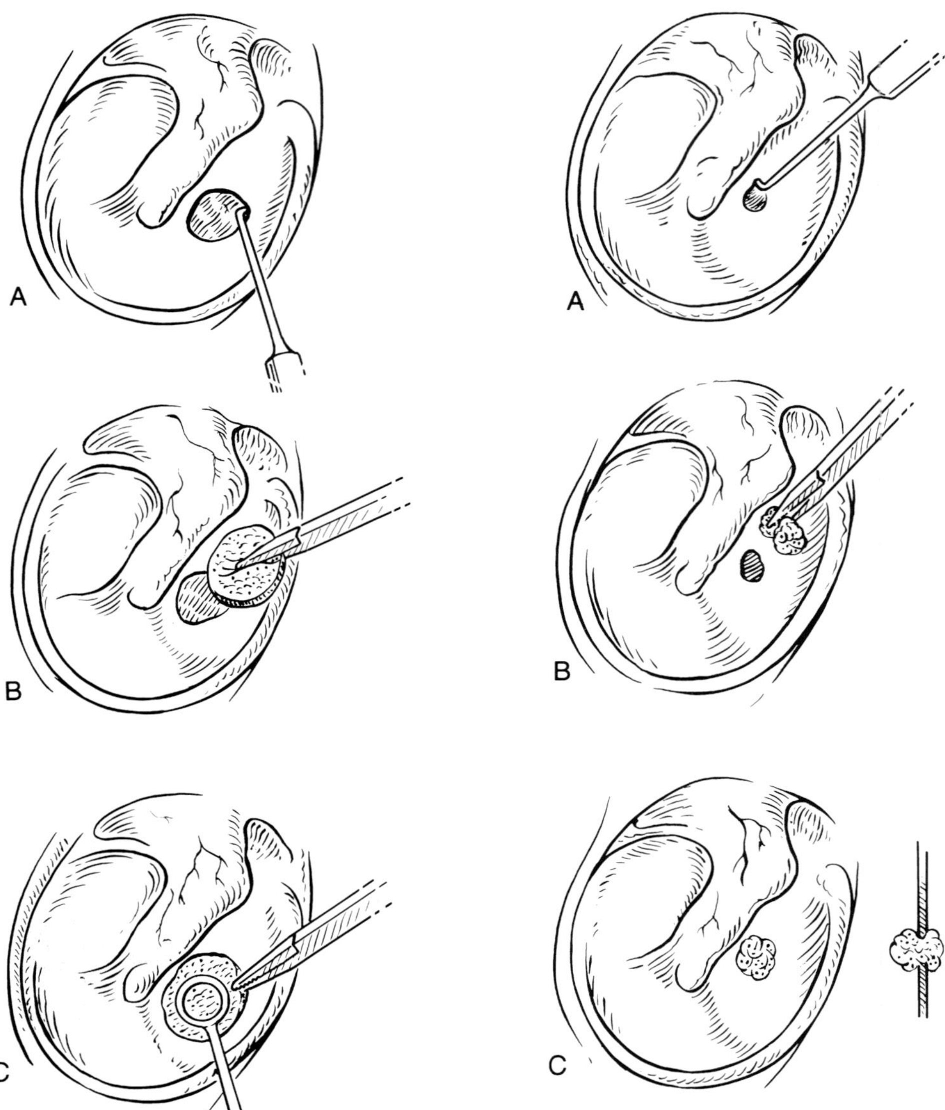

FIG. 1. Steristrip patch. **(A)** Edges of perforation freshened with 1-mm stapes hook. **(B)** Steristrip patch positioned with alligator forceps. **(C)** Patch pressed into position with ring curette.

FIG. 2. Fat graft. **(A)** Edges of perforation freshened with 1-mm stapes hook. **(B)** Fat from earlobe brought into surgical field. **(C)** Fat wedged into perforation. Side view shows it protruding, dumbbell-like, on either side.

graft through the perforation directly, a simpler technique. This is appropriate for a larger but fresh perforation wherein there is no concern for middle ear scarring or ossicular dysfunction (Fig. 3). The edges are again freshened, which is accomplished either with a stapes hook or with a needle and alligator forceps. Tragal perichondrium is harvested by injecting directly over the tragus and incising down to perichondrium. The perichondrium can be lifted off the lateral surface of the cartilage *in situ* or, if more perichondrium is needed, the

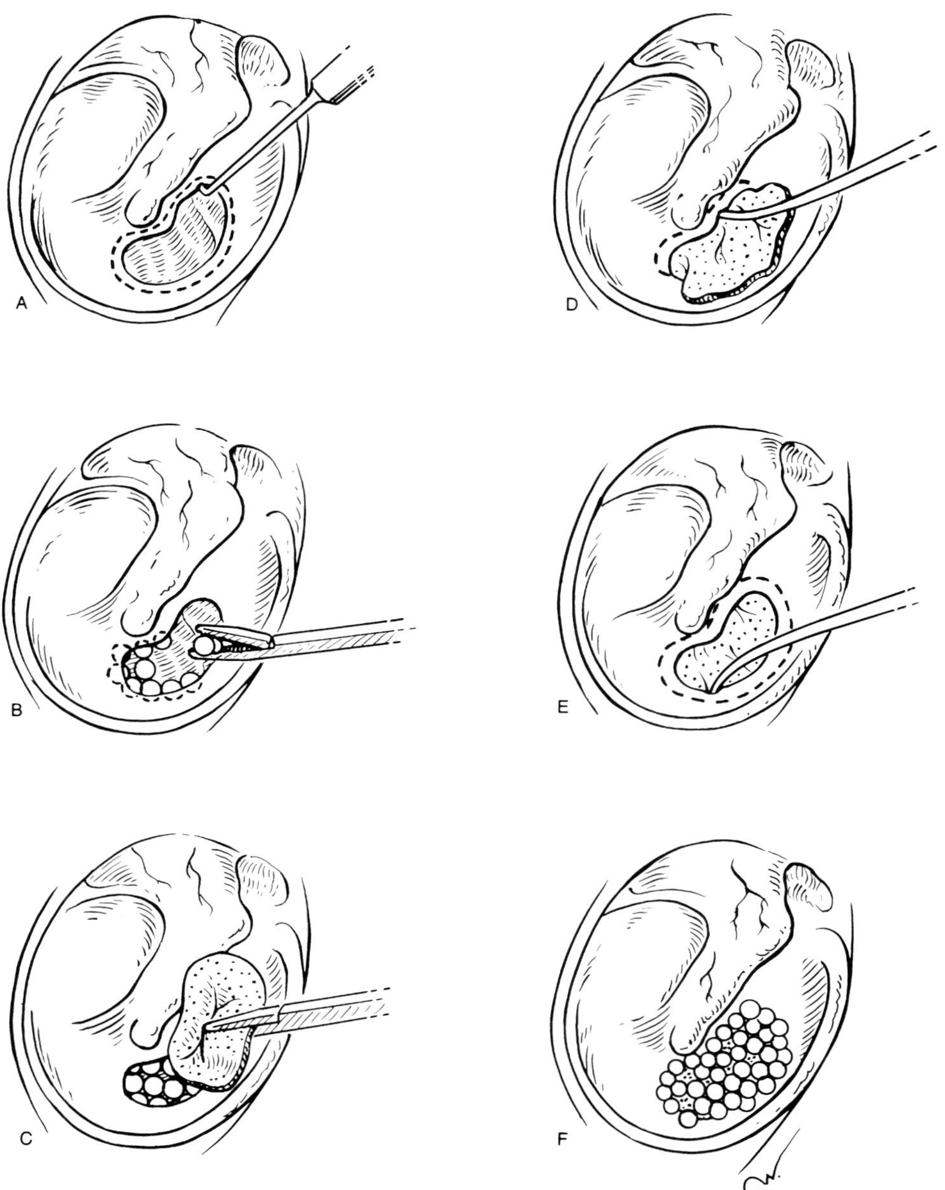

FIG. 3. Perichondrial underlay graft. **(A)** Edges of perforation are freshened, undersurface is roughened (extent indicated by *dotted lines*). **(B)** Middle ear is filled with saline-saturated collagen microdots. **(C)** Perichondrial graft is applied over perforation. **(D)** Edges of graft are tucked under using a Rosen needle. **(E)** Final adjustment of graft: circumferentially tucked under edges of perforation. **(F)** Graft site covered with thrombin-saturated collagen microdots.

entire tragus can be excised and perichondrium stripped off both surfaces. The cartilage is replaced in the surgical pocket, and the incision is closed with 4-0 nylon sutures. The middle ear is prepared by filling it through the perforation with saline-saturated collagen microdots. If preferred, the microdots can be saturated with nonototoxic ophthalmic antibiotic drops, such as sodium sulamyd. Care is taken to pack the anterior middle ear and ET area first, then the rest of the mesotympanum and hypotympanum. Although the size and location of the perforation limits visibility, the parts under and around the perforation are easily packed. The graft is trimmed to a size 3–4 mm larger than the perforation in every direction (ie, 6–8 mm larger in diameter). The graft is moistened with saline and placed on the lateral surface of the perforation, and the edges are circumferentially tucked under the perforation, using a Rosen needle. The latter surface is covered with collagen microdots saturated with either thrombin, antibiotic, or steroid drops. The ear canal is then filled with Bacitracin ointment (Glaxo Wellcome, Research Triangle, NC), a cotton fluff placed in the meatus, and an eye pad taped over the auricle.

This technique has advantages and disadvantages compared with conventional underlay tympanoplasty. The main disadvantages are the lack of a full middle ear exploration and reliance on the undersurface of the perforation to provide adherence and vascularization to the graft. The advantages are a simpler surgical set-up (small plastic set plus middle ear hook, Rosen needle, and elevator), graft available within the surgical field (no need for postauricular shave and incision), and shorter time required.

Myringoplasty and Ventilation Tube

With any of the above techniques, the surgeon may consider simultaneous placement of a ventilation tube. This may be useful if preoperative ET function is questionable (4). Even if ET function is close to normal, in the postoperative period there is often a temporary ET insufficiency due to middle ear mucosal edema or packing. A simultaneous tube can be placed if there is adequate tympanic membrane remaining at some distance from the perforation (5). Patients with questionable ET function who have failed office myringoplasty or have inadequate drum remnant for a conventional ventilation tube should probably be re-grafted with the simultaneous implantation of a subannular ventilation tube, a procedure requiring a tympanomeatal flap, and, hence, better performed in the operating room.

POSTOPERATIVE CARE

Oral antibiotics can be given perioperatively, at the surgeon's discretion. If used, they are probably most effective if begun the night prior to surgery, and continued for 5 days following surgery. The patient is given the usual postoperative instructions, cautioning against lifting, straining, sneezing, and nose-blowing. Follow-up visits should be done according to the surgeon's preferred routine.

REFERENCES

1. Belucci R: Basic considerations for success in tympanoplasty. *Arch Otolaryngol* 90:732, 1969.
2. Yanagisawa E: Infections of the ear. In: Lee KJ, ed. *Essential otolaryngology*, 4th ed. New York: Medical Examination Publishing Co., 1987.
3. Riedel CL, Wiley TL, Block MG: Tympanometric measures of ET function. *J Speech Hear Res* 30(2): 207–214, 1987.
4. Jahn AF: Chronic otitis media: Diagnosis and treatment. *Med Clin North Am* 75:1277–1291, 1991.
5. El-Gundy A: Manometric and endoscopic study of tubal function in drum perforation. *Am J Otol* 14(6):580–584, 1993.

PART 6

The Skin and Hair

Office-Based Surgery of the Head and Neck
Edited by Yosef P. Krespi, MD
Lippincott–Raven Publishers, Philadelphia © 1998

21

Double Eyelid Blepharoplasty: A Newly Modified Technique

Jeffrey M. Ahn and Philip T. Ho

Double eyelid blepharoplasty is the most commonly performed facial plastic surgery in Asian patients. Although traditionally thought of as a procedure done predominantly in the Far East (Korea, Japan, Hong Kong, Taiwan), Asian eyelid surgery has gained increasing popularity in the United States with the great influx of Asian immigration. According to United States Department of Commerce estimates, the Asian population in the United States has grown a consistent 4%–5% yearly, with a total projected Asian population of 12 million in the year 2000 and 17 million by 2010 (1). With such a population growth, it is incumbent on today's facial plastic surgeon to understand the many nuances of the Asian eyelid, including the varying anatomy, the various operational techniques, and the often subtle aesthetic goals that need to be achieved.

Double eyelid blepharoplasty involves the creation of an upper eyelid supratarsal fold or crease in an otherwise creaseless eyelid. This condition of having a single eyelid is reported to exist in almost 50% of the Asian population (2). Although extensively discussed in the Asian literature, the first article in the English literature discussing Asian eyelid surgery was in an article by Millard in 1955 that detailed field surgery in the Korean War (3). Later, in 1963, Fernandez, borrowing predominantly from Korean techniques, introduced the incisional double eyelid method to the English literature (4). He also mentioned, but did not advocate, the Japanese method of suture-only.

Double eyelid surgery has often been incorrectly labeled as "Westernization" of the Asian eyelid. Although it was true in the past that certain racial groups (Koreans) desired more round eyes like their European counterparts (3), the concept of dramatically changing the shape and ethnicity of eyelids is largely outdated in contemporary times. Instead, modern Asian blepharoplasty procedures attempt to create a greater aesthetic, more natural look within the context of individual and racial features. In Asian cultures, there is an appeal to have a subtle but definitive eyelid crease, which lends the appearance of a wider, brighter eye.

DIFFERING UPPER EYELID ANATOMIES: ASIAN VERSUS CAUCASIAN

The difference in appearance between Asian and Caucasian (Occidental) eyelids, and the various surgical techniques used to create eyelids, require an understanding of the anatomic differences in the upper eyelids (5–8). The Caucasian upper eyelid, from anterior to posterior just above the tarsal plate, consists of the following layers: skin, orbicularis oculi muscle, preseptal fat pad, orbital septum, preaponeurotic fat pad, levator palpebri superioris muscle, and aponeurosis, the Müllers muscle attaching superiorly to the tarsal plate, and conjunctiva. There is minimal subcutaneous tissue below the skin and minimal preseptal fat. The upper eyelid crease is formed just superior to the level (2–3 mm) of the tarsal plate, where the orbital septum and levator aponeurosis merge and levator fibers insert into the pretarsal orbicularis muscle, dermis, and skin. This fusion point also limits the preseptal (brow) and preaponeurotic fat to the upper lid above the crease.

In contrast, Asian eyelids differ in several anatomic areas that lend to the more full, fatty eyelid appearance that seemingly lacks the suprapalpebral fold. The usually scant subcutaneous layer is often more pronounced. Both the preaponeurotic fat and the preseptal fat (sometimes called retro-orbicularis oculi fat, or ROOF) layers are much more thick in Asians (9). Both fat layers also extend more prominently down into the pretarsal eyelid region because of the attenuation and lower fusion point of the levator aponeurosis with the orbital septum. This eyelid fullness is felt to obscure the appearance of any supratarsal folds present in Asians. Thus, when addressing the Asian eyelid for double eyelid blepharoplasty, the fullness created by the fat pads must often be reduced to create a distinctive supratarsal crease. The general lack of double eyelids in Asians is attributed to the diffuse and variable insertion of the levator aponeurosis in the orbicularis muscle and dermal layers of the pretarsal eyelid. Instead of crossing and inserting onto the anterior eyelid just above the level of the tarsal plate, the levator fibers become thin and often end blindly in the pretarsal layers with no definitive band attachment. Thus, no distinctive fold is usually found.

OTHER TECHNIQUES: INCISIONAL METHOD VERSUS SUTURE TECHNIQUE

Traditionally, there have been two main approaches to double eyelid blepharoplasty: the full incisional method and the suture technique. As the name implies, the incisional technique involves a nearly full-length incision in the upper eyelid skin, with resection of various combinations of eyelid skin, orbicularis muscle, and fat (preseptal or preaponeurotic) (2–4,10–20). The tarsal plate or levator aponeurosis is then sutured, usually permanently, to the pretarsal subcutaneous layers. Sometimes, various methods of epicanthoplasty (Z-plasty, M-flaps, skin incision extensions, and so forth) are integrated with the incisional blepharoplasties. Proponents of incisional methods believe that the various tissue layer resections are critical in creating permanent, aesthetically pleasing supratarsal folds. Resection of fatty and muscle tissue layers allows for better tarsal-dermal adhesion formation and better visualization of the newly formed creases. Drawbacks to these techniques include fairly invasive operations, long postoperative recoveries, greater potential for complications (such as asymmetry, scar formation, infection, and hematoma), and near-irreversibility. In addition, overly aggressive surgeons can create very unnatural-appearing eyelids, with deflated contours, abnormal wrinkling, and overly prominent creases.

The suture technique involves placing interrupted permanent sutures to allow the tarsal plate or levator aponeurosis to adhere to the pretarsal dermis, thereby creating supratarsal folds (10,11,13,21). Variations in methods have included the number of sutures and the use of various incisions in the skin or conjunctiva to facilitate suture placement. No tissue or skin resection is involved. Positive aspects of the suture methods include minimal invasiveness, ability to reverse or modify in the future, and speed of both the operation and postoperative recovery. Criticisms have focused on the long-term failure rate, the inability to address tissue excesses, and the resultant shallow folds created.

NEWLY MODIFIED TECHNIQUE: STEP-BY-STEP

In this chapter, we introduce a newly modified technique of double eyelid blepharoplasty that combines the strong points of both incisional and suture methods. Our method is recommended primarily for younger patients and those with minimal excess eyelid skin and fat. This modified method is not recom-

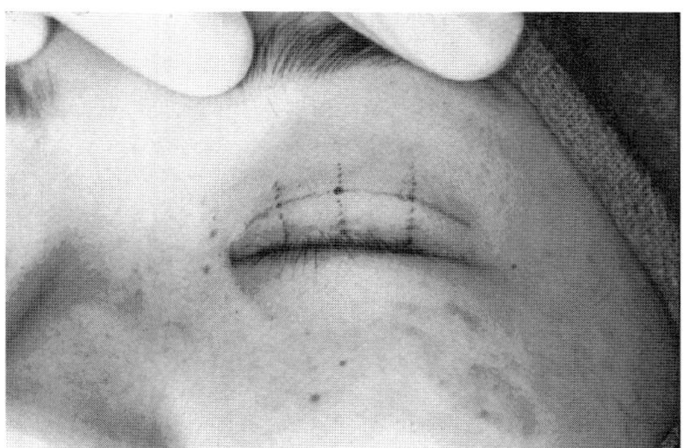

FIG. 1. Marking of supratarsal fold.

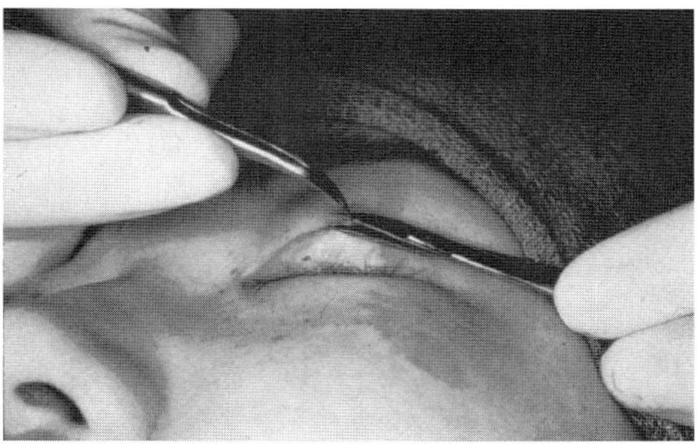

FIG. 3. Incision and dissection of the subcutaneous layer.

mended for older patients with prolapsing tissue layers, or for patients who have excessively thick or redundant eyelid tissues. Patients are fully evaluated preoperatively with a thorough history and physical examination. The patient's expectations and surgical options are fully discussed. The eyelids are evaluated and measured with the patient sitting upright (Fig. 1).

A thin wire is used to delineate the level of the new supratarsal folds with the patient's eyes both open and closed. This usually ranges between 5 and 10 mm above the ciliary border. The measured line is extended from above the level of the medial canthal corner to just medial of the lateral canthus, with a slightly higher height laterally. Instead of a complete linear skin incision, however, three to six interrupted stab incisions are made along the planned eyelid crease (Fig. 2). These incisions measure approximately 10–15 mm horizontally, and are often centered over the medial, central, and lateral limbus. Careful blunt dissection with tenotomy scissors is made through the subcutaneous layer and any excess fat is sparingly removed (Fig. 3). Orbicularis oculi muscle is spread apart along the fibers to reveal the preseptal or retro-orbicularis fat layer, which is usually prominent in Asians. By gently pushing on the eyelid small amounts of fat are extruded and then conservatively removed. Dissection is then continued deep to the orbital septum, which can be carefully transected. This exposes the preaponeurotic fat pads (medial and central), which can be sparingly removed (Fig. 4). The total amount

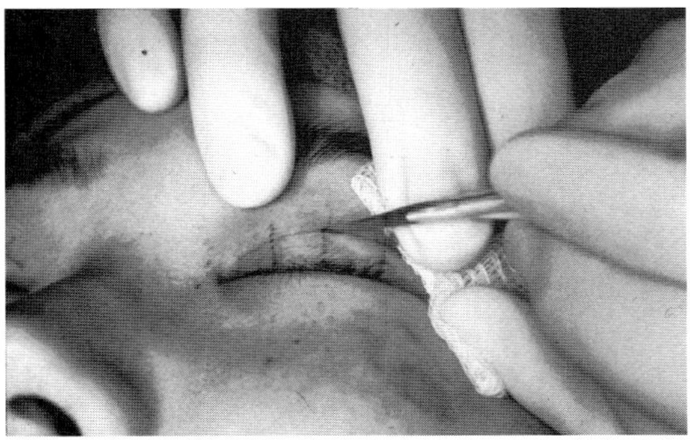

FIG. 2. Stab incision along the planned eyelid crease.

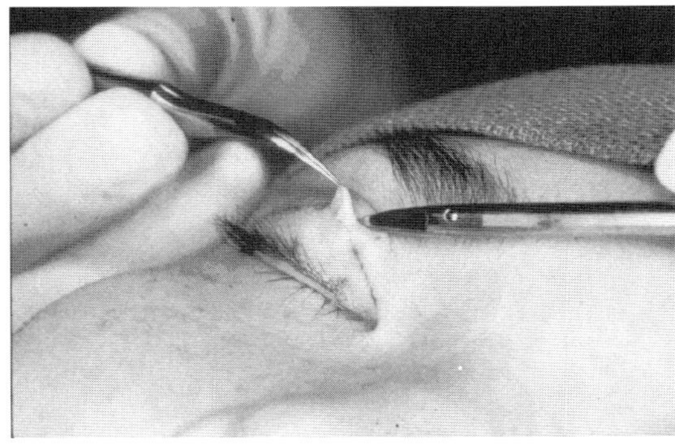

FIG. 4. Dissection and removal of excess fat.

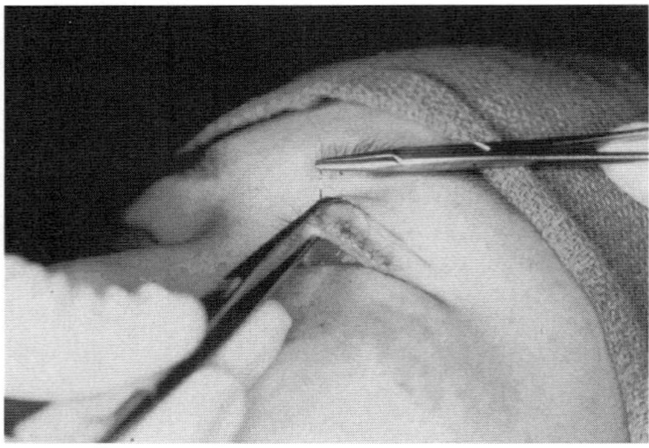

FIG. 5. Placement of interrupted permanent sutures at the new supratarsal fold.

of fat and muscle resected depends on careful preoperative and intraoperative evaluation. The levator aponeurosis is neither dissected nor violated.

Once sufficient soft tissue resection is completed through the skin stab incisions, the new supratarsal folds are created by using interrupted permanent sutures (Fig. 5). Interrupted 7-0 monofilament nylon sutures are passed through the skin incisions, through all layers of the upper eyelid, and out the conjunctiva. These sutures are then passed back through the conjunctiva and out the same skin incisions. The suture knots are secured and buried in the subcutaneous layer (Fig. 6), and the skin incisions are not closed.

No incisions are made in the conjunctiva. There are no reports of corneal abrasion or eye infection.

There are several subtle advantages of the newly modified method:

More aesthetic wound healing
Easily modified, extended, and possibly reversed
Less bleeding
Shorter operative time
Quicker postoperative recovery

Compared with incisional methods, the newly modified method involves less invasiveness and reduces chances of complications. The small skin stab incisions with no closure minimizes scarring and decreases operative and postoperative recovery time. Judicious excision of fat and soft tissue enhances the final eyelid appearance and improves adhesion of the new folds. The overall procedure incurs few complications. When compared with suture-only methods, the key advantage of the newly modified technique is the ability to resect fat and muscle. As previously noted, resection allows for better fold adhesions and better aesthetic lid contouring of the usually fatty Asian eyelid.

Overall, we have performed this modified double eyelid blepharoplasty on more than 100 patients with excellent results. With 6–24 months of follow-up, no loss of supratarsal folds has occurred, nor have there been reop-

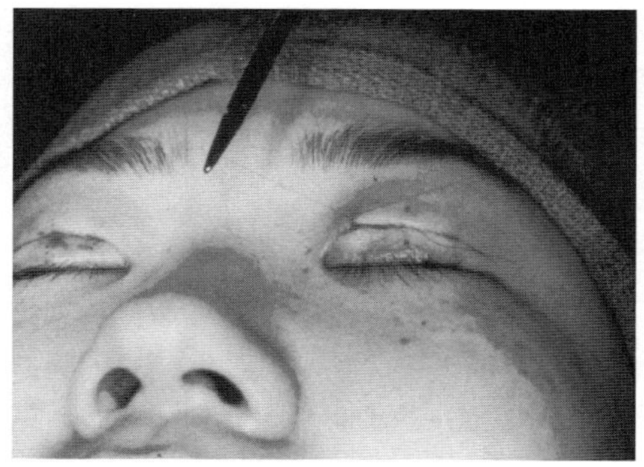

FIG. 6. Subcutaneous closure.

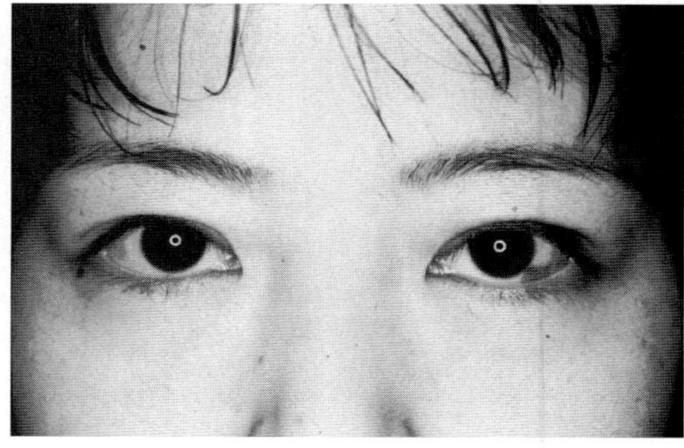

FIG. 7. Delayed subconjunctival hemorrhage.

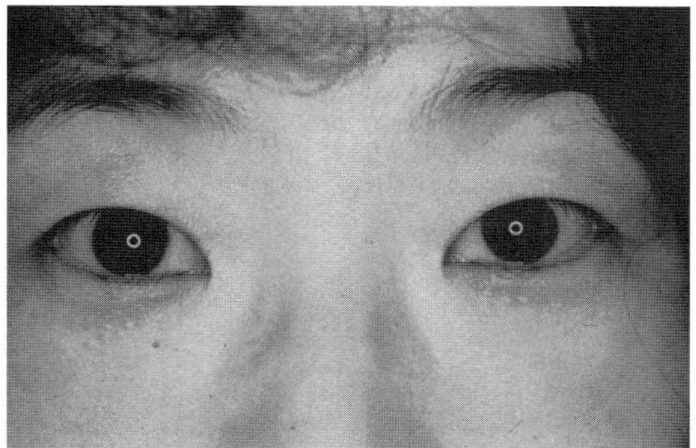

FIG. 8. Patient before double eyelid blepharoplasty.

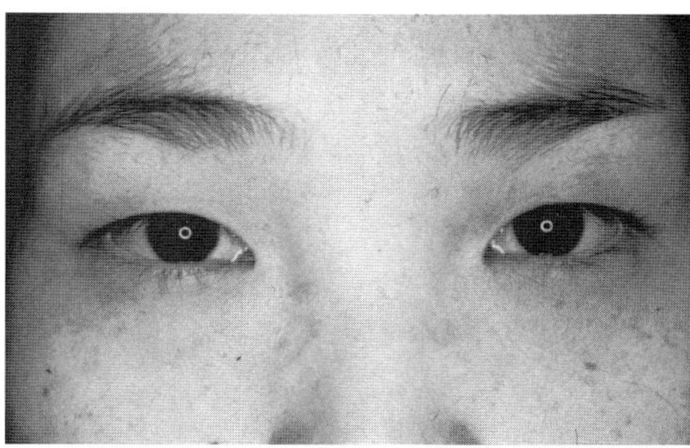

FIG. 10. Patient before double eyelid blepharoplasty.

erations for unsatisfactory results. Less than 10 complications have been reported, including one suture extrusion, approximately three cases of prolonged postoperative edema >2 weeks, and two episodes of delayed subconjunctival hemorrhage (Fig. 7). Preoperatively, as with any other blepharoplasty procedure, the potential complications are fully discussed; they include:

Suture extension
Prolonged postoperative edema
Subconjunctival hemorrhage
Asymmetry
Loosening of folds
Hematoma
Infection
Corneal abrasion

Before and after photos (Figs. 8–13) show that natural-appearing supratarsal folds are created with no abnormal wrinkles and contours. Although the eyes do appear wider and brighter with new supratarsal folds, the patient's ethnic characteristics are not lost.

CONCLUSION

Double eyelid blepharoplasty, the most common aesthetic operation among Asians, involves creating a natural-appearing, aesthetically pleasing, well-defined supratarsal eyelid fold. In contrast to the Caucasian double eyelid, the Asian single eyelid has attenuated, variable insertion of the levator aponeurosis into the pretarsal tissues, and increased

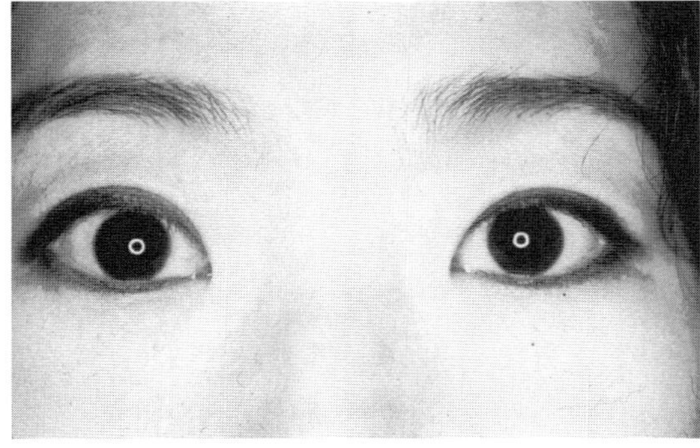

FIG. 9. Patient after double eyelid blepharoplasty has been performed.

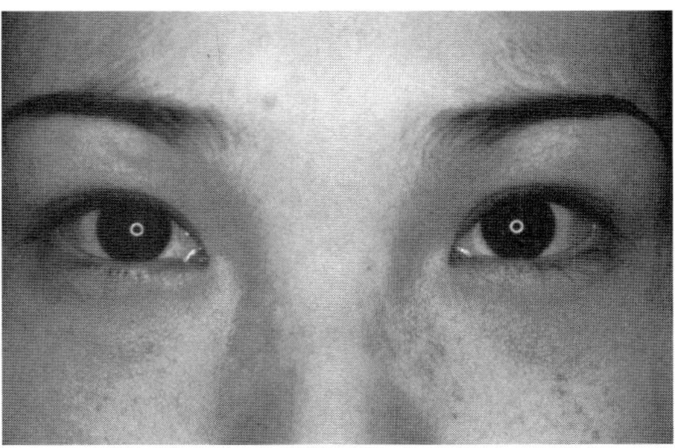

FIG. 11. Patient after double eyelid blepharoplasty has been performed.

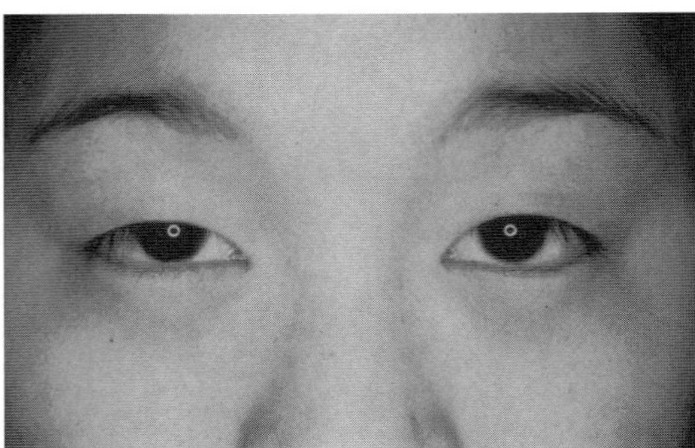

FIG. 12. Patient before double eyelid blepharoplasty.

amounts of fat tissue layers lower in the eyelid. Although all such surgery must be individually tailored, most double eyelid techniques reported in the literature have been generalized as either an incision method or a suture technique. We have introduced a new modified technique for double eyelid blepharoplasty that combines positive elements of both of these general methods. This is a rapid technique requiring only three small skin incisions, which allows for fat and soft tissue resection, and only three sutures to create natural, permanent, effective supratarsal folds. Because this method is minimally invasive, we believe it is ideal for double eyelid surgery in younger Asian patients with minimal eyelid fat.

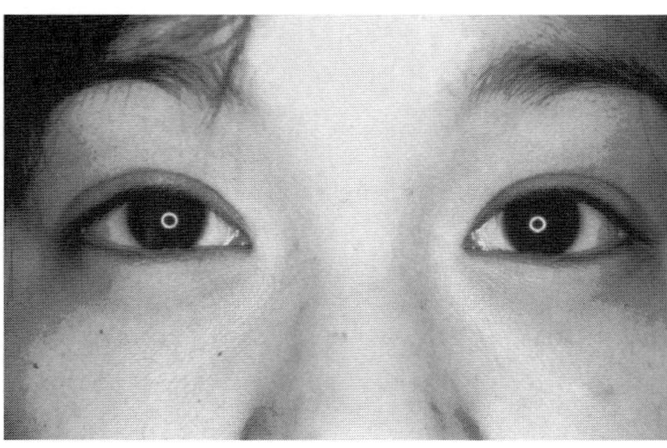

FIG. 13. Patient after double eyelid blepharoplasty has been performed.

REFERENCES

1. *Demographic profiles: A portrait of New York City's community districts from the 1980 and 1990 censuses of population and housing.* New York City: City of New York Department of City Planning, 1992.
2. *Statistical abstract of the United States.* Washington, DC: The United States Department of Commerce, 1995.
3. Amrith S: Oriental eyelids: Anatomical and surgical considerations. *Singapore Med J* 32:316–318. 1991.
4. Baek SM, et al: Oriental blepharoplasty: Single-stitch, nonincisional technique. *Plast Reconstr Surg* 83(2): 236–242, 1989.
5. Bang YH: The double-eyelid operation without supratarsal fixation. *Plast Reconstr Surg* 88(1):12–17, 1991.
6. Carraway JH: Surgical anatomy of the eyelids. *Clin Plas Surg* 14(4):693–701, 1987.
7. Castanares S: Classification of baggy eyelids deformity. *Plast Reconstr Surg* 59(5):629–633, 1977.
8. Chen WP-D: *Asian blepharoplasty.* Boston:Butterworth-Heinemann, 1995:192.
9. Choi AK: Oriental blepharoplasty: Nonincisional suture technique versus conventional incisional technique. *Facial Plastic Surgery* 10(1):67–83, 1994.
10. Constantinides MS, Adamson PA: Aesthetics of blepharoplasty. *Facial Plastic Surgery* 10(1):6–17, 1994.
11. Doxanas MT, Anderson RL: Oriental eyelids. *Arch Ophthalmol* 102:1232–1235, 1984.
12. Fernandez LR: Double eyelid operations in the Oriental in Hawaii. *Plast Reconstr Surg* 25(3):257–264, 1960.
13. Fernandez LR: The East Asian eyelid: Open technique. *Clin Plast Surg* 20(2):247–253, 1993.
14. Flowers RS: The art of eyelid and orbital aesthetics: Multiracial surgical considerations. *Facial Aesthetic Surgery* 14(4):703–721, 1987.
15. Flowers RS: Upper blepharoplasty by eyelid invagination. *Clin Plast Surg* 20(2):193–207, 1993.
16. Flowers RS, Flowers SS: Precision planning in blepharoplasty. *Clin Plast Surg* 20(2):303–310, 1993.
17. Hin LC: Oriental blepharoplasty: A critical review of technique and potential hazards. *Ann Plast Surg* 7(5): 362–374, 1981.
18. Hin LC: Unfavorable results in Oriental blepharoplasty. *Ann Plast Surg* 14(6):523–534, 1985.
19. Hiraga Y: The double eyelid operation and augmentation rhinoplasty in the Oriental patient. *Clin Plast Surg* 7(4):553–567, 1980.
20. Jelks GW, Jelks EB: Preoperative evaluation of the blepharoplasty patient. *Clin Plast Surg* 20(2):213–224, 1993.
21. Kanter WR, Wolfort FG: Blepharoplasty of the Asian eyelid. In: Wolfort FG, Kanter WR, eds. *Aesthetic blepharoplasty.* Boston: Little, Brown and Company, 1995:121–142.
22. Kontis TC, Papel ID, Larrabee WF: Surgical anatomy of the eyelids. *Facial Plastic Surgery* 10(1):1–5, 1994.
23. Matsunaga RS: Westernization of the Asian eyelid. *Arch Otolaryngol* 111:149–153, 1985.
24. May JW Jr: Retro-obicularis oculi fat (ROOF). *Plast Reconstr Surg* 86:682, 1990.
25. McCurdy JA Jr: Westernization of the Oriental eyelid. *Otolaryngol Head Neck Surg* 90:142–145, 1982.
26. McCurdy JA Jr: Cosmetic surgery of the Asian eye. In: *Cosmetic surgery of the Asian face.* New York: Thieme Medical Publishers, 1990:3–38.

27. McCurdy JA Jr: Upper lid blepharoplasty in the Oriental eye. *Facial Plastic Surgery* 10(1):53–66, 1994.
28. Millard DR Jr: Oriental peregrinations. *Plast Reconstr Surg* 16:319–336, 1955.
29. Millay DJ: Upper lid blepharoplasty. *Facial Plastic Surgery* 10(1):18–26, 1994.
30. Murakami CS, Plant RL: Complications of blepharoplasty surgery. *Facial Plastic Surgery* 10(2):214–224, 1994.
31. Mutou Y, Mutou H: Intradermal double eyelid operation and its follow-up results. *Br J Plast Surg* 25:285–291, 1972.
32. Sheen JH: A change in the technique of supratarsal fixation in upper blepharoplasty. *Plast Reconstr Surg* 59(6):831–834, 1977.
33. Shirakabe Y, et al. The double-eyelid operation in Japan: Its evolution as related to cultural changes. *Ann Plast Surg* 15(3):224–241, 1985.
34. Siegel RJ: Contemporary upper lid blepharoplasty: Tissue invagination. *Clin Plast Surg* 20(2):239–245, 1993.
35. Siegel RJ: Essential anatomy for contemporary upper lid blepharoplasty. *Clin Plast Surg* 20(2):209–212, 1993.
36. Watanabe K: Measurement method of upper blepharoplasty for Orientals. *Aesthetic Plast Surg* 17:1–8, 1993.
37. Weng CJ, Noordhoff MS: Complications of Oriental blepharoplasty. *Plast Reconstr Surg* 83(4):622–628, 1989.
38. Zubiri JS: Correction of the Oriental eyelid. *Clin Plast Surg* 8(4):725–737, 1981.

Office-Based Surgery of the Head and Neck
Edited by Yosef P. Krespi, MD
Lippincott–Raven Publishers, Philadelphia © 1998

22

Midface Lift

Z. Paul Lorenc

Ever since the beginning of the 20th century when Hollander and Lexer (1) performed the first-described rhytidectomies, an ever-increasing search for the perfect solution to the aging of the face has continued. More specifically, patients seek the solution to midface aging, primarily the descent of the malar fat pad, and the deepening of the nasolabial fold.

With recent advances, including aggressive lipectomy of the neck as well as the incorporation of the SMAS-platysma in recontouring of the face, an excellent result can be achieved. A straight jaw line with elimination of the jowls and a well-defined neck with a newly recreated acute cervicomental angle can be achieved. The rejuvenation of the upper third of the face, including standard blepharoplasties, transconjunctival lower blepharoplasties accompanied by laser resurfacing, and endoscopic brow lifts can control the aging process extremely well. Despite these successes in the upper and lower thirds of the face, even with up-to-date techniques, correction of the aging process of the midface has not proved to be consistently obtained or long-lasting. Several techniques used today include injection of fat into the nasolabial fold and redistribution of the SMAS flap (2); subperiosteal dissection of the midface with its suspension (3); and a technique used at our institution for the last 2 years that includes repositioning of the malar fat pad via limited facelift incisions. Our technique involves a limited retrotragal facelift incision, aggressive contouring of the neck using a suction cannula, wide SMAS flap undermining of the lower face to address the jowls and the neck contour, and repositioning plus suspension of the malar fat pad with suspension sutures.

MIDFACE ANATOMY

It is of paramount importance that a thorough understanding of the anatomy of the midface be grasped to adequately correct the aging forces of the midface. Since the original description by Mitz and Peyronie in 1976 (4), the SMAS has had a long history as a pertinent structure in correcting the aging face and neck. Based on the original article, the SMAS is defined as a tissue plane comprised of fibrous or muscle tissue that lies in direct continuity with the platysma muscle and lacks direct bone insertions. The SMAS was believed to be part of the fascia superficialis of the face that invests the muscles of facial expression.

Close approximation of the SMAS to the parotid fascia, however, has recently been questioned because it exhibits significant variation in consistency in different areas of the face. Two questions are of great clinical importance. Does the SMAS truly exist beyond the nasolabial fold? If so, where does it insert?

Recent anatomic studies support the concept that the medial extension of the SMAS beyond the nasolabial folds is contiguous with the superficial portion of the orbicularis oris muscle. This finding is of extreme surgical importance, because it means that unrestricted lateral pull on the SMAS actually will deepen the appearance of the nasolabial fold. This may be prevented if its insertion into the orbicularis oris muscle is interrupted, or the prolapsed malar fat pad is repositioned in a superolateral direction.

The second anatomic question of great importance in the midface is that of the extent

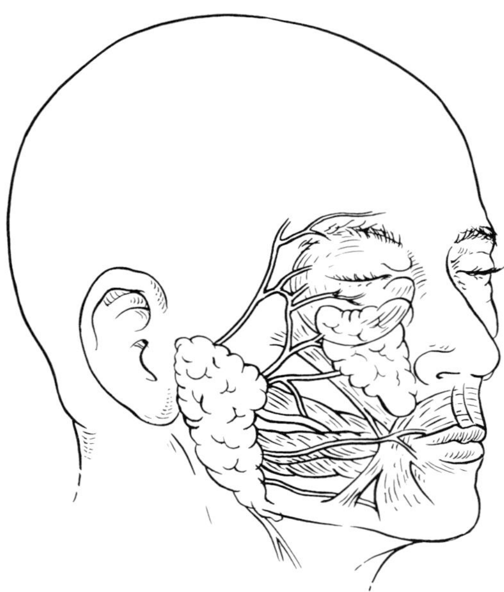

FIG. 1. Anatomic boundaries of the malar fat pad.

and the location of the malar fat pad. This thickened collection of subcutaneous fat is triangular in shape (Fig. 1) The base of the triangle is along the nasolabial crease. The superficial portion of the triangularly oriented malar fat pad is just deep to the inferior edge of the orbicularis oculi muscle. The lateral edge of the triangle is just medial to the zygomaticus major muscle. In a young patient, the apex of the triangular malar fat pad overlies the body of the zygoma. The superolateral location of the malar fat pad in youth accounts for the flat nasolabial fold as well as the aesthetically pleasing prominence of the zygomatic areas.

AGING OF THE MIDFACE

Aging of the face results from many complex interactions of internal and external forces. Among those most commonly attributed as external aging factors is the effect of sun exposure on the skin. As one ages, atrophy occurs in the skin, subcutaneous fat, connective tissue, and muscles. Ptosis of the soft

tissues of the face relative to that of the bony framework is the result of the downward pull of gravity. Facial folds and creases that develop as the patient ages result from obstruction of vertical descent of the soft tissue by stout fibrous attachments connecting the skin and fat to the underlying skeleton.

Facial muscle atrophy with age seems to play a relatively insignificant part in the aging of the midface. To reverse midface aging and achieve an overall youthful appearance, three factors must be carefully examined and addressed. These are:

1. Recognizing the importance of malar fat pad ptosis.
2. Correcting the prominent nasolabial fold.
3. Reversing the downturning of the oral commissure.

Unless all three factors are recognized and corrected the results of midface surgery will be short-lived. One also has to recognize that to redistribute the SMAS and the overlying fat and skin in an appropriate way, both must be addressed as two separate yet intimately involved units (5).

If the differential aging of the fascial component of the face as compared with the fat and skin components is not taken into account, midface ptosis will not be eliminated but only repositioned. As one ages, the malar fat pad, previously located in a lateral position, descends in an anterior medial and inferior direction. As the aging process continues, gravity draws the malar fat pad further down, stretching the network of its fibrous attachments. The malar fat pad is bunched up along the barrier present at the nasolabial crease, creating an even more pronounced nasolabial fold. At the same time, a tear trough is created, owing to the inferior descent of the malar eminence. With superior lateral repositioning of the malar fat pad, the aging changes can be reversed.

In the technique used at our institution, both wide undermining of the SMAS platysma flap and its repositioning in a superolateral direction allows for recontouring of the neck and elimination of the jowls. Addressing the malar

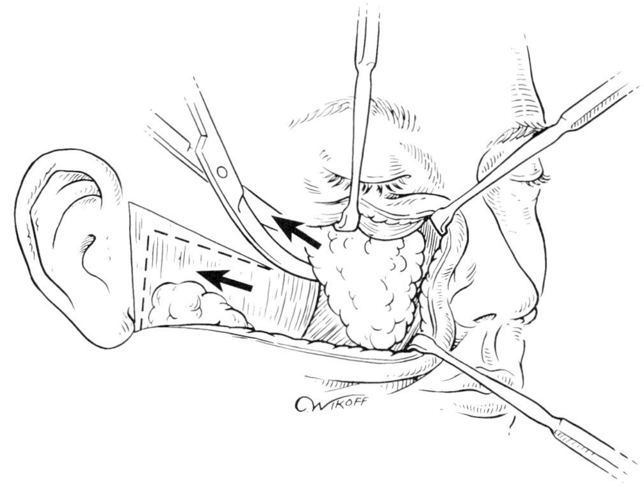

FIG. 2. Multi-vector midface lift. The malar fat pad is repositioned in a superolateral vector, different from the vector of pull on the SMAS-platysma flap.

fat pad as a separate entity and dissecting it separately from that of the SMAS allows for a multi-vectorial redraping of the midface (6). The multi-vectorial approach allows the forces of the pull vectors to be directed perpendicular to the tissues being elevated (Fig. 2). In the neck, the platysma is pulled more laterally than superiorly, and in the midface the malar fat pad is pulled more vertically than laterally. This differential pull results in a more uniform and natural rejuvenation of the midface, and allows for a more exact correction of midface ptosis.

SURGICAL PLANNING

Demand has recently increased for correction of the facial aging without the telltale signs of standard facelift scars. Surgical correction of midfacial ptosis is ideally suited to meet this demand. Owing to its limited incision and limited surgical dissection, the midface lift is ideally suited to be performed in the office on an outpatient basis. The technique described in this chapter is ideally suited for patients aged 45–50 years. In that particular subset of patients, midfacial ptosis with prominent nasolabial folds can be a concern. Typically in that age group, severe aging of the neck (ie, prominent medial platysma bands) is not found. Correction of the mild neck deformity, therefore, can be addressed via a limited lateral incision combined with aggressive suction lipectomy of the neck.

The procedure is typically performed in the office setting on an outpatient basis. After the preoperative markings have been made with the patient in an upright position, intravenous sedation is administered. Routinely, the face is injected with 0.5% of lidocaine solution with epinephrine (1:200,000). With the recent introduction of propofol in outpatient surgery, the patient can be maintained at a comfortable level throughout the procedure. Because no subperiosteal dissection is performed in the midface, no deeper anesthesia is necessary. Postoperatively, the patient is discharged from the office after being monitored by the nursing staff. Standard facelift dressing with accompanying Jackson Pratt drains are used; they are removed on the first postoperative visit at 24 hours. Routine use of a Medrol dose pack (The Upjohn Co., Kalamazoo, MI) together with antibiotics and oral pain medication is employed.

SURGICAL TECHNIQUE

The midface lift is performed using a standard incision extending from within the temporal hairline anterior to the helical rim, inferiorly in a retrotragal position, and circumscribing the ear lobule (see Fig. 2). No conchal sulcus incision is necessary unless marked laxity of the neck is present. Via the standard retrotragal incision, the skin is undermined widely using scissors. A temporal incision is made down to the subtemporoparietal fascial plane, where blunt, bloodless dissection is executed. Thus, a mesotemporalis that contains the frontal branch of the facial nerve is created.

Subcutaneous dissection extends to the lateral orbital rim. The lateral fibers of the orbicularis oculi muscle are elevated with the skin flaps. With scissors, the dissection continues over the malar fat pad and extends to the nasolabial crease as well as beyond the jowl and inferior to the angle of the mandible. In the neck, the dissection is elevated above the level of the platysma muscle down to the level of the inferior cervical crease. Suction-assisted neck lipectomy is performed as needed. The lateral border of the platysma muscle is identified and incised approximately 5 cm below the angle of the mandible. Dissection of the SMAS begins with a 4-cm transverse incision through the SMAS 1 cm below the inferior border of the zygomatic arch. This is continued as a vertical incision in the SMAS parallel to and approximately 0.5 cm anterior to the tragus (see Fig. 2). The incision is then carried inferiorly where it joins the previous platysma dissection. The SMAS flap is elevated medially to the anterior border of the parotid gland. After medial dissection of the platysma, the SMAS-platysma flap is advanced and rotated in a superolateral direction, excess tissue is excised, and the flap is sutured in place with absorbable sutures. The vector of the SMAS-platysma flap pull is parallel to the body of the mandible. Orienting the SMAS-platysma vector in this manner eliminates the jowls and redefines the cervicomental angle. Of interest is the observation that even an extremely strong pull of the SMAS-platysma flap does not correct midface ptosis.

Malar fat pad ptosis is then addressed. At the level of the malar prominence just superior to the origin of the zygomaticus major muscle and inferior to the lateral edge of the orbicularis oculi muscle, facelift scissors are inserted and spread in a vertical direction. After creating a wide portal of entry into the deep plane of the face, the malar fat pad is dissected from its deep attachments utilizing a combination of scissor and finger dissection. This is a well-defined, bloodless plane that can be followed medially to the nasolabial fold extending from the orbital rim to the nasal ala. This dissection is just superficial to the periosteum of the midface, and no motor branches of the facial nerves are encountered. With this maneuver, complete mobilization of the malar fat pad is accomplished. Using 3-0 Polydioxanone sutures, the apex of the malar fat pad is elevated and restored to the more superior and lateral position of youth. The vector of pull of the malar fat pad is perpendicular to the nasolabial fold. The divergence of the vectors of pull of the SMAS and the malar fat pad is apparent. The malar fat pad is sutured to the fascia of the malar eminence, which eliminates midface ptosis and corrects the downturning of the oral commissure. Once the SMAS-platysma and the malar fat pad flaps have been suspended in their proper positions, redraping, excision, and closure of the skin flaps are done in a standard manner. Jackson Pratt drains and facelift dressings are routinely used for 24 hours.

DISCUSSION

Because the face ages in a harmonious fashion, aging changes should be corrected in the same manner. Nothing is more distressing than a partially rejuvenated face that only magnifies the disharmony that is present. This disharmonious effect only accentuates the "facelifted" appearance. Procedures described in this chapter enable correction of midface ptosis to an extent similar to that of the upper and lower face.

Because laxity in the aging skin, fat, fibrous tissue, and muscle is unequal, these layers need to be separated and dealt with on an

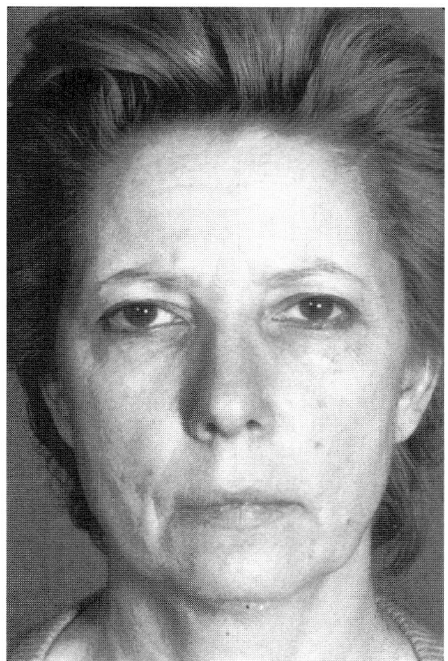 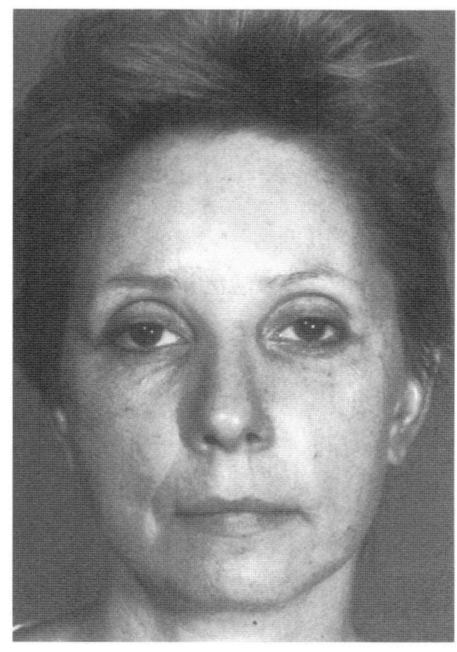

FIG. 3. (A) Preoperative and **(B)** 1-year postoperative photograph of a 53-year-old woman after a midface lift procedure and a blepharoplasty.

individual basis. In the procedure described, muscles, fat, fibrous fatty tissues, and skin ptosis correction is addressed on an individual basis. With this technique, the surgeon can vary the vectors and adapt them appropriately based on the aging of the face that has taken place.

Midface rejuvenation by repositioning the malar fat pad can achieve a youthful appearance that is routinely obtained in the upper and lower thirds of the face and neck. The ptotic midface is mobilized and repositioned along vectors to recreate a youthful appearance. The malar eminence is re-established, the deepened nasolabial folds are corrected, and the downturned oral commissure is raised. Except for a slight increase in midfacial edema, the complication rate as compared with a standard facelifting procedure has not increased. The aesthetic improvements are dramatic and patient satisfaction is high (Fig. 3).

REFERENCES

1. Larson DL: An historical glimpse of the evolution of rhytidectomy. *Clin Plast Surg* 22:207, 1995.
2. Robbins LB, Brothers DB, Marshall DM: Anterior SMAS plication for the treatment of prominent nasomandibular folds. *Plast Reconstr Surg* 96:1279, 1995.
3. Ramirez OM: Endoscopic full facelift. *Aesthetic Plastic Surg* 18:363, 1994.
4. Mitz V, Peyronie M: The SMAS in the parotid and cheek area. *Plastic Reconstr Surg* 58:80, 1976.
5. Ivy EJ, Lorenc ZP, Aston SJ: Is there a difference? A prospective study comparing lateral and standard SMAS face lifts with extended and composite rhytidectomies. *Plast Reconstr Surg* 98:1135, 1996.
6. Owsley JQ: Lifting the malar fat pad for correction of prominent nasolabial folds. *Plast Reconstr Surg* 91:463, 1993.

Office-Based Surgery of the Head and Neck
Edited by Yosef P. Krespi, MD
Lippincott–Raven Publishers, Philadelphia © 1998

23

Endoscopic Forehead Plasty

Z. Paul Lorenc

Facial expressions in the human play an integral part in conveying messages and feelings, and aesthetic surgeons have to be keenly aware of this. Surgical procedures that specifically alter the patient's appearance should only be performed when the benefits far outweigh the possible drawbacks and complications. This is especially true when a proven and accepted technique such as a coronal brow lift has been performed successfully since its original description in 1926 by Hunt (1).

Unless we can promise our patients that the results of a new technique will be the same as or better than those obtained with a standard technique, we should refrain from using that technique. Ideally, a new technique also should decrease the surgical time, decrease trauma to the tissues, reduce expense, and make the postoperative recovery easier on the patient.

We have used endoscopes in aesthetic surgery of the face at our institution since 1993 with excellent results. Because the endoscopic set-up has become much more compact and simple to operate, it is ideally suited to use in an office-based surgical facility.

Endoscopy (in Greek, meaning "to look within") was first described by Hippocrates for the examination of the rectum with a very primitive endoscope-speculum. Much has changed since the time of the first endoscope; yet, it is difficult to understand why endoscopic techniques were not introduced into aesthetic surgery sooner. The basic concepts of endscopy (ie, observation and manipulation of tissues at a distance from the incision site) remain the same regardless of the surgical specialty. Endoscopic techniques have many advantages. Minimized incisions markedly lessen disruption of the blood vessels and disruption of the lymphatic channels, which, in turn, decreases postoperative edema and reduces recovery time. The access incisions can be placed distal to the area of surgery, resulting in their being easily camouflaged. They can be placed in a hair-bearing area, which provides a significant aesthetic advantage. Because of the decreased amount of dissection and flap elevation, less raw surface is created, thereby decreasing the chances of seroma formation. The intense illumination and magnification of the endoscope enhances visualization of vital structures, such as the supratrochlear and supraorbital nerves, thus making it easier to preserve them, when required.

A number of unique requirements present themselves when endoscopic aesthetic surgery of the face is performed. Because most of the aesthetic surgical procedures of the face take place in the subcutaneous tissue, creating an optical cavity is of paramount importance. Insufflation of facial tissues with gas or instillation of fluid, as is done in the joint, is not practical or feasible in the face. Creating an optical cavity, therefore, must be done either with internal supports, such as an endoretractor, or by external traction, such as traction sutures. The simple concept of traction and counter-traction that is taken for granted when open techniques are utilized must be carefully studied and examined when applied to endoscopic facial surgery. Graspers, hooks, dissectors, cannulas, elevators, or external sutures can be used to create an optical cavity.

FUNCTIONAL ANATOMY OF THE FOREHEAD

Surgeons must be extremely familiar with the anatomy of the area on which they operate. In-depth knowledge of the anatomy is helpful and necessary when using open techniques, but it becomes even more important when performing endoscopic surgery. The forehead anatomy is relatively simple, yet no reference was made in the literature to the complex spatial relationship of the sensory nerves until 1993 (2). Unlike the sensory innervation, forehead musculature anatomy has been well described (3).

In general, the muscles of facial expression are referred to as cutaneous muscles that lie within the layers of the superficial fascia. These muscles originate from the underlying bone or fascia and insert onto the deep surface of the skin. The frontalis muscles are two thin paired quadrilateral muscles without bony attachments. These two muscles are integral parts of the occipitofrontalis muscle complex. The medial fiber extensions of the frontalis muscles are continuous with those fibers of the procerus muscle; the lateral fibers blend with the corrugator supercilii and the orbicularis oculi muscles. This muscular complex is relatively superficial and is located deep to the subcutaneous tissue of the forehead with sensory innervation interposed between. The orbicularis oculi muscle arises from the nasal part of the frontal bone and the frontal process of the maxilla. Muscle fibers from the orbital part of the orbicularis oculi muscle insert into the eyebrow skin, becoming the depressor supercilii muscle. The procerus muscle is a musculofascial slip that arises from the fascia of the lateral aspect of the nasal bones, inserting into the skin of the lower forehead as well as interdigitating with the caudal portion of the frontalis muscle. The paired corrugator supercilii muscles, which are pyramidal in shape, are located deep to the frontalis and the orbicularis oculi muscles. The corrugator muscles arise from the periosteum of the medial portion of the superciliary arch and insert into the deep surface of the eyebrow skin (3).

The corrugator supercilii muscles are interposed between the two main sensory nerves of the forehead, the supraorbital and the supratrochlear. A study of 20 consecutive patients undergoing a coronal lift was undertaken at our institution (4). The results showed a remarkably constant spatial relationship between the supraorbital and the supratrochlear nerves with respect to each other and to the midline. The average distance from the midline to the exit of the supraorbital nerve from the skull was 2.7 cm. The distance from the midline to the exit of the supratrochlear nerve was 1.7 cm; its point of exit from the skull averaged 0.8 cm anterior to that of the supraorbital nerve (Fig. 1). This spatial relationship is of great importance, specifically when an endoscopic forehead lift is performed. Knowing the nerves' location allows quick identification and preservation.

The frontal branch of the facial nerve provides the motor innervation of the forehead musculature. The frontal branch of the facial nerve is different in that, unlike the others that lie beneath the facial fascial layers, it assumes a rather superficial course once it crosses over the zygomatic arch. The frontal branch traverses the zygomatic arch at a point represented approximately as the midpoint of a line drawn from the tragus to the lateral canthus. At that point, the frontal branch is superficial, running within the substance of the SMAS just on the deep surface of the temporoparietal fascia. In its distal course, it pierces through the temporoparietal fascia to innervate the frontalis muscle on its deep surface. With wide undermining of the lateral forehead tissues, it is apparent that extreme care must be taken not to injure the frontal branch of the facial nerve. The vascular supply of the forehead is one of axial classification; it is composed of the supraorbital, supratrochlear, and superficial temporal arterial vessels.

The process of aging is one of constant change that begins with the first breath. To understand the aging process, one has to comprehend the function of the facial muscles. A very complex dynamic interplay occurs between the actions of the static forces, such as

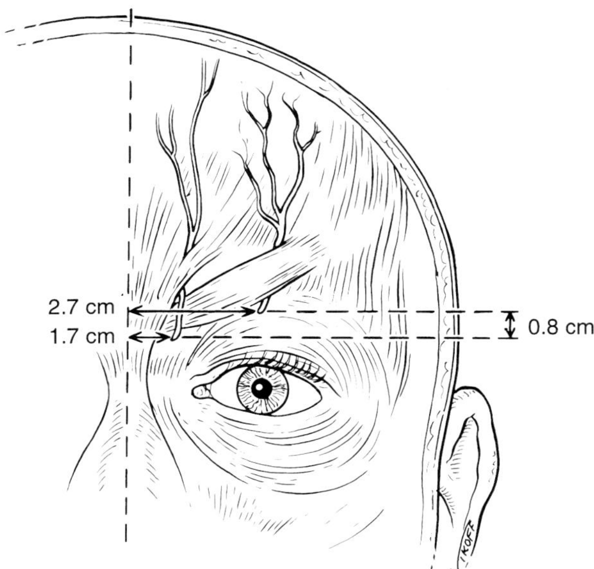

FIG. 1. A representation of the constant spatial relationship between the supraorbital and supratrochlear nerves.

gravity, and the periosteal attachments versus those of the actively contracting muscles of the forehead. This is coupled with the aging process and its constant changes to the elasticity of the eyebrows and the forehead skin. In the forehead, the frontalis muscles are the dominant elevators of the brow. The other previously described muscles act as strong depressors of the medial, mid, and lateral portions of the eyebrows. The presence and function of strong periosteal attachments at the level of the orbital rim must be recognized. It is necessary that these be completely released to elevate the forehead and the brows. As the aging process continues, the skin of the forehead undergoes changes that cause the position of the eyebrows to descend. This is consciously and subconsciously counteracted by the patient actively contracting the frontalis muscles to elevate the brow and maintain unobstructed vision. This constant dynamic battle results in transverse forehead rhytids present only during active contraction, but eventually leads to permanent transverse grooving of the forehead. Excessive activity of the corrugator supercilii muscles causes vertical rhytids of the glabella. Contraction of the procerus muscle results in horizontal rhytids at the root of the nose. As the activity of the depressor muscles becomes more accentuated, the brow descends further and the patient attempts further contraction of the frontalis muscle, which results in increasingly deeper rhytids of the forehead.

Based on recently increased knowledge of the physiology and dynamics of the forehead, one would have to assume that ablation of the depressor muscles of the eyebrows would result in a more cephalad resting position. Depressor muscle ablation, in conjunction with a radical and complete release of periosteal attachments at the level of the orbital rim and complete freeing of the temporal line of fusion, allows a more cephalad positioning of the eyebrows. These techniques also markedly improve the rhytids of the forehead and glabella (5).

EQUIPMENT AND INSTRUMENTATION

Minimally invasive surgical techniques require equipment that is new and relatively expensive. The recent exponential growth and development of endoscopic equipment, and its decreased size and more compact appear-

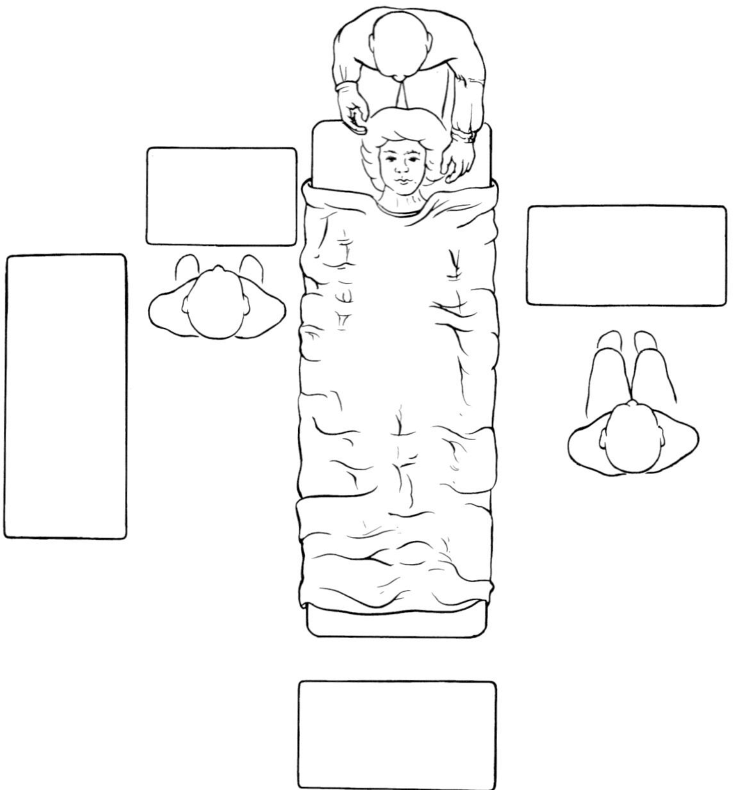

FIG. 2. Operating room set-up. Video monitor is positioned at the foot of the surgical table.

ance, make endoscopic equipment easily incorporated into office-based surgery. Furthermore, market forces have markedly decreased the price of endoscopic instrumentation.

Endoscopic equipment can be divided into two major groups: equipment needed to visualize structures and equipment needed for instrumentation of structures. Instruments included in a compact unit necessary for visualization are: video camera, camera control unit, light source, 13-in monitor, fiberoptic cable, 5-mm 30° endoscope with its encasing cannula, and documentation devices, such as a photographic camera or a videocassette recorder. Instrumentation devices include scalp dissectors, periosteal elevators, neurovascular dissectors, endoscopic scissors, endoscopic graspers, and endoscopic suction devices. With these instruments and a contact

diode laser, one can execute a complete endoscopic forehead plasty.

All of the visualizing equipment is placed on a compact mobile stand at the foot of the operating table for easy visualization. Endoscopic dissectors are positioned routinely on a mayo stand (Fig. 2).

SURGICAL TECHNIQUE

Skin Markings

After the patient has been placed in a supine position, a marking pen is used to outline the procedure area, including the midline of the forehead and the trajectory of the frontal branch of the facial nerve. At the level of the orbital rim, the proposed exit of the supraorbital and the supratrochlear nerves are outlined at 2.7 and 1.7 cm from the midline, respectively. The more anterior point of emergence of the supratrochlear nerve (0.8 cm) is also indicated. Next, the incision sites and the area to be undermined are marked. Two longitudinal paramedian incisions, which are used in this technique, are marked 2 cm lateral to the midline just within the hairline, extending 2 cm in a posterior direction. The temporal incisions are then marked. These transverse temporal incisions are marked approximately 2 cm within the temporal hairline and measure 2–3 cm in length. They are placed just lateral to the temporal line of fusion. If midfacial dissection is planned, an incision in a lateral crow's foot measuring 1.0 cm is also marked.

ANESTHESIA

Because endoscopic forehead plasty is routinely performed on an ambulatory basis, monitored intravenous sedation is used. After preoperative sedation by the anesthesiologist, an intravenous propofol drip is started. The incision sites as well as the posterior scalp are then injected using a solution of 0.5% lidocaine with epinephrine (1:200,000). Routine injection of the orbital rim is avoided because tissue staining can result from local infiltration. The surgeon sits at the head of the table. The anesthesiologist is to the patient's left, the scrub nurse is on the patient's right, and the monitor is at the foot of the bed (see Fig. 2).

DISSECTION

After the patient has achieved a proper level of sedation, previously outlined incisions are made. The paramedian incisions are carried down to the subperiosteal level. At this point, blind dissection of the posterior scalp in the subperiosteal plane is carried out using a wide scalp dissector.

A wide complete release of the posterior scalp to the level of the vertex is made to facilitate instrumentation through minimized in-

cisions. The temporal incisions are then made down to the temporalis muscle fascia. In this avascular plane, blunt dissection is made anteriorly and posteriorly using a blunt elevator. Blind dissection of the anterior forehead is performed carefully in a subperiosteal plane extending to approximately 1 cm above the level of the orbital rim. At this point, a 30°, 5-mm endoscope with its cannula sleeve is introduced. To achieve complete mobilization of the forehead and the scalp, a wide scalp elevator is used to release the temporal line of fusion. The dissection is always carried out in a lateral to medial direction with the endoscope being placed through the paramedian incision and the elevator through the temporal ones. This is done to avoid entering the bloody subtemporalis muscle fascia plane if dissection proceeds from medial to lateral. Next, the temporal line of fusion of the right and left sides of the patient is released. Through the two paramedian incisions, the subperiosteal plane is completely dissected to the level of the orbital rim under direct vision. Routinely, this is a highly illuminated avascular bloodless plane that separates without difficulty.

Next, the periosteal attachments at the level of the orbital rim extending from the left to the right frontozygomatic suture must be completely released. This can be done using either endoscopic scissors or a diode laser (Cynosure, Boston, MA). Using a malleable endoscopic waveguide, a 600 μ flexible fiber is introduced. With a continuous setting of 12 W, the periosteum is completely released in a bloodless atraumatic fashion (Fig. 3). After a complete periosteal release, with the laser in the OFF position, the waveguide can be used to separate the edges of the periosteum to achieve an approximate 1.0-cm gap. Lateral dissection of the orbital rim extending to the level of the zygoma is then done under direct vision using periorbital subperiosteal dissectors. After complete visualization of the supraorbital and the supratrochlear nerves bilaterally, the diode laser is used to ablate the interposed corrugator muscles and the medially located procerus muscle. Care is taken to ablate the muscles to the point where subcuta-

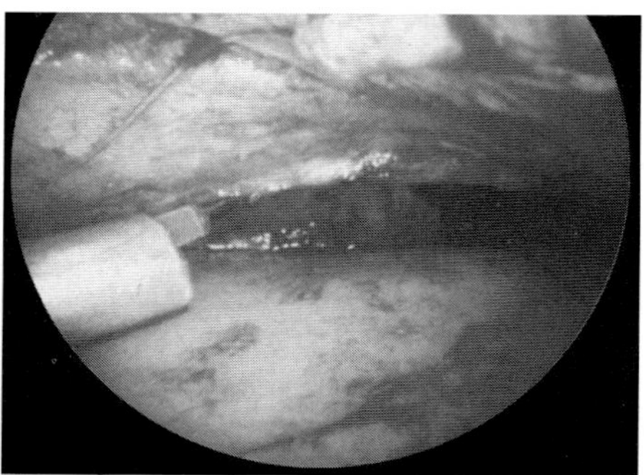

FIG. 3. Endoscopic view of periosteal release using the diode laser.

neous tissue is visualized through the endoscope. If any bleeding occurs during this maneuver, the laser is used for coagulation.

Thorough and complete ablation of the depressor muscles is necessary, because a mere myotomy of the depressor muscles would result in recurrent activity within several months and recurrent brow ptosis. The endoscope is withdrawn after completing release of the periosteal attachments and ablation of the depressor muscles. At this point, one can observe that with digital manipulation the forehead and the brow position can be markedly elevated without exerting significant force.

During the initial developmental stages of endoscopic forehead lift, it became apparent that fixation of the forehead and brows in a more cephalad position is of paramount importance. Several methods can be used for fixation, including temporary transcortical titanium screws, absorbable Polydioxanone Kirschner wires, and internal suspension sutures via cortical bone tunnels (Fig. 4). Any of the three methods will provide adequate fixation of the brow until sufficient healing has taken place and the brow is maintained in its new position. Typically, an elevation of 3–4 mm of the brow is achieved. Depending on the desired vector of pull, medial or lateral,

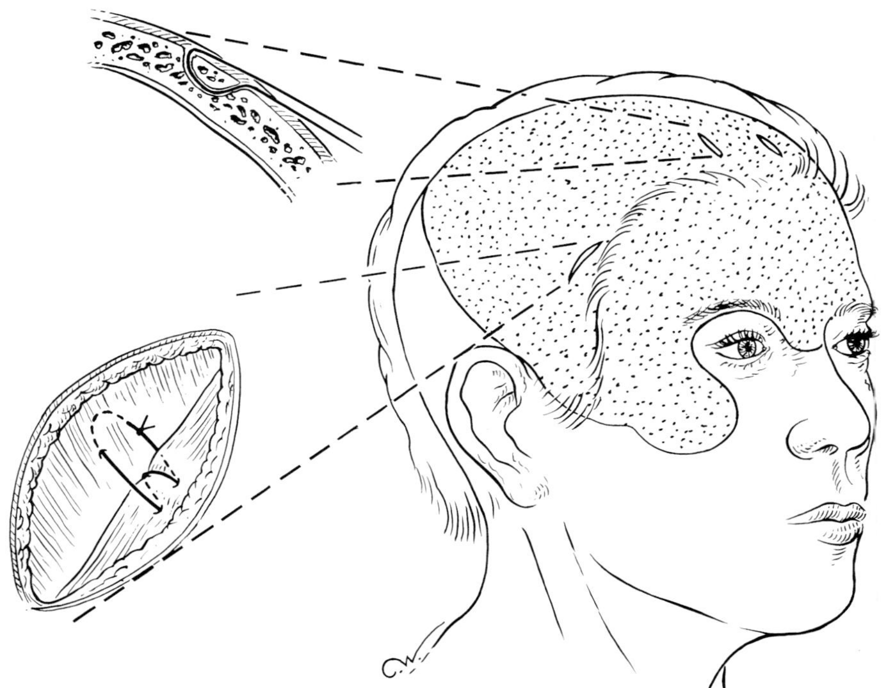

FIG. 4. Drawing depicting the extent of subperiosteal undermining plus techniques of brow suspension.

elevation can be done in a preferential manner. If more lateral elevation of the tail of the eyebrow is required, a stronger pull is applied perpendicular to the temporal incision.

Before the temporal incisions are approximated, a figure-of-eight suture is placed from the galea to the temporalis muscle fascia proper (see Fig. 4). This maneuver elevates the lateral portion of the brow, and it can be adjusted accordingly. All scalp incisions are then closed using subcutaneous 3-0 plain gut sutures. No drains are used. At the completion of the operation, opthalmic ointment is placed into the conjunctival sacks and a standard facelift dressing is applied.

POSTOPERATIVE CARE

Patients are maintained in the recovery area for 1–2 hours postoperatively with continuous ice packs to the forehead and periorbital area. Patients are then discharged from the office and placed on oral antibiotics, pain medication as needed, and a Medrol dose pack (The Upjohn Co., Kalamazoo, MI). Patients are instructed to ambulate the day of surgery and maintain head elevation at 30°. The first postoperative visit is at 48 hours, at which time the dressing is removed and bacitracin ointment is applied to the incision sites. Full activity, except for strenuous exercise, is resumed within 3–5 days after surgery (Fig 5).

COMPLICATIONS

Currently, long-term results of endoscopic forehead plasty are similar to those performed by conventional methods. Early results appear to have been less long-lasting due to the fact that approaches to the endoscopic forehead lift were performed initially in the subgaleal plane. The importance of complete periosteal attachment release as well as rigid "fixation" of the brow in a more cephalad position were not initially fully understood. Since endoscopic forehead plasty has moved to the subperiosteal plane and routine radical release of the periosteal attachments is performed, elevation is maintained without difficulty. Major complications as experienced with coronal forehead lifts (eg, areas of alopecia, pruritus, and difficult wounds) have not been seen with minimal access surgery. Of the initial 100 cases treated, we observed 2 of temporary weakness of the frontal branch of the facial nerve that completely resolved within 6 weeks. This was likely due to the aggressive undermining in the area of the zygomatic

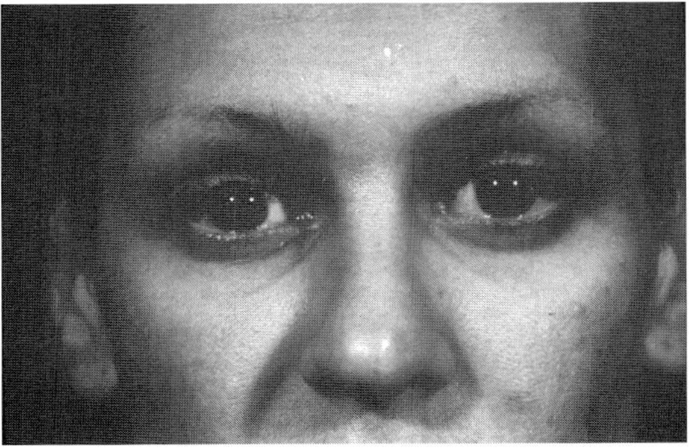
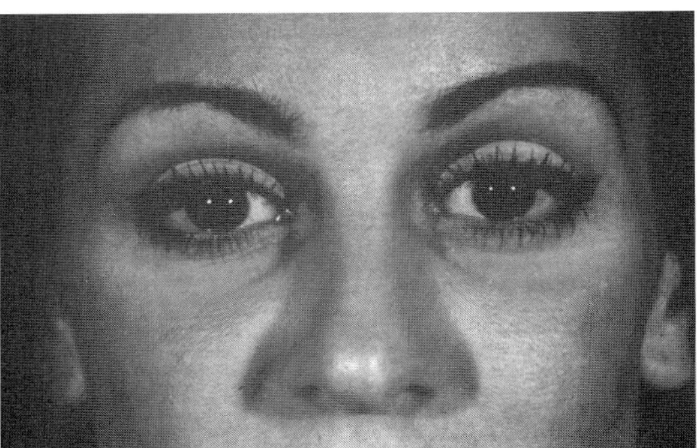

A   B

FIG. 5. (A) Preoperative and **(B)** postoperative photos of a 36-year-old woman who underwent an endoscopic laser forehead plasty. No blepharoplasty was performed.

arch. Interestingly, although the access incisions have been markedly minimized, moderate forehead edema persists owing to the aggressive subperiosteal undermining. Because new fixation methods have evolved and cortical tunnels are used, difficulties with alopecia have been eliminated.

Overall, endoscopic laser-assisted forehead plasty is a rewarding procedure for the patient with minimal risks. It can be performed without any difficulty on an outpatient basis in an office setting.

REFERENCES

1. Connell BF, Lambros VS, Neurohr GH: The forehead lift techniques. *Aesthetic Plast Surg* 13:217, 1989.
2. Lorenc ZP, Ivy EJ, Aston SJ: *The course and relations of sensory nerves of the forehead: Study in vivo.* Presented at the 26th Annual Meeting of the American Society for Aesthetic Plastic Surgery, Boston, MA, 1993.
3. Clemente CD: *Anatomy: A regional atlas of the human body.* Philadelphia: Lea & Febiger, 1975.
4. Lorenc ZP, Ivy EJ, Aston SJ: Neurosensory presentation in endoscopic forehead plasty. *Aesthetic Plast Surg* 19:411, 1995.
5. Ramirez OM: Endoscopic techniques in facial rejuvenation. *Aesthetic Plast Surg* 18:141, 1994.

Office-Based Surgery of the Head and Neck
Edited by Yosef P. Krespi, MD
Lippincott–Raven Publishers, Philadelphia © 1998

24

Laser Blepharoplasty and Laser-Assisted Endoforehead Lift

Gary J. Nishioka and Wayne F. Larrabee, Jr

A variety of lasers have been used successfully in blepharoplasty surgery, including the carbon dioxide (CO_2), potassium-titanyl phosphate (KTP), and sculptured-tip neodymium: yttrium-aluminum-garnet (Nd:YAG) lasers (1–9). The decision to perform blepharoplasty surgery using either conventional techniques (augmented with fine-tipped cautery or radio frequency devices) or laser is a decision made according to surgical preference. The controversy regarding lasers in blepharoplasty revolves around their advantages and disadvantages when compared with conventional cold steel techniques, which still serve as the gold standard. The advantages of the laser are improved hemostasis, reduced operative time, and reduced pain, swelling, and ecchymosis in the early postoperative period. An obvious economic advantage is marketability. Disadvantages over cold steel techniques include cost, moderate learning curve, proper operating room facility, appropriately trained staff, issues of patient and staff protection, anesthesia considerations, and possible slower wound healing and worse scarring of skin incisions. Based on a recent survey, it is clear that there is a strong recent trend toward laser blepharoplasty with the CO_2 laser as the most commonly used laser. As laser technology continues to evolve and as new generations of lasers and laser instrumentation are developed, the laser may eventually become the universally preferred technique.

Laser surgery requires a properly equipped operative suite that satisfies the American National Standards Institute's guidelines for laser safety, a formal laser protocol for patient and staff safety, trained personnel including a laser nurse, and an anesthesiologist experienced in laser cases if anesthesia is administered. Selection of the specific laser to be used is not discussed in this chapter. However, the CO_2 laser is the most commonly employed laser using either the conventional continuous wave or the newer high-peak power, short-pulsed laser.

Patient evaluation and selection is the same as for the conventional blepharoplasty patient. However, for the lower eyelid the surgical technique best suited for the laser is transconjunctival. A small to moderate amount of excess skin can be removed with the pinch technique. If rhytids without excess skin are the principal problem they can be removed by resurfacing with either a 35% trichloroacetic acid (TCA) chemical peel or with a CO_2 skin resurfacing laser. Some surgeons use phenol but we prefer the former modalities. Recently, development of the erbium:YAG skin resurfacing laser now provides another option. If a significant amount of lower lid skin and muscle must be removed we perform a standard cold steel transcutaneous blepharoplasty. Laser application in this setting can be and is done by some authors, but it is more awkward owing to the eyelashes and angle of dissection.

UPPER BLEPHAROPLASTY TECHNIQUE

The patient is marked preoperatively and if intravenous sedation is used a topical local anesthetic is administered to the conjunctiva. After the patient is prepared and draped local infiltrative anesthesia is given. A David-Baker or modified Erhardt lid clamp is then placed to retract the eyelid and protect the cornea (Fig. 1). It should be noted that these clamps tend to flatten and compress the eyelid structures. This creates a different operative feel compared with conventional surgery, steepening the learning curve. Using nonreflective metal eye shields eliminates this effect. We are currently using a Sharplan 150XJ surgipulse CO_2 laser (Sharplan Lasers Inc.,

Allendale, NJ) on continuous wave set at 6 W using an 0.2-mm spot size. Authors using the surgipulse mode use a setting of 400 mJ at 6–8 W. Settings for other CO_2 lasers such as the Ultrapulse 5000 (Coherent Inc., Palo Alto, CA), LX-20P (Luxar Inc., Bothell, WA), and others are available from the manufacturers.

If an eye shield is used, the assistant provides light inferior countertraction on the eyelid at the ciliary margin while the incision is made with a laser. One author (7) believes that cold steel provides more rapid wound healing and a smaller scar than do lasers,

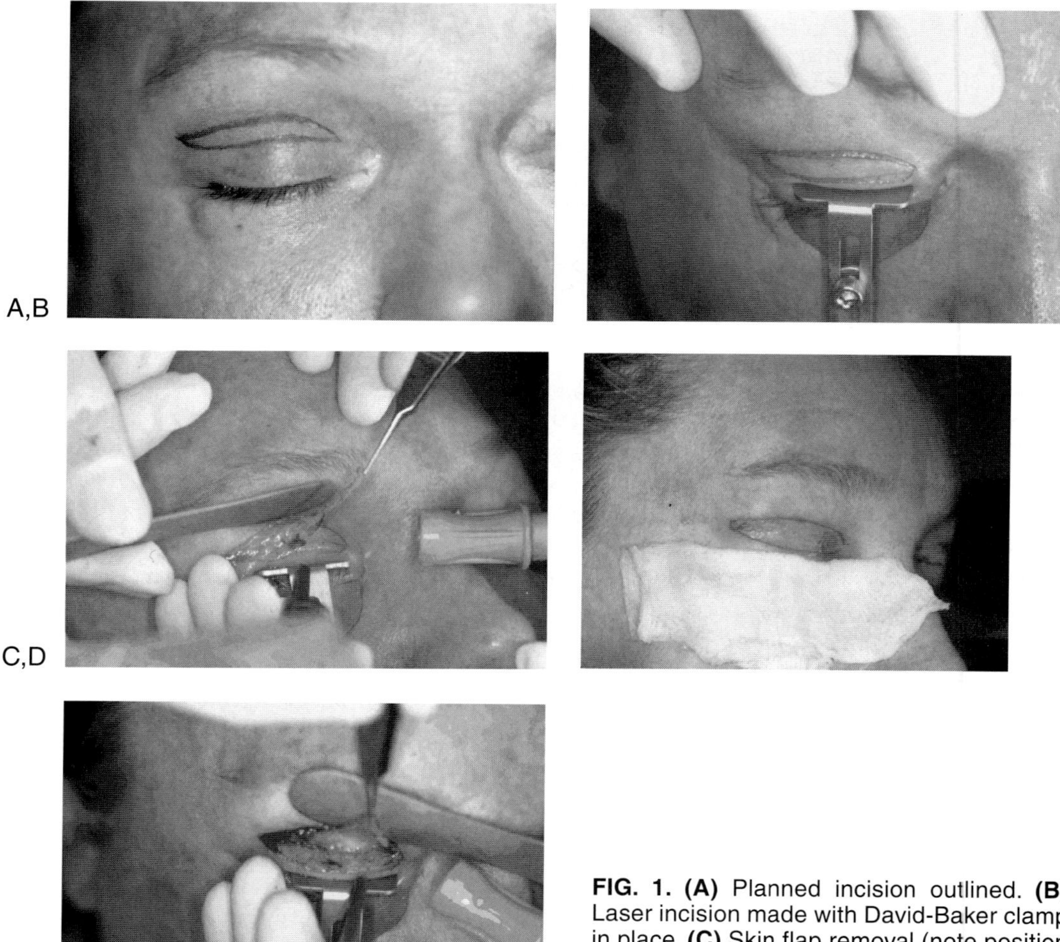

FIG. 1. (A) Planned incision outlined. **(B)** Laser incision made with David-Baker clamp in place. **(C)** Skin flap removal (note position of shield and high-speed suction). **(D)** Skin flap removed. **(E)** Removal of preaponeurotic fat.

whereas others believe they are equivalent (3,8). This point remains unresolved. It is our preliminary opinion that wound healing is somewhat slower and the initial scar is slightly more dense with lasers using continuous wave than with lasers using cold steel. At present, we are making the skin incision with a scalpel and then using continuous wave laser for the remainder of the procedure. Using the surgipulse mode for making the skin incision could theoretically resolve these potential problems, as the effects of charring and collateral thermal injury are greatly reduced. However, no clinical data are available and with loss of the hemostatic properties of continuous wave, the surgipulse mode may offer no advantage over cold steel.

UPPER LID BLEPHAROPLASTY

When making the skin incision for an upper lid blepharoplasty, it is important to use smooth movement of the handpiece to control the depth of the incision. Any pause can result in making an incision too deep, especially when using an eyelid clamp. Furthermore, with the laser there is a loss of tactile sensation compared with the conventional technique. This requires the surgeon to develop a greater reliance on visual landmarks when performing the dissection along a tissue plane. Using cold steel instruments, the planes of tissue dissection can be discriminated; however, the laser does not provide this ability. Hemostasis is excellent with the laser on continuous wave. However, when a bleeding site is encountered, it can be controlled by defocusing the laser, or by using bipolar or fine-tipped cautery. Depending on the degree of orbicularis muscle resection needed, a separate skin and muscle flap is performed or a combined skin-muscle flap is removed.

The orbital septum is opened with the laser and the desired amount of fat is removed using a nonreflecting metal shield or wet tongue blade or cotton tip applicator as a protective backdrop. The incision is closed according to the surgeon's preference. Postoperative care is the same as with the conventional technique. Ophthalmic antibiotic ointment, cold packs, head elevation, and avoidance of squinting are important features of postoperative care to minimize swelling and ecchymosis. When the skin incision is made with the continuous wave laser, we prefer to use a subcuticular closure and remove the sutures at 7 days postoperatively.

LOWER LID BLEPHAROPLASTY

For lower lid blepharoplasty, the laser is best suited for the transconjunctival approach. With the transcutaneous approach, we prefer using cold steel; however, it can be performed with a laser (9).

After local anesthesia is placed and adequate time for hemostasis has elapsed, a cotton tip applicator is gently pressed against the eye shield, moving the globe posteriorly and exposing the conjunctiva. A Jaeger plate can also be used as a substitute for eye shields if desired. When placed into the cul-de-sac, this instrument provides good exposure of the conjunctiva. The lower lid can be everted by digitally retracting the lower eyelid inferiorly or by placing a Desmarres lid retractor or small rake if the lid is too tight. An incision is made 6–10 mm below the eyelid margin or midway between the tarsal plate and fornix beginning medially at about the level of the punctum and moving laterally. The lateral extent is dictated by the position of the temporal fat pad determined preoperatively. The first pass of the laser makes an incision just through the conjunctiva. The second pass divides the inferior retractors. The fat pads come into view at this point. If there is any uncertainty, careful scissor dissection to confirm orientation is recommended. The Desmarres lid retractor is then inserted into the incision to provide anterior and inferior retraction.

The encapsulating fasciae of the fat compartments are opened and the inferior oblique muscle is identified (Fig. 2). If the procedure is being performed with intravenous sedation, then local anesthesia of the fat pads is

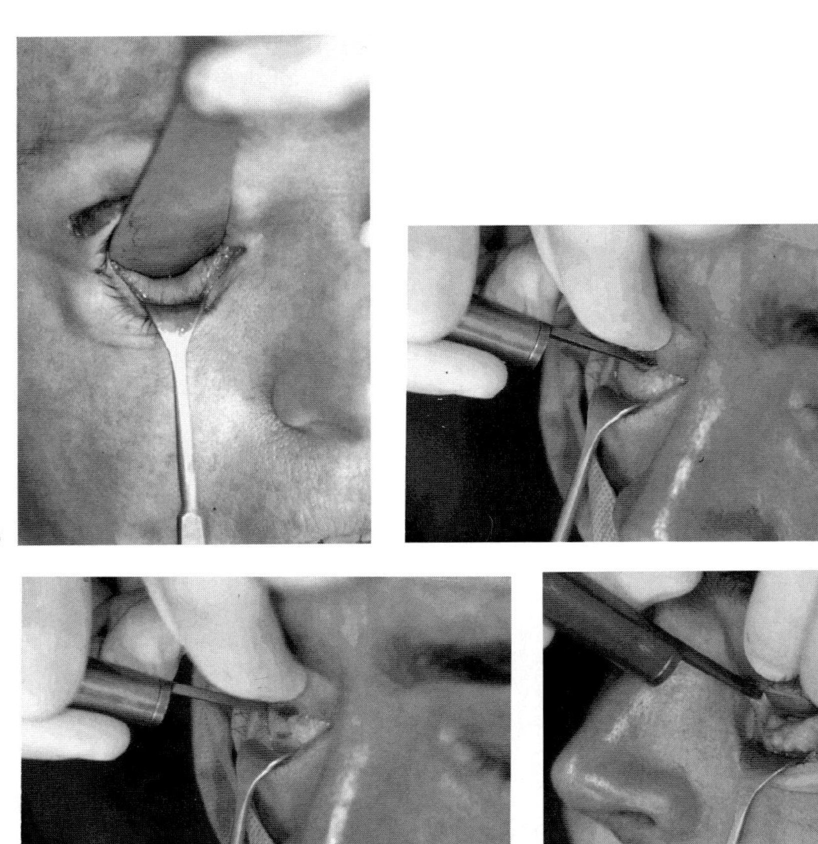

FIG. 2. **(A)** Jaeger plate placed in the cul-de-sac with anterior inferior retraction of the lower eyelid with the Desmarres retractor. **(B)** Nonreflective metal eye shield for corneal protection. **(C)** Laser incision of the conjunctiva. **(D)** Exposure of the middle fat compartment. **(E)** Laser excision of fat (note position of Desmarres retractor serving as a protective background).

required. The fat is removed using the laser with either a nonreflecting metal shield or some other protective backdrop. Carefully positioning the Desmarres retractor works well. Once adequate fat resection has been performed and verified, attention can then be directed toward management of the eyelid skin. The incision can be left open or closed with a single 6-0 mild chromic gut suture with the knot placed away from the conjunctiva to prevent irritation.

Any required skin resurfacing of the lower eyelids for rhytids can be done with either a 35% TCA chemical peel or by CO_2 laser resurfacing. Excess skin can be removed by a pinch technique. Using local anesthetic with Wydase (Wyeth-Ayerst, Philadelphia, PA) (hyaluronidase), a small amount of solution is injected along the lower lid margin. After adequate spreading has occurred, a fine forceps is used to pinch and weld excess skin into an upright position 1–2 mm below the eyelashes. This ridge of skin is then excised with scissors along its base. The wound is closed using a 6-0 running subcuticular suture or adhesive. Taping the suture ends with Mastisol (Ferndale Laboratories Inc., Ferndale, MI) and steristrips prevents displacement of the sutures. Using a pull-out suture makes suture removal pleasant for the patient. Interrupted sutures of 6-0 or 7-0 monofilament are used otherwise. These are removed in 4–5 days. Some surgeons will also perform a TCA chemical peel beginning just below the incision line if skin resurfacing is needed. Until further experience is acquired, concomitant laser skin resurfacing is not recommended for use simultaneously with a pinch procedure. Postoperative care is the same as with the conventional technique.

Laser blepharoplasty is a well-accepted procedure. Potential risks specific to laser blepharoplasty beyond conventional blepharoplasty include increased fire hazard, ocular injury to staff, injury to patient eyelashes and skin from misdirected fire, and possible slower wound healing and worse scarring of incisions compared with the cold steel procedure. Despite these potential risks, the laser remains an excellent tool for blepharoplasty and may become the new gold standard in the near future.

LASER ENDOSCOPIC FOREHEAD LIFT

This procedure is discussed in detail in Chapter 23. Any new or innovative surgical technique or tool that facilitates achieving the desired surgical result, reduces the risk of complications, and minimizes postoperative morbidity is a significant advancement. We have found that using the CO_2 laser to release the arcus marginalis and resect the corrugators, procerus, and depressor supercilii muscles results in a significant reduction in postoperative edema and ecchymosis compared with endoscopic scissor resection and bipolar cautery. The key to this technique was the development of a flexible laser fiber delivery system. Sharplan developed this system for the 150XJ surgipulse known as Fiberlase.

Fiberlase is a hollow optical fiber with an outer diameter of 2 or 3 mm and an internal diameter of 1 mm that produces a spot size of 0.8 mm. The fiber length employed for the endoscopic forehead lift is 120 mm and maintains ≥95% efficiency. Lasering is noncontact with the tip placed 2–3 mm from the target point. A helium-neon aiming beam guides the surgeon. Debris is kept clear of the fiber tip by an argon gas purging system. Argon gas also assists in cooling, permitting higher wattage without fiber degradation. This fiber is fitted into a sheath and attached to a launch coupler. The sheath with fiber can be bent to conform to the contour of the forehead (Fig. 3). Laser plume evacuation is performed with a high-speed vacuum connected to an appropriately sized metal tip suction instrument.

Incision with the surgipulse mode, which has a waveform consisting of two energy pulses delivering 400 mJ of energy at 20 W. Each pulse is <600 µs (below the thermal relaxation time of skin); pulses are separated temporally by a span >600 µs. We have achieved excellent results by incising the arcus marginalis using the surgipulse mode, followed by resection of desired musculature with the continuous wave mode set at 20 W

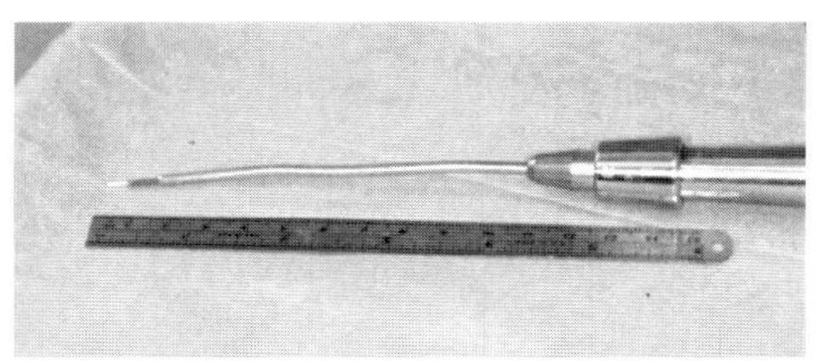

FIG. 3. Fiberlase flexible laser fiber delivery system.

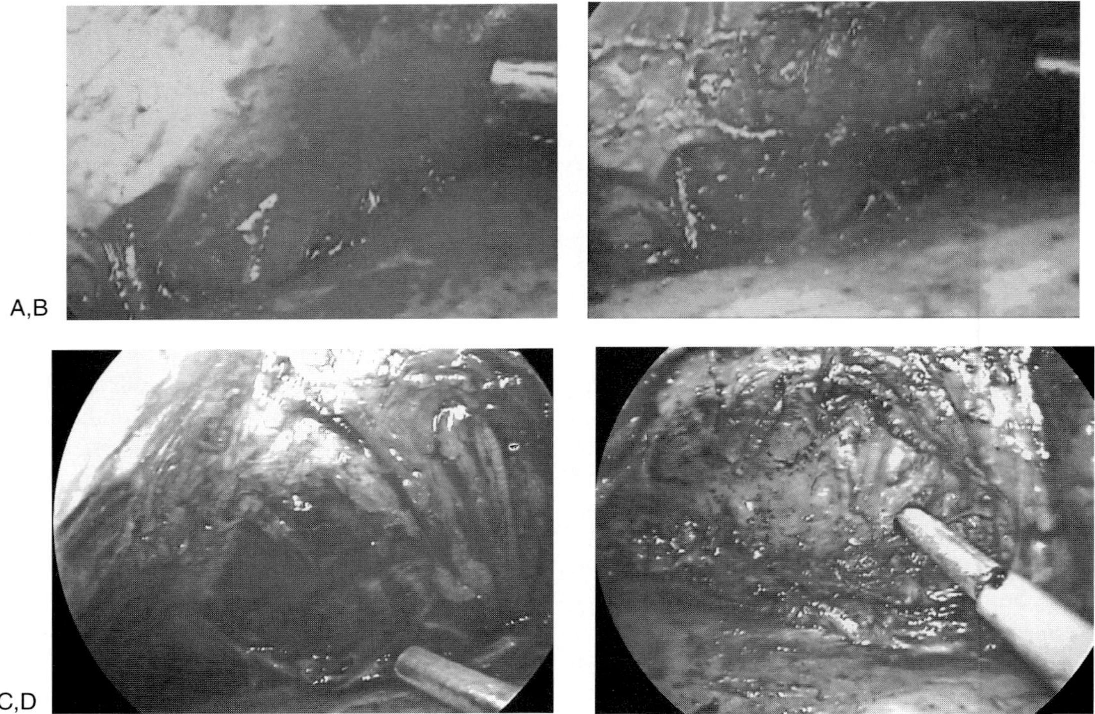

FIG. 4. (A) Arcus marginalis with the supraorbital nerve exiting at the orbital rim. **(B)** Laser incision of the arcus marginalis using surgipulse (suprapulse) mode until the ROOF (retro-orbicularis oculi fat) level is reached. **(C)** Right corrugator muscle exposed. Note CO_2 laser fiber tip and supraorbital nerve fibers. **(D)** Right corrugator muscle ablated with CO_2 laser on continuous wave. Supraorbital and supratrochlear nerve fibers are preserved.

(Fig. 4). Continuous wave permits coagulation of very small vessels found within the musculature. However, if brisk oozing occurs from a small vessel, bipolar cautery is sometimes necessary. In our hands, the laser has reduced swelling and ecchymosis compared with the endoscopic scissor technique and bipolar cautery.

As laser technology continues to expand and more refined and sophisticated delivery systems are developed, the versatility and importance of the laser in performing surgery will grow dramatically.

ACKNOWLEDGMENT

We would like to acknowledge the technical assistance provided by Valerie Steffers, RN, in developing these techniques.

REFERENCES

1. Baker SS, Muenzler WS, Small RG, Leonard JE: Carbon dioxide laser blepharoplasty. *Ophthalmology* 91(3): 243–283, 1984.
2. Baker SS: Carbon dioxide laser upper lid blepharoplasty. *Am J Cosm Surg* 9:141–145, 1992.
3. David LM, Sanders G: CO2 laser blepharoplasty: A comparison to cold steel and electrocautery. *J Dermatol Surg Oncol* 13:110–114, 1987.
4. David LM, Abergel RP: Carbon dioxide laser blepharoplasty: conjunctival temperature during surgery. *J Dermatol Surg Oncol* 15:421–423, 1989.
5. David LM, Goodman G: Blepharoplasty for the laser dermatologic surgeon. *Clin Dermatol* 13:49–53, 1995.
6. Glassberg E, Babapour R, Lask G: Current trends in laser blepharoplasty. *Dermatol Surg* 21:1060–1063, 1995.
7. Mittlelman H: The use of lasers for blepharoplasty. *Facial Plast Surg Clin North Am* 4(2):257–265, 1996.
8. Morrow DM, Morrow LB: CO2 laser blepharoplasty: A comparison with cold-steel surgery. *J Dermatol Surg Oncol* 18:307–313, 1992.
9. Seckel BR: Blepharoplasty: Operative procedures. In: Seckel BR. *Aesthetic laser surgery*. New York: Little, Brown & Company, 121–155, 1995.

Office-Based Surgery of the Head and Neck
Edited by Yosef P. Krespi, MD
Lippincott–Raven Publishers, Philadelphia © 1998

25

Cutaneous Laser Resurfacing

M. Morad Khosh, Gary J. Nishioka, and Wayne F. Larrabee, Jr.

Cutaneous laser resurfacing is a new and exciting modality for treating the effects of chronologic and photo aging of the skin. Visible skin changes that result from aging include rhytids, lentigines, telangiectasis, dyschromias, keratoses, loss of translucency, decreased elasticity, and sallow color (1–3). Histologically, aged skin shows a compact and laminated stratus corneum without a clear transition to the underlying stratus lucidum. The epidermis further exhibits some degree of dysplasia with atypical keratinocytes, variable cell necrosis, epidermal vaculization, and decreased numbers of Langerhans' cells. Homogenization of the upper papillary dermis ground substance occurs, and loss of collagen results in dermal thinning (1).

Historically, the most widely practiced methods of treating aging and photo-damaged skin have been chemical peeling and dermabrasion. Each of these modalities, however, has certain limitations and shortcomings. Medium depth peels, such as with trichloroacetic acid, may not achieve the depth necessary for the desired results. Deeper peels using phenol result in hypopigmentation, and carry a risk of cardiac toxicity. Chemical peeling is technique-sensitive and operator-dependent with regard to precise control of peel depth. All peeling agents pose a risk around mucous membranes and eyes. Dermabrasion is also operator-dependent, and poses a potential hazard around the mouth and the eyes. Possible spread of blood-borne pathogens represents another criticism of dermabrasion. These shortcomings have fueled a search for better techniques in the management of aging skin.

Cutaneous laser resurfacing offers advantages over chemical peeling and dermabrasion in that it permits precise layered ablation of superficial skin in a bloodless manner with minimal collateral damage to deeper skin.

SCIENTIFIC BASIS

A carbon dioxide (CO_2) laser with a wavelength of 10.6 μ is preferentially absorbed by water. It therefore serves as an excellent tool for cutting or evaporating skin because of the high cellular and interstitial water content. Although CO_2 lasers have been used for the past 30 years in the field of medicine, skin resurfacing with conventional lasers was not possible owing to an unacceptable high rate of scarring. This was the result of collateral thermal damage to papillary dermis and adnexal skin structures. Recent advances in laser technology and a better understanding of tissue interaction with laser thermal energy has allowed development of lasers that cause minimal surrounding thermal damage.

According to Beer's Law, laser energy heats a critical tissue volume until the tissue temperature exceeds the vaporization threshold (4). Thermal conductance from the laser impact site to adjacent areas causes coagulative necrosis and collateral tissue damage. Thermal conductance can be minimized by delivering an ablative dose of laser energy faster than the tissue thermal relaxation time. In this situation, laser-treated areas will vaporize before thermal energy can be conducted to adjacent structures. Tissue ablation can thus be achieved to a depth of tens of microns.

In human skin, the thermal relaxation time has been determined to be 695 μs, and this is typically approximated to <1 ms (5). Minimal energy density for char-free vaporization has been calculated as 5 J/cm². Therefore, to vaporize human skin effectively without inducing significant collateral tissue necrosis, a laser must generate and deliver 5 J/cm² in <1 ms. Medical laser companies have achieved this by building powerful lasers capable of generating high-energy outputs with a short pulse duration, or alternatively, by focusing a less powerful beam of laser energy into a small spot size (thereby increasing the energy density) and rapidly scanning the spot size over a relatively large area.

INSTRUMENTATION

The recent surges in medical laser utilization have spurred the growth of multiple manufacturing companies offering a variety of lasers for CO_2 laser skin resurfacing. A list of lasers currently available for skin resurfacing is shown in Table 1. The first two companies to provide lasers for skin resurfacing were Sharplan and Coherent.

Sharplan (Allendale, NJ) developed a microprocessor-controlled optomechanical flashscanner compatible with the ordinary CO_2 laser, called SilkTouch. This system uses a focusing handpiece to concentrate the laser energy into a 0.20-mm diameter spot. Because the laser energy is being focused into a small spot size, the resulting energy density is great. For example, at an energy setting of 20 mJ with a 0.20-mm spot size, an energy density of 63 J/cm² can be generated. This focused

beam is rapidly scanned in a spiral fashion over a 2–9-mm diameter area. The rapid movement of the beam over the tissue ensures <695 microsecond exposure of individual sites. Thus, char-free vaporization is easily performed even with low-power lasers.

Coherent UltraPulse (Palo Alto, CA) is a powerful laser capable of generating 500 mJ of energy in individual 1-ms pulses. This laser incorporates radiofrequency gas-slab technology, which eliminates the factors that limited the maximal energy output of conventional high-voltage DC-excited lasers (2). When used with a 3-mm diameter handpiece, this method can deliver an energy density of 7 J/cm². The laser energy is delivered in a collimated fashion, and obviates the necessity of keeping the handpiece within a specified distance from the skin. A computer pattern generator (CPG) is available that enhances the speed and precision of surface ablation (6).

Studies comparing tissue effects of Sharplan SilkTouch and Coherent UltraPulse indicate that at similar power density settings, depth of laser ablation and surrounding thermal damage are comparable (7). Single passes at 7 W showed vaporization depth of 70 μ with thermal subcrater damage <150 μ (8). Wound healing after pulsed laser ablation has been demonstrated to be similar to that after dermabrasion and chemical peels. Epidermal regeneration from adnexal structures results in complete cutaneous re-epithelization in 7–10 days. Histologically, the laser-treated skin shows a normalized epidermis without evidence of previous actinic damage, although minimal solar elastosis in the papillary dermis may persist. After laser treatment, new bands of compact and horizontally oriented collagen are seen within the dermis (2,9,10).

TABLE 1. *Available Lasers for Skin Resurfacing*

Coherent, UltraPulse 5000C
Sharplan, SilkTouch 150XJ
Sharplan, SilkTouch 40C
Sharplan, SilkTouch Jr
Lucar Nova Pulse, LX-20SP
Tissue Technologies, TruePulse
Laser Sonics-Heraeus Surgical, Paragon ClearPulse

PATIENT SELECTION

Ideal patients for cutaneous laser resurfacing have fine static rhytids, perioral or periorbital wrinkles, or full-face photo aging and have lightly pigmented skin. Glogau's photo aging classification (Table 2) divides patients into different categories of photo aging and provides a simplified approach to assess response to chemical peeling. This categorization can be extended to patients undergoing laser resurfacing (11). Type 1 patients do not need deep peeling or laser resurfacing and do best with a skin care program. Type 4 patients would not benefit from superficial peeling, but may do well with multiple laser resurfacing. Type 2 and 3 patients represent those expected to demonstrate the most benefit from laser resurfacing (11).

Degree of skin pigmentation is one of the most important factors affecting resurfacing outcome. Fitzpatrick's scale of skin pigmentation (Table 3) is most commonly used to classify degree of skin pigmentation and determine suitability for laser resurfacing. Patients with type 1 and 2 skin respond better to chemical peeling and laser resurfacing. Patients with Fitzpatrick 3 or 4 skin type are at risk for post-treatment hyperpigmentation. Laser resurfacing in this group of patients should be undertaken cautiously with vigilant pre- and postoperative bleaching regimens.

Use of isotretonin within the previous year represents a contraindication to laser skin resurfacing. Laser treatment should not be undertaken until the patient has had a full recovery to the normal degree of moisture and oiliness of skin. To proceed earlier while the sebaceous glands are still suppressed by the isotretinoin increases the risk of poor healing and hypertrophic scarring. Prior history of radiation therapy with resultant loss of dermal appendages may similarly represent a risk of postoperative complications.

Patients who plan to have laser treatment of the periorbital area must have careful assessment of lower lid laxity. Poor lid tone can contribute to the development of excessive scleral show or ectropion after periorbital resurfacing. This group of patients should undergo a lid tightening procedure prior to laser resurfacing.

Laser resurfacing will not have a significant effect on dynamic rhytids and cutis laxa. In general, it is not a replacement for blepharoplasty or rhytidectomy, but rather an adjunct. We routinely perform laser resurfacing simultaneously with other facial rejuvenation procedures, such as rhytidectomy, transconjunctival blepharoplasty, and endoscopic subperiosteal forehead plasty. However, we carefully avoid laser resurfacing of any area that has been undermined during rhytidectomy.

Psychological readiness to endure a 7–10-day period of skin re-epithelization, and a willingness to accept prolonged post-treatment erythema are important in patient selec-

TABLE 2. *Glogau's Classification of Photo Aging*

Type 1
  No wrinkles
  Early photo aging
  Mild pigmentary changes
  Twenties and thirties
Type 2
  Wrinkles in motion
  Early to moderate photo aging
  Early lentigines
  Parallel smile lines
  Late thirties or forties
Type 3
  Wrinkles at rest
  Advanced photo aging
  Dyschromia, telangiectasia
  Fifties or older
Type 4
  Wrinkles throughout, no normal skin
  Yellow-gray skin color
  Severe photo aging
  Sixties and seventies

TABLE 3. *Fitzpatrick Classification of Skin Types*

Skin Type	Skin Color	Hair Color	Tanning Response
1	White	Red	Always burns, never tans
2	White	Blonde	Usually burns, difficult to tan
3	White	Brown	Sometimes burns, average tan
4	Brown	Brown/black	Rarely burns, tans with ease
5	Dark brown	Black	Very rarely burns, tans very easily
6	Black	Black	No burn, tans very easily

tion. Patients should be questioned regarding personal or familial history of keloid formation to assess proclivity for scar formation. Past history of herpatic outbreaks should also be sought, although perioperative treatment with antiviral therapy is recommended regardless of prior herpes infection.

Although laser resurfacing technology has gained prominence in aesthetic rejuvenation of skin (eg, treatment of perioral and periorbital rhytids, treatment of acne scarring, or elimination of weathered and aged epithelium), numerous other applications exist in treating benign or premalignant skin lesions. Conditions amenable to laser resurfacing include seborrheic keratosis, actinic keratosis, syringoma, xanthelasma, lentigines, pigmented macules, rhinophyma, and actinic cheilitis.

PREOPERATIVE MANAGEMENT

Laser skin resurfacing involves three distinct phases of care: prelaser skin preparation, laser resurfacing, and postlaser care. All three of these phases are continually undergoing modification as clinical and basic science research produces new ideas and innovations.

Prelaser skin preparation plays an important role in postlaser healing, and it reduces the incidence of hyperpigmentation. A variety of regimens is available, all using some combination of one or more of the following: glycolic acid, tretinoin (Retin-A, Ortho Pharmaceutical Corp., Raritan, NJ), kojic acid, hydroquinone, and sunscreen. Both glycolic acid and tretinoin are skin exfoliants, with tretinoin also providing increased cellular activity, which may promote more rapid healing following resurfacing. Kojic acid and hydroquinone both lighten the skin by targeting melanocytes.

Although most clinicians implement some type of prelaser skin program from 3 to 6 weeks prior to the laser date, some believe it best not to pretreat, citing the fact that the degree of postlaser erythema is proportional to the final result. No clinical data have been published to support this claim, however. Interestingly, other clinicians believe that pretreatment with tretinoin significantly reduces the healing time.

Medications dispensed prior to lasering include a first-generation cephalosporin (7 days), an antiviral agent (acyclovir; 800 mg twice a day for 7 days), and a schedule II or III narcotic, depending on the procedure. Although a number of antiherpetic agents are available, we use acyclovir, as it is the only agent approved by the U.S. Food and Drug Administration for prophylaxis. Although newer generation antiherpetic agents would probably work as well, they remain unapproved for this role. Antibiotics and acyclovir are started the day before the scheduled laser date.

OPERATIVE PROCEDURE

The approach to anesthesia remains widely varied, and is largely dependent on the background of the clinician and the type of facility where the procedure is performed. In general, if only one aesthetic subunit is addressed, local infiltrative anesthesia with or without oral sedation is recommended. When two aesthetic subunits are addressed, such as the periorbital plus the perioral area, local anesthesia with intravenous sedation is performed. Full-face laser resurfacing is best done under general anesthesia.

General anesthesia using laryngeal mask airway (LMA) is a relatively new method of controlling the airway that seems ideal for lasering. When using LMA, the patient is maintained in an anesthetic level light enough to continue spontaneous respiration. Because the laryngeal mask rests over the larnyx, it is much less stimulating than an endotracheal tube. The amount of anesthetic agent required is much reduced, which translates into rapid emergence and recovery. Patients can often be discharged from the recovery area in 30–45 minutes. Local infiltrative anesthesia is still recommended with LMA in order to reduce the need for general anesthetic agents. Furthermore, local anesthesia enhances comfort during the early postlaser period.

The importance of skin preparation remains an unanswered issue. Because lasering vaporizes the outer surface of the skin while leaving the deep skin intact to serve as a first line barrier against microorganisms, the value of skin preparation may be minimal to none. What is important is that if skin preparation is performed, nonflammable agents be used.

After the laser has been successfully test fired and the patient is ready for lasering, patient eye protection is addressed. The eyes must be protected regardless of where the face is being lasered. External eye shields or corneal shields are used, depending on whether periorbital lasering is being done. During local anesthesia or intravenous sedation, a topical ophthalmic anesthetic is instilled to facilitate eye shield placement with minimal patient discomfort.

We perform skin resurfacing with a Sharplan 150XJ laser using the superpulse mode. Laser setting parameters for SilkTouch are tabulated in Table 4. For other CO_2 resurfacing lasers such as the Coherent (UltraPulse 5000C, Palo Alto, CA), Luxar Nova Pulse (LX-20SP, Bothel, WA), Tissue Technologies (TruePulse, Beverly, MA), and Laser Sonics-Heraeus Surgical (Paragon ClearPulse, San Jose, CA), consult the manufacturer for the recommended settings.

Our preference is to use the 200-mm handpiece with a 6-mm spot size for full-face and perioral lasering. For periorbital lasering, we prefer the spot size to be 4 mm.

Lasering is performed in a controlled manner with minimal overlap of adjacent areas. The periorbital area is treated with a single pass at 12 W, while the rest of the face is treated with one or more passes at 16–18 W. After each pass with the laser, the skin should be wiped with a moist gauze, and the lasering depth assessed.

Clinical parameters that aid in determining the depth of lasering include skin color, status of wrinkles, and skin shrinkage. A pink to red color, which is usually encountered after the first laser pass, indicates an epidermal depth. Yellow to gray coloration is indicative of papillary dermal depth. Chamois color correlates with reticular dermal depth, and the maximal safe depth of lasering. Loss of skin shrinkage on laser impact, and ablation of wrinkles are other indications to stop further lasering. Above all, it is important to exercise conservatism and err on the side of undertreatment rather than risk excessively deep lasering.

In general, laser skin resurfacing involves one of three facial subunit combinations, periorbital or perioral, both periorbital and perioral, and full face. When lasering both periorbital and perioral regions, serious consideration should be given in recommending full-face laser resurfacing. Postoperative erythema is more conspicuous when these regions are treated in isolation, which makes camouflage with make-up more difficult.

POSTOPERATIVE MANAGEMENT

Skin re-epithelization following laser resurfacing typically takes 7–10 days. Clinically, this corresponds to a period of oozing and crusting that can be difficult for the patient to manage. Patients often require extra reassurance and encouragement during this period.

To facilitate postoperative skin care, different dressings have been proposed. Dressings can be broadly classified into two categories: ointments and occlusive dressings. In our opinion, occlusive dressings for the first 3–5 days significantly facilitate healing and re-

TABLE 4. *Start Safe Laser Parameters for Sharplan SilkTouch*

Handpiece (mm)	Scan Size (mm)	Scan Time (seconds)	Power (watts)
125	3.0–6.0	0.13–0.52	7
200	4.0–9.0	0.08–0.52	18
260	5.0–12.0	0.04–0.51	34

duce pain. The two occlusive dressings we are using at this time are Silon-TSR (Bio Med Sciences Inc., Bethlehem, PA) and Flexzan (Dow Hickams Pharmaceuticals Inc., Sugar Land, TX), although many others are available. Ointments include plain petroleum jelly, various antibiotic-based products, or bovine collagen. We currently use bovine collagen (Catrix, Donell DerMedex, New York, NY) to cover areas not covered by the occlusive dressing, and all lasered areas following removal of the occlusive dressing until the skin has re-epithelized. During this period, patients are instructed to maintain good hydration, and to moisten the skin as frequently as possible. During the first 2 weeks, pruritis may be a source of complaint. This usually responds to 1%–2.5% hydrocortisone ointment. Patients should be cautioned to avoid direct sun exposure, and to apply sunscreen for the first 6 months.

The most problematic aspect of the post-laser period, following initial oozing and crusting, is erythema. Erythema may take up to 6 months to resolve. No standard therapy currently exists for this problem, and patients are encouraged to use make-up as camouflage. Ongoing research regarding methods to avoid or reduce erythema involves altering laser pulse parameters. Variations include significant reductions in pulse duration and increase in the power density to further reduce collateral thermal damage.

EFFICACY

Overall treatment results from laser resurfacing have been very favorable (7,10,12, 13–18). Patient satisfaction is typically good to excellent. Although most reported studies have follow-up periods of <1 year, longer follow-up periods are not expected to affect patient satisfaction adversely. Female patients with fine static rhytids, diffused actinic photo aging, Glogau photo aging types 2 and 3, and Fitzpatrick skin types 1 and 2 report the best results (Figs. 1–3). Static facial rhytids and pigmentary changes show more significant improvement than acne scars (13). Among various facial subunits, the periorbital region demonstrates the best results. The periorbital

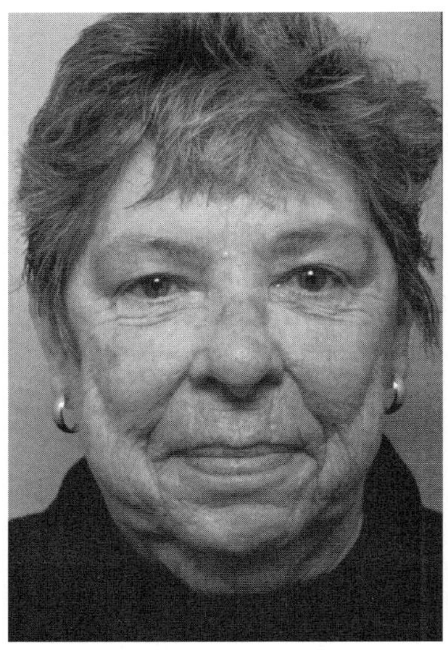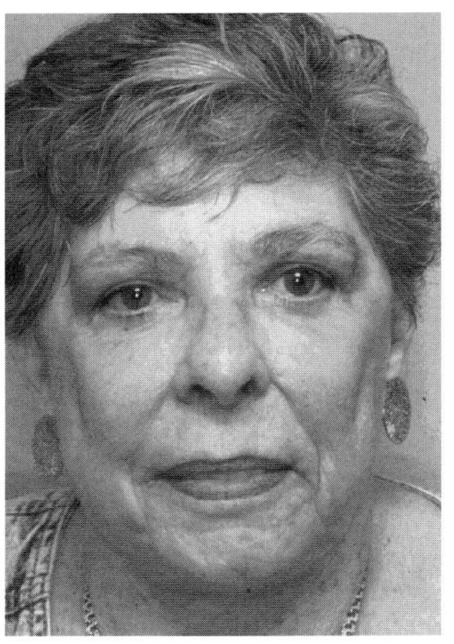

A,B

FIG. 1. (A) A 65-year-old woman with aging face and diffuse sun-damaged skin. **(B)** Six months following full-face laser resurfacing, which was preceded by rhytidectomy, upper and lower blepharoplasty, and chin implantation 8 weeks later.

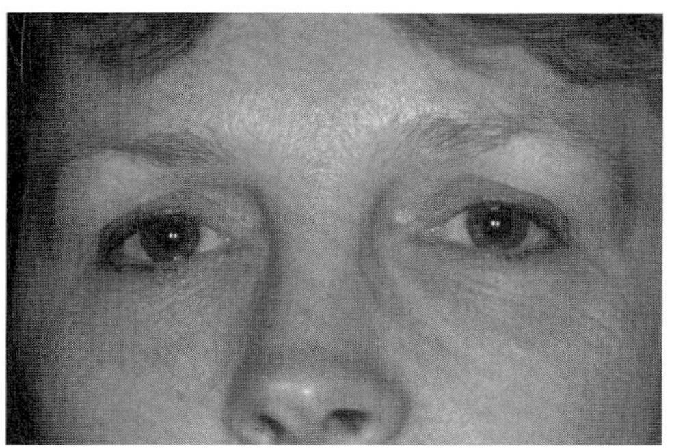 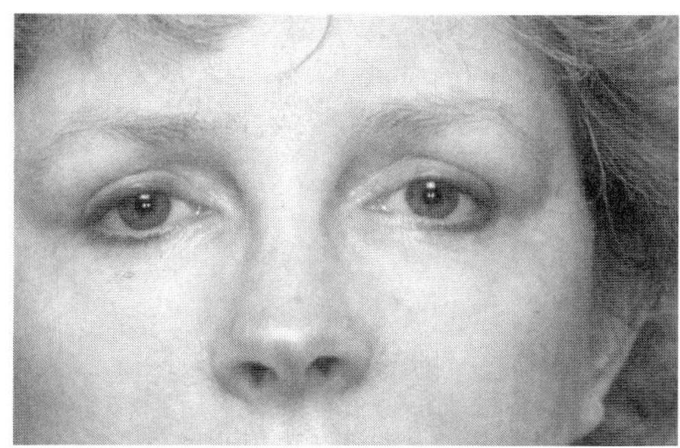

A,B

FIG. 2. (A) A 41-year-old woman with fine periorbital rhytids. **(B)** One year following periorbital lasering.

area is also the easiest to camouflage during the erythema phase.

COMPLICATIONS

Postlaser erythema is considered a normal part of the healing process, not a complication. Increased skin sensitivity to soaps and cosmetics, itching, telangiectasis, and acne are some of the other transient sequelae of laser resurfacing. Reported incidence of persistent postoperative complications with laser resurfacing is low (7,10,12,14,16,17). The incidence may increase, however, as the numbers of physicians performing the procedure increase rapidly. Postoperative scarring and ectropion are considered major postoperative complications, whereas transient pigmentary changes, herpes labialis, infection, and milia are thought of as minor complications (Table 5).

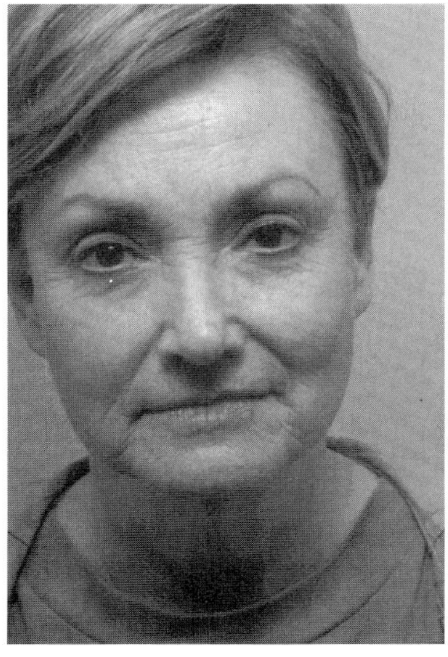 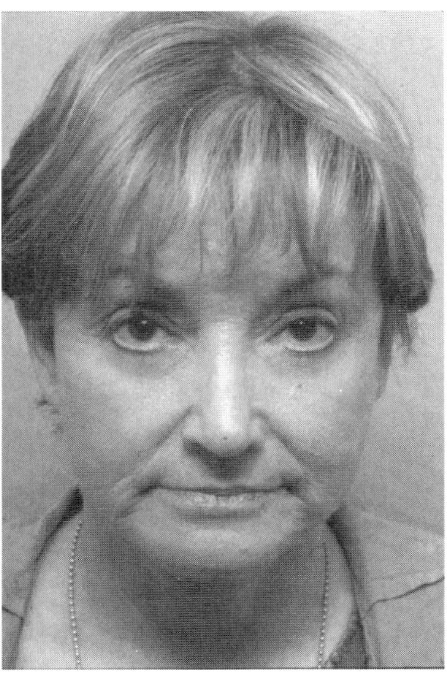

A,B

FIG. 3. (A) A 62-year-old woman with aging face. **(B)** Six months following endoscopic forehead lift, rhytidectomy, and laser resurfacing of the periorbital and perioral area.

TABLE 5. *Complications of Laser Resurfacing*

Transient hyperpigmentation
Milia
Herpes simplex
Hypertrophic scarring
Transient induration
Ectropion
Hypopigmentation
Cracks in teeth
Infection

Development of postoperative ectropion is unique to eyelid resurfacing. The incidence has been reported as 0%–0.8% (2,10). This complication can be minimized by careful preoperative evaluation for lower lid laxity. If lid laxity exists, then a tightening procedure should be performed prior to laser resurfacing. Corneal abrasion or globe injury have not been reported in the literature.

Scarring has not been encountered in most of the published reports (12,16,17). A single episode of scarring was reported by Fitzpatrick et al. (10) in 38 laser treatments in the periorbital area. The scarring resolved in 4 months with local steroid treatment. Scarring results from excessively deep lasering, and the eyelid skin is most prone to scarring. Adherence to guidelines outlined for assessment of depth of lasering must be followed diligently. In patients with prior phenol peeling, visible color changes in the skin are less reliable, and conservative judgment should be exercised. Patients with recent (<1 year) history of isotretonin application are at increased risk for scar development.

Transient hyperpigmentation has been reported as 17%–33% (9,11,15,16). This tends to occur more commonly in patients with greater skin pigmentation (Fitzpatrick types 3 and 4). The incidence may be decreased by preoperative use of hydroquinone or Retin A, which is resumed postoperatively once re-epithelization is completed. Hyperpigmentation generally develops in the third or fourth postoperative week, and resolves within 4 months. Hypopigmentation is much less common (0%–3%) (3,7,10,12,17). The decrease in pigmentation is only moderate, and not as severe

as that encountered with phenol peels. It is postulated that hypopigmentation results from melanocyte damage owing to excessive depth in lasering.

Herpes labialis is rare if prophylactic antiviral therapy is employed (0%–2%) (10,12,16, 17). Herpes infection can be seen even in patients without a prior history of fever blisters. Most clinicians are now in agreement that prophylactic antiviral therapy should be used in any patient undergoing laser resurfacing on the face. Milia has been reported in 0%–14% of patients (12,16,17). Bacterial infection has not been reported, perhaps due to routine use of prophylactic antibiotics. Cracking of teeth is a theoretical complication of heat-induced expansion. It is recommended, therefore, that teeth be covered with a moist gauze during laser resurfacing (3).

CONCLUSION

Cutaneous laser resurfacing offers several advantages over previously available skin exfoliation techniques. It allows uniform, precise, and accurate superficial skin ablation with minimal damage to adjacent skin structures. Laser resurfacing can be combined with other facial plastic procedures to enhance cosmetic results. When performed in appropriately selected patients, good to excellent results can be expected with minimal risk of complications.

REFERENCES

1. Blain AK, Pratt L: Physiological consequences of human skin aging. *Cutis* 43:431–436, 1989.
2. Chernoff WG, Schoenrock LD, Cramer H, Wand J: Cutaneous laser resurfacing. *Int J Aesthetic Reconstr Surg* 3:57–68, 1995.
3. Roberts TL, Ellis LB: CO$_2$ laser resurfacing: Recognizing and minimizing complications. *Aesthetic Surg Quarterly* 16:142–148, 1996.
4. Reid R: Physical and surgical principles governing CO$_2$ laser surgery on the skin. *Dermatol Clin* 9:297, 1969.
5. Hruza GJ: Skin resurfacing with lasers. *Fitzpatrick's Journal of Clinical Dermatology* 3:30–41, 1995.
6. David LM, Sarne AJ, Unger WP: Rapid laser scanning for facial resurfacing. *Dermatol Surg* 21:1031–1033, 1995.

7. Lask G, Keller G, Lowe N, Gormley D: Laser skin resurfacing with the SilkTouch Flashscanner for facial rhytids. *Dermatol Surg* 21:1021–1024, 1995.
8. Chernoff G, Slatkine M, Zair E, Mead D: SilkTouch: A new technology for skin resurfacing in aesthetic surgery. *Lasers Surg Med*; accepted for publication April 1995.
9. David LM, Lask GP, Glassberg E et al: Laser abrasion for cosmetic and medical treatment of facial actinic damage. *Cutis* 43:583–587, 1989.
10. Fitzpatrick RE, Goldman MP, Satur NM, Tope WD: Pulsed carbon dioxide laser resurfacing of photoaged facial skin. *Arch Dermatol* 132:395–402, 1996.
11. Glogau RG, Matarasso SL: Chemical face peeling: Patient and peeling selection. *Facial Plastic Surgery* 11:1–8, 1995.
12. Waldorf HA, Kauvar AN, Geronemus RG: Skin resurfacing of fine to deep rhytids using a char-free carbon dioxide laser in 47 patients. *Dermatol Surg* 21:940–946, 1995.
13. Ho C, Nguyen Q, Lowe NJ, Griffin ME et al: Laser resurfacing in pigmented skin. *Dermatol Surg* 21:1035–1037, 1995.
14. Lowe NJ, Lask GP, Griffin ME, Maxwell A et al:. Skin resurfacing with the Ultrapulse carbon dioxide laser: Observations on 100 patients. *Dermatol Surg* 21:1025–1029, 1995.
15. Apfelberg DB: The Ultrapulse carbon dioxide laser with computer pattern generator automatic scanner for facial cosmetic surgery and resurfacing. *Ann Plast Surg* 36:522–529, 1996.
16. Alster TS, West TB: Resurfacing of atrophic facial acne scars with a high-energy, pulsed carbon dioxide laser. *Dermatol Surg* 22:151–155, 1996.
17. Felder DS, Mayl N: Periorbital dioxide laser resurfacing. *Seminars in Ophthalmology* 11:201–210, 1996.
18. Alster TS, Garg S: Treatment of facial rhytids with a high energy pulsed carbon dioxide laser. *Plast Reconstr Surg* 98:791–794, 1996.

Office-Based Surgery of the Head and Neck
Edited by Yosef P. Krespi, MD
Lippincott–Raven Publishers, Philadelphia © 1998

26

Management of Facial Wrinkles With Botulinum Toxin Injections

Andrew Blitzer, William J. Binder, and Mitchell F. Brin

Hyperfunctional facial lines are common cosmetic deformities involving the forehead, glabellar area, nasolabial creases, and lateral orbital region. These excessively prominent lines may be misinterpreted as anger, anxiety, fear, fatigue, and melancholia, as well as aging. Such lines have been treated with surgical excision, a procedure that often has minimal effect on the lines and leaves unsightly scars. Other options include collagen, silicone, or fat injection in an effort to balloon out the skin and flatten the folds (1–3).

Most facial rejuvenation procedures do not address the cause of the hyperfunctional lines, which appear to result from functional pull of the underlying mimetic facial musculature. Patients who have Bell's palsy have been observed to have smooth skin without deep hyperfunctional lines. In our previous work utilizing injections of botulinum toxin (BTX) for facial dystonia or hemifacial spasm, we noted a reduction or absence of these deep hyperfunctional lines and an improved cosmetic appearance (4,5). BTX weakens the overactive underlying muscle contraction, causing facial skin flattening and an improved cosmetic appearance (6–9).

BOTULINUM TOXIN

BTX is produced by the bacteria *Clostridium botulinum*. Eight serologically distinct toxins designated A, B, C1, C2, D, E, F, and G have been described (10). Botulinum toxin exerts its effect at the neuromuscular junction by inhibiting the release of acetylcholine, and this in turn causes weakness or flaccid paralysis. Pharmacologic and morphologic studies suggest that the toxin enters the nerve ending via a receptor-mediated endocytosis. This process appears to be energy dependent, but independent of Ca^{2+} concentration or nerve stimulation (11–13). Botulinum toxin does not affect the synthesis or storage of acetyl choline, but rather the release of vesicle-bound acetyl choline. The therapeutic effect is related to the peripheral blockade of neuromuscular activity through an enzyme-related interference in neurotransmitter exocytosis (14,15).

No long-term adverse effects of significant health hazard have been reported with the use of BTX-A (6–8,14). Muscle biopsies taken from patients after repetitive injections have failed to show any long-term evidence of permanent degeneration or atrophy, and those patients have received dosages that were two to five times those we have used for aesthetic improvement (16,17). Patients receiving very high doses of toxin may also develop antibodies to the toxin; however, the antibodies are not dangerous, but render the patient unresponsive to further treatment. The factors predisposing patients to the development of antibodies are unknown, but some experience has shown that the risk is increased with the use of >300 U (14). Therefore, we have developed and used an electromyographically (EMG) guided technique to increase the accuracy of the injection, which may therefore minimize the dose and antigenic exposure.

Botulinum toxin A has been approved by the U.S. Food and Drug Administration as safe and effective therapy for blepharospasm, strabismus, and hemifacial spasm since December 1989. The National Institutes of Health consensus conference of 1990 also included this toxin as safe and effective therapy in the treatment of adductor spasmodic dysphonia, oromandibular dystonia, and cervical dystonia (14). There are many other "off-label" uses, such as spasticity, sphincter dysfunction, and tremor disorders that have been successfully managed with botulinum toxin. In this chapter, we report our ongoing clinical observations regarding the use of BTX for hyperfunctional facial lines.

MATERIALS AND TECHNIQUE

Lyophilized botulinum toxin A (BOTOX, Allergan, Irvine CA) was obtained and stored frozen as recommended (-20°C) until reconstitution with sterile saline at the time of injection. One international unit of Botulinum toxin is defined as the LD_{50} in mice. The LD_{50} in humans is estimated to be approximately 3000 IU (18).

In our clinical studies, the toxin was reconstituted with normal saline to a concentration of 25–50 U/mL. BTX was injected via a monopolar hollow bore teflon-coated electromyography needle connected to an EMG recorder. Using a technique we have previously described (4,5,19–27), the needle is placed through the skin overlying the exaggerated facial line into the muscle associated with the hyperfunctional line. Once the needle is in the muscle, the patient is instructed to accentuate the line with a smile or frown, until the maximal EMG signal is achieved. The needle may be moved until it is in the most active part of the muscle complex. Toxin is then injected in 0.1-mL aliquots. By using an initial low dose, a graded weakening can be achieved over sequential visits.

Patients are first evaluated with a thorough review of their medical history, medications, and prior facial plastic surgery. Excluded from treatment are patients with a history of sensitivity to toxin or a neuromuscular disorder, such as myasthenia or Eaton-Lambert syndrome, or those who cannot complete the protocol. Preliminary photographs are taken for each patient and for each site, both at rest and while active. All photographs are standardized by using the same camera, lens system, flash system, and film. Photographs are repeated at 2 weeks and 6 weeks postinjection.

Aside from the photographs, patients and doctors independently rate hyperfunctional lines with a 0–3 rating scale (0 reflecting no facial wrinkles, 1 signifying mild facial wrinkles, 2 denoting moderate facial wrinkles, and 3 representing severe facial wrinkling at rest and during function, before injection, and at 2 and 6 weeks after injection).

We are reporting (28) a series of 210 injected sites in 162 patients. The injection sites included 40 forehead, 89 glabella, 72 crow's feet, 4 platysma, 4 nasolabial, and 1 mentalis.

The doses used in our study were based on our previous experience, and they were modified for some patients depending on response. The dose for forehead lines was 5–25 U with a mean of 17.3 U; glabellar lines was 5–20 U with a mean of 11.1 U; crow's feet was 5–15 U with a mean of 6.2 U; nasolabial was 2.5–5 U with a mean of 3.12 U; and platysma was 10–20 U with a mean of 15 U. A beneficial response was found in 199 of 210 (95%) facial sites. All of the patients had toxin effect within the first 24–72 hours.

Overall, the best average beneficial change in function (based on the 0–3 rating scale) was noted in the forehead (1.84%–46% improvement), followed by the glabellar area (1.5%–37.5% improvement), and then in crow's feet (1.36%–34% improvement). The rating difference at rest were forehead 1.45; glabella 0.97; and crow's feet 0.9. The p value for a one-tailed Student's t-test was $p = 0.00005$ (Figs. 1 and 2).

The adverse effects of the toxin injections were minimal and included temporary droop of the eyelid or brow or droop of the upper lip (nasolabial fold injection) in seven patients. No systemic reactions were noted. The effects

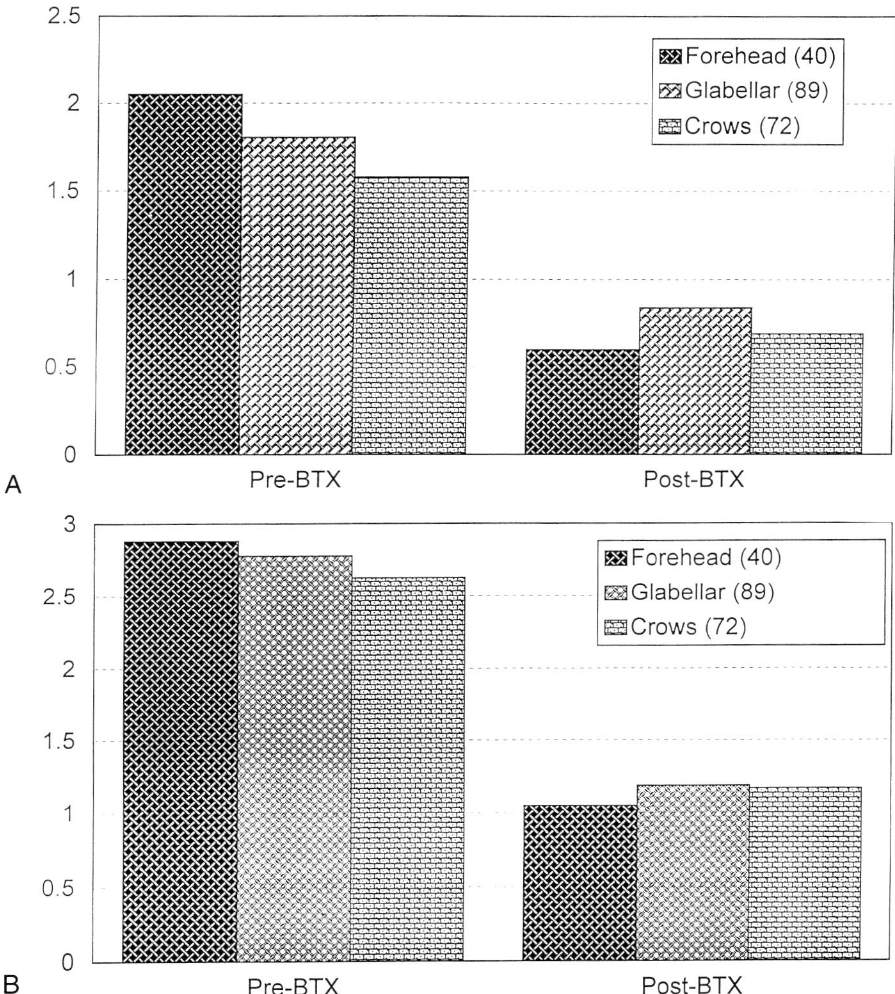

FIG. 1. Overall, the best average beneficial change in function was noted in the forehead, followed by the glabellar area and then in crow's feet **(A)** at rest (one-tailed $p = 0.00005$ for each) and **(B)** in action (one-tailed $p = 0.00005$ for each). BTX, facial lines ($n = 201$ regions).

of the injection lasted an average of 3–6 months, whereupon most patients returned for re-evaluation and treatment.

DISCUSSION

BTX has several advantages over other techniques in the management of hyperfunctional facial lines. BOTOX injections can be administered during a routine office visit, with minimal discomfort. The injections may be given serially with small doses to titrate the results while a patient's treatment strategy is being formulated. The only morbidity is related to temporary mild weakness of other adjacent facial muscles. The EMG technique allows for accurate placement of the needle electrode in the more active portions of the muscle, which may achieve maximal effect with minimal dose. Accurate EMG placement and minimal dose is likely responsible for a very low incidence of morbidity with our technique, and for the overwhelmingly successful effects of the injections.

Continued work is necessary to determine the exact mechanism of the toxin, the short- and long-term effects on muscle, and adjuvants or other mechanisms to obtain longer periods of benefit. BTX may also provide a useful laboratory tool to explore the various factors that contribute to facial line formation. It is our experience that BTX is a safe and important adjunctive technique for the management of patients with symptomatic hyperfunctional facial lines.

REFERENCES

1. Newmank, Dolsky R, Nguyen A: Facial profile plasty by liposuction extraction. *Otolaryngol Head Neck Surg* 93(6):718–731, 1988.
2. Pitanguy I: Indications for treatment of frontal and glabellar wrinkles in an analysis of 3,404 consecutive cases of rhytidectomy. *Plast Reconstr Surg* 67(2):157–166, 1981.
3. Pollack SV: Silicone, fibril, and collagen implantation for facial lines and wrinkles. *J Dermatol Surg Oncol* 16:957–961, 1990.
4. Blitzer A, Brin MF, Keen MS, Aviv JS: Botulinum toxin for the treatment of hyperfunctional lines of the face. *Arch Otolaryngol Head Neck Surg* 119:1018–1023, 1993.
5. Brin MF, Fahn S, Moskowitz C et al: Localized injections of botulinum toxin for the treatment of focal dystonia and hemifacial spasm. *Mov Disord* 2:237–254, 1987.
6. Tosoy EA, Bukley EG: Treatment of blepharospasm with botulinum toxin. *Am J Ophthalmol* 99:176, 1985.
7. Scott AB, Kennedy RA, Stubbs HA: Botulinum toxin A injection is a treatment for blepharospasm. *Arch Ophthalmol* 103:347, 1984.
8. Maoriello JA Jr: Blepharospasm Meige's Syndrome and hemifacial spasm: Treatment with botulinum toxin. *Neurology* 35:1499, 1985.
9. Lang DH, Brin MF, Fahn S, Lovelace RE: Distal effects of locally injected botulinum toxin: Incidences and effects. *Adv Neurol* 50:609–613, 1988.
10. Simpson LL: The origin, structure, and pharmacological activity of botulinum toxin. *Pharmacol Rev* 33:155–188, 1981.
11. Simpson LL: Kinetic studies on the interaction between botulinum toxin type A and the cholinergic neuromuscular junction. *J Pharmacol Exp Ther* 212:16–21, 1980.
12. Simpson LL, Dasgupta BR: Botulinum neurotoxin type E: Studies on mechanism of action and on structure activity relationships. *J Pharmacol Exp Ther* 224:135–140, 1983.
13. Black JD, Dolly JO: Interaction of 125I-labelled botulinum neurotoxins with nerve terminals. I. Ultrastructural autoradiographic localization and quantitation of distinct membrane acceptors for types A and B on motor nerves. *J Cell Biol* 103:521–534, 1986.
14. National Institutes of Health Consensus Development Conference: *Clinical use of botulinum toxin.* 8:1–20, 1980.
15. Hambleton P, Moore AP: Botulinum neurotoxins: Origin, structure, molecular actions, and antibody. In: Moore P, ed. *Handbook of botulinum toxin treatment.* Oxford: Blackwell Science, Ltd, 1995:15–27.
16. Borodic GE, Ferranter R: Orbicularis muscle histology after repetitive injections of botulinum A toxin on orbicularis oculi muscle. *J Clin Neurol Opthalmol* 12:121–127, 1992.
17. Scott AB, Kennedy RA, Stubbs HA: *Botulinum toxin.* Presented at the Annual Meeting of the American Academy of Ophthalmology, Altanta, Georgia, 1990.
18. Brin MF, Fahn S, Moskowitz CB et al: Injections of botulinum toxin for the treatment of focal dystonia. *Neurology* 36(suppl 1):176, 1986.
19. Brin MF, Fahn S, Moskowitz CB et al: Localized injections of botulinum toxin for the treatment of focal dystonia and hemifacial spasm. *Adv Neurol* 599–608, 1988.
20. Blitzer A, Brin MF, Fahn S, Lovelace RE: The use of botulinum toxin in the treatment of focal laryngeal dystonia (spastic dysphonia). *Laryngoscope* 98:193–197, 1988.
21. Blitzer A, Brin MF, Fahn S: Botulinum toxin injection for the treatment of oromandibular dystonia. *Ann Otol Rhinol Laryngol* 98:93–97, 1989.
22. Brin MF, Blitzer A, Fahn S, Lovelace RE: Adductor laryngeal dystonia: Treatment with local injections of botulinum toxin (botox). *Neurology* (suppl 1):244, 1988.
23. Brin MF, Blitzer A, Fahn S et al: Adductor laryngeal dystonia (spastic dysphonia): Treatment with local injections of botulinum toxin (botox). *Mov Disord* 4:287–296, 1989.
24. Blitzer A, Brin MF: Laryngeal dystonia: A series with botulinum toxin therapy. *Ann Otol Rhinol Laryngol* 100:85–90, 1991.
25. Brin MF, Blitzer A, Greene PE, Fahn S: Botulinum toxin therapy for the treatment of oromandibulolingual dystonia (OMD). *Neurology* (suppl 1):294, 1988.
26. Blitzer A, Brin MF, Stewart C, Fahn S: Abductor laryngeal dystonia: A series treated with botulinum toxin. *Laryngoscope* 102:163–167, 1992.
27. Blitzer A, Brin MF, Fahn S: Botulinum toxin injections for lingual dystonia. *Laryngoscope* 101:799, 1991.
28. Blitzer A, Binder WJ, Keen MS et al: The management of hyperfunctional facial lines with botulinum toxin injections: A multicenter study of 210 sites in 162 patients. *Arch Otolaryngol Head Neck Surg*; in press

Office-Based Surgery of the Head and Neck
Edited by Yosef P. Krespi, MD
Lippincott–Raven Publishers, Philadelphia © 1998

27

Hair Transplantation

David S. Orentreich and Steven J. Pearlman

HISTORY OF THE PROCEDURE

In 1939, Okuda, a Japanese dermatologist, described, in a report virtually unrecognized in the English-speaking world, the use of small full-thickness autografts of hair-bearing skin to correct alopecia of the scalp, eyebrow, and mustache areas (1,2). This method was almost the same as Orentreich's, reported in 1959 (3). Okuda constructed special metal trephines (circular punches) with diameters of 2–4 mm and used these to bore out grafts from hair-bearing areas of the scalp. A similar instrument was used to prepare recipient sites in the area of alopecia into which the grafts were placed. Okuda noted that better cosmetic results were achieved if slightly smaller trephines were used for the recipient holes. A total of 200 patients, most of whom had cicatricial alopecia, were successfully treated in this fashion. Okuda did not, however, specifically note use of this treatment in patients with male pattern baldness (androgenetic alopecia).

Unfortunately, because of World War II, Okuda's work was not recognized outside Japan until many years later. This was generally true for other relevant publications and for the proceedings of various Japanese dermatological societies and societies of plastic surgery, which were written entirely in Japanese. Thus, knowledge and trial of these techniques outside Japan were long delayed (4). However, in 1970, Friederich mentioned Okuda's significant contribution and designated the free punch graft method as the Okuda-Orentreich technique (5).

More than 40 years have elapsed since the first controlled experiments with autografts in 1954 that led to the 1959 publication of *Autografts in Alopecias and Other Selected Dermatological Conditions* (6). Hair-bearing scalp punch grafts transplanted into areas of male pattern baldness androgenetic (7) or andro-chronogenetic alopecia (8) continue to grow hair more than four decades later. In the interim, there have been hundreds of lectures, symposia, workshops, papers, books (9), and other works published on this and related techniques of hair replacement surgery. Some 200 physicians have observed the basic transplant technique at our medical facility, and today hair transplantation is one of the most commonly performed office-based plastic surgical procedures in the United States.

THE PRINCIPLE OF HAIR TRANSPLANTATION

The success of hair-bearing autografts (hair transplants) to correct androgenetic alopecia (AGA) and certain other alopecias depends on the principle of donor and recipient dominance, terms introduced by Orentreich (3) in 1959. Donor-dominant grafts retain the characteristics of the donor site after transplantation to a new site, whereas recipient-dominant grafts take on the characteristics of the tissue at the recipient site. These concepts of dominance were developed out of studies investigating the localization of various dermatoses, including several types of alopecia. The research use of such autografts, with appropriate multiple controls, helped to further our understanding of certain physiological and pathological cutaneous phenomena.

With the 1959 publication of *Autografts in Alopecias and Other Selected Dermatological Conditions* came Orentreich's realization that AGA could be treated surgically. The 1959 article illustrated the aesthetic placement of grafts in the frontal scalp in a pattern that reconstructed the anterior hairline, with allowance for an appropriate degree of temporal recession and frontal peaking. The hairline continued to recede, and the grafts aesthetically placed in front of the pre-existing hairline continued to show stable hair growth, increasingly anterior to the receding hairline.

The results of the 1954 experiment with autografts for the treatment of AGA corroborated that "the capacity for development of baldness appears to be controlled by factors resident in localized areas of the scalp"(9) (ie, the pathogenesis of AGA is inherent in each individual hair follicle). The phenomenon explained the occasional clinical finding of singular, normally growing terminal hairs in a sea of male pattern baldness. The results of the study published in 1959 also refuted the then-popular theory that AGA resulted from ischemia, secondary to the chronic activity of the scalp muscles by branches of the facial nerves, causing shearing stresses in the scalp dermis (10).

Since the development of punch graft hair transplantation for AGA and other alopecias, many improvements have been made in both instrumentation and technique. Physicians with different surgical training have entered the field of hair replacement surgery and expanded the surgical options to modalities other than punch grafting. Some innovations have endured, some have been abandoned, and others remain controversial. A review of some of the more significant advances follows.

Saline infiltration of the donor area (11) improved graft harvesting, as did the introduction of sharper and motorized punches (12). The closure of donor sites with sutures, instead of allowing them to heal by secondary intention, reduced both healing time and patient discomfort in addition to improving the cosmetic appearance of the donor site scar (13,14). Although the strip graft method introduced by Vallis (15) never became fully established, it may have been the first use of a double-bladed knife to obtain a strip of donor graft tissue, which is now a popular technique of donor harvesting.

The past 5 years have been a period of tremendous innovation and expansion in the field of hair replacement surgery. New techniques and improvements in surgical instrumentation have greatly increased the quality of the end aesthetic result as well as the skill and speed with which the transplant surgeon can operate. Surgical skills, techniques, and instrumentation have been so improved and refined that the transplantation of hundred, and indeed thousands, of mini and micro grafts in a single session is not an unrealistic goal for the 1990s transplant surgeon (Arnold J: *500 Micro and Mini Grafts Before or After Lunch*; instructional video).

Strip donor harvesting, mini and micro grafting techniques, and laser surgery are the developments that have revolutionized office-based hair transplant surgery. The technique of harvesting conventional grafts containing 10–15 hairs with a motorized punch and placing them in neat rows in the bald recipient area has been largely replaced by the method of strip harvesting, followed by the random planting of hundreds of mini and micro grafts in the bald recipient area in an attempt to mimic the natural, scattered appearance of hair growth.

The application of laser technology to hair transplantation was first introduced by Grevelink and Brennick (16) in 1994. The goal was to reduce bleeding from graft recipient sites using a carbon dioxide (CO_2) laser flashscanner. Bleeding is rarely a risk to the patient. However, it can cause extrusion of grafts with subsequent increased handling and potential trauma to the grafts. The need to apply pressure and replace grafts due to bleeding is reduced by use of lasers, thereby shortening surgical time (17). An additional benefit of the hemostatic nature of the CO_2 laser is a reduced need for vasoconstrictive agents.

The CO_2 laser is well suited to creating controlled recipient sites in the scalp. The tissue penetration of the CO_2 laser is less than 100 μm in a high-energy pulsed mode (18). When tissue is treated with a high enough power density for a very short time, controlled tissue ablation is achieved without significant heating of the surrounding tissue (19). Therefore, a critical volume of tissue can be vaporized in this manner by either a high power, short pulse mode or the rapid sweep with a continuous beam (20).

The flashscanner creates a collimated beam with a cylindrical cross section, which is well suited to creating a recipient site for hair transplantation. Pulsed collimated beams have a bell-shaped cross-section with higher power in the center, which may promote more char along the walls of the recipient site. The Sharplan SilkLase flashscanner (Sharplan, Allendale, NJ) generates a spot size of <0.15 mm in diameter in a controlled spiral pattern at a power of 40–80 W. This power density is higher than the threshold of vaporization necessary for precise ablation. Reducing collateral thermal damage with the flashscanner preserves the integrity of the surrounding tissue and reduces char to better support a micro or mini hair graft.

PATIENT EVALUATION

Most men and women with an area of significant balding and an adequate source of donor hair in the occipito-temporal region of the scalp are good candidates for hair transplants. The procedure can be performed in people of all races (21). However, not all hair loss is androgenetic or of a type suitable for autograft correction. It is essential that an accurate diagnosis be made by patient history and by clinical and laboratory evaluation (22). Laboratory studies of differential, contributory, and pathogenic factors operative in an AGA diagnosis include complete blood count with differential; venereal disease research laboratory testing; bilirubin; alkaline phosphatase; cholesterol; triglycerides; serum glutamic oxaloacetic transaminase; uric acid and creatinine levels; adrenal function tests, in-

cluding cortisol and dehydroepiandrosterone sulfate; androgen function tests, including testosterone, sex hormone binding globulin, and free testosterone index; and thyroid function tests, including free thyroid index (T_4 and T_3 uptake), and possibly T_3 and thyrotropic hormone. If menstrual irregularities or signs of virilization are also present in the prospective female hair transplant patient, then determination of follicle-stimulating hormone, luteinizing hormone, and prolactin levels may be indicated. Screening for human immunodeficiency virus and hepatitis B are recommended for all hair transplant candidates.

Based on the aforementioned principle of autograft dominance, hair transplantation is not suitable for patients with active hair loss caused by alopecia areata, lupus erythematosus, psuedopelade of brocq, lichenplano pilaris, folliculitis or scleroderma and its variants, morphea, and coup de sabre. On the other hand, "burnt out" lupus, morphea, and other cicatricial alopecias (23) can often be successfully treated with hair transplants. In these latter cases, we recommend performing a test procedure involving a small number of grafts. Permanent baldness secondary to burns, trauma, or radiation can be corrected with transplants if adequate donor hair remains.

Patient evaluation requires that the general medical status of the patient is good with particular emphasis given to identifying any bleeding diathesis or tendency to keloid formation. The recipient and donor site sizes, and the density, color, texture, and curl of the hair available for correction are evaluated to determine what degree of improvement is feasible. These findings, a proposed hairline, and the amount of bald scalp to be covered are then discussed with the patient.

Hair transplantation must never be urged on unenthusiastic patients. If one is already satisfied with his or her appearance, the coaxing of an accompanying spouse or friend should not be allowed to sway the patient's feelings. If the patient is young and actively losing hair, a family history may provide some insight into his or her eventual degree of baldness. The decision to start hair transplants early, even while the hair loss is progressing, is made with an awareness of the emotional makeup and needs of the patient. To prevent disappointment, both the patient and physician should have a realistic expectation of what is surgically possible. Sufficient time should be spent with patients to allay any fears and to correct misunderstandings. Patients should be fully informed about the procedure, including its immediate and long-term postoperative consequences. The physician should avoid accepting the psychiatrically disturbed patient for surgery. If one is in doubt, postponing the procedure is a sensible decision. Alternatively, single test transplants to an inconspicuous area can be performed. This test is recommended for patients with keloid tendencies and is useful for an apprehensive patient; it does more with a few minutes of surgery than can be done with prolonged verbal reassurances.

PLANNING THE PROCEDURE

After determining that a patient can be helped with transplants, other options for correction are also discussed, including flap and scalp reduction techniques. If a hairpiece is worn, the patient is advised that it can be used postoperatively as long as the attachment sites do not rest on any transplanted grafts. The social, recreational, cosmetic, and occupational limitations imposed by hair transplantation surgery and the postoperative healing period are reviewed. The approximate number of transplants for optimal correction, the cost, the number of grafts per procedure, the sites and the frequency of procedures, and the time required for appearance of first growth and then final regrowth are estimated and discussed with the patient in detail. The reasons for performing the transplants for each area in several or multiple procedures are explained. This is because avascular necrosis might result if all the grafts required were performed in one session. Intergraft spacing must therefore be planned so that an adequate blood supply reaches all the grafts.

In planning the procedure, a brief description of the sequence of events that the actual surgery will follow are reviewed with the patient. Local anesthesia, hair trimming of the donor sites, punch and strip harvesting techniques, and the placement of grafts are explained to the patient. Of greatest importance is the establishment of the hairline. The patient should be given a mirror to hold at eye level while a hairline is drawn in, which is then reviewed with the patient and agreed upon. This is one of the most important decisions in patient care after determining that a hair transplant is indicated. Artfully re-establishing the frontal hairline is essential to avoid an unnatural appearance. Besides exhibiting a natural widow's peak, the hairline must be suitable for both the present and the future. The direction, color, texture, and density of the hair to be transplanted may need review at this time. To avoid hairs going awry, all grafts in the recipient area are oriented so that the hair follicles follow a natural pattern. This is usually centripetal on the dome of the scalp and frontal on the anterior scalp (Fig. 1). In the past, when re-establishing the frontal hairline with conventional grafts, 3.0–4.0 mm in diameter, the overlapping of grafts reduced the appearance of a scalloped edge. Presently, smaller diameter mini or micro grafts may be used exclusively along the frontal hairline or interspersed between conventional grafts to produce a more natural appearance (Fig. 2).

Mini grafting is an established concept with a new name. In 1970 Orentreich (24,25) described the use of small circular punch grafts to refine the frontal hairline. These mini and micro grafts were reincarnated in the early 1980s when Marritt (26) used them in eyelash transplantation, and Nordstrom (27) subdivided 4-mm punch grafts into micro grafts, each containing two to four follicles, and inserted them into stab incisions. This work was further discussed by Marritt (28), Bradshaw (29), and Stough et al. (30), who bisected or quadrasected larger punch grafts and placed them into small punch holes or stab incisions.

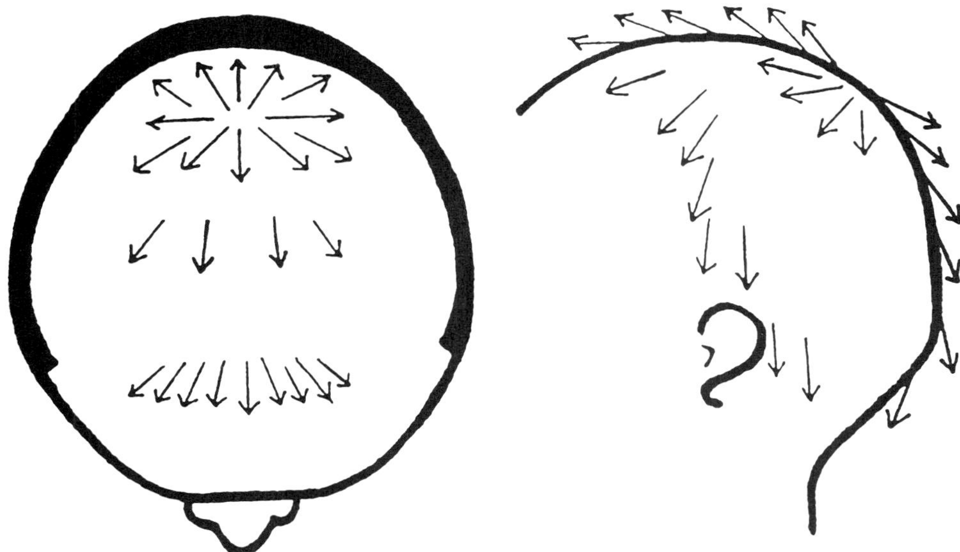

FIG. 1. Natural direction of hair growth. (Adapted from Orentreich DS, Orentreich N: Hair transplantation. *J Dermatol Surg Oncol* 11:323, 1985.)

Mini grafts consist of three to four hairs obtained by meticulously cutting a circular 4.0–4.5-mm punch graft into quadrants, or by cutting a long strip of donor skin into multiple grafts, each bearing three to four hairs. The mini grafts are then placed into 2.0-mm holes cut with a punch or into stab incisions made with a no. 15 scalpel blade (8). Micro grafts containing one to two hairs can be placed into 1.25-mm punch recipient sites or into stab incisions. Micro grafts are essential to optimize the natural appearance of the frontal hairline.

Before the procedure, the total number of grafts, the optimal number of grafts to be trans-

planted per session, the frequency of sessions, the total number of sessions, and the type of grafts to be used depend on the unique characteristics of each patient and should be determined with the transplant surgeon.

When a decision to proceed is made, photographs of the recipient sites are taken and the patient is advised to wear appropriate clothing for the day of surgery, the removal of which will not disturb the graft sites and postoperative dressings (ie, no turtlenecks or clothing that must be pulled over the head). The patient is advised to shampoo the morning of the transplant procedure because

FIG. 2. Smaller diameter plugs—mini grafts or micro grafts at frontal hairline. (Adapted from Orentreich DS, Orentreich N: Hair transplantation. *J Dermatol Surg Oncol* 11:323, 1985.)

shampooing is contraindicated for 4–5 days postoperatively. Styling product use is contraindicated immediately prior to surgery. The patient is advised not to take anticoagulants or aspirin in any form for 14 days before and 2 days after surgery. Tylenol (McNeil Consumer, Fort Washington, PA) can be substituted. In addition, garlic supplements are thought to have anticoagulant properties, and this popular dietary supplement should be discontinued 14 days prior to and 2 days after surgery. No alcohol is advised for 1–2 days pre- and postsurgery, and strenuous exercise in the 48-hour period prior to surgery is best avoided. The patient is advised to let the hair grow long in advance of the surgery date to allow for adequate combing over of the operative sites. The patient should be instructed not to fast prior to surgery and to eat a normal breakfast or lunch.

PROCEDURE

Hair transplants can be performed with the patient in a recumbent or sitting position. If vasovagal syncope occurs, it is recomended to have available a motorized chair that can reposition the patient from the sitting position into the supine position. The upper clothing is removed and the patient is draped for comfort and to avoid soiling. The operative sites and proposed hairline are reviewed with the patient.

Preoperative Medication and Anesthesia

Each surgeon chooses a preferred method of sedation. Because we perform the procedure with the patient in a sitting position, we use oral Valium (Roche Pharmaceuticals, Nutley, NJ) or intramuscular Versed (Roche Pharmaceuticals), with or without nitrous oxide analgesia prior to the injection of local anesthetic, usually 2% lidocaine with 1:100,000 epinephrine. Epinephrine is excluded in patients with cardiac conditions. Although allergy to lidocaine is extremely rare, a skin test is appropriate if the patient

believes that he or she is allergic. Administering the lidocaine slowly through a 30-gauge needle with or without refrigeration of the injection site minimizes patient discomfort. To avoid overdosing with lidocaine, especially when operating on large areas, the donor site is anesthetized and harvested first. This removes some of the injected anesthetic and allows time for some metabolism of the lidocaine before the recipient site is injected. Vasovagal bradycardia can induce syncope, and should be anticipated, especially on the first visit. At any time that syncope is imminent, the patient should be placed in the supine position and, if necessary, the legs should be elevated. Injecting epinephrine with the lidocaine helps counteract bradycardia and reduces bleeding. Carbonated colas or orange juice should be offered to the patient because they quickly correct the hypoglycemic effect of epinephrine.

Although large volumes of anesthetic sometime make the procedure more tolerable for the patient, unnecessarily large volumes of fluid should be avoided in the frontal area. Large injected volumes may contribute to the formation of surgical edema and subcutaneous bleeding, and generally cause postoperative care problems involving forehead and eyelid swelling. Elasticized bandaging of the forehead overnight and a short course of corticosteroids may ameliorate this problem should it arise.

Harvesting the Grafts

When selecting the donor site, the density, color, thickness, texture, and curl of the hair are considered to facilitate blending with the hair at the recipient sites. The hair covering that portion of the donor site to be excised is clipped to a 3-mm length, but not shaved, to allow visualization of the implied angle and direction of the hair follicles in relation to the skin surface. This allows proper angling of the punch or multibladed scalpel when punching or strip harvesting the grafts. Cutting across the hair follicles injures them and reduces the number of hairs that will grow from each graft (Fig. 3).

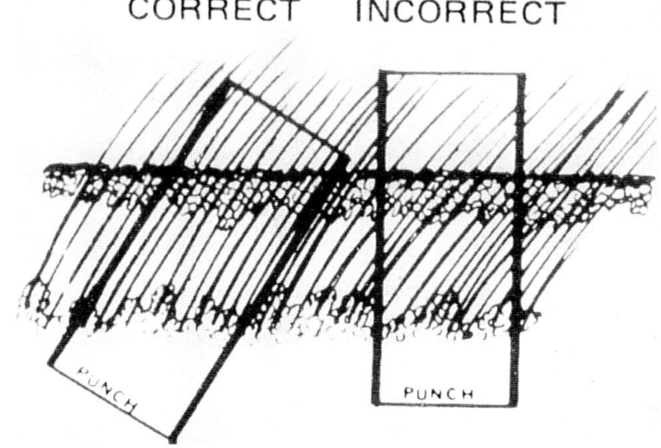

FIG. 3. Proper angling of punch or multibladed scalpel. (Adapted from Orentreich DS, Orentreich N: Hair transplantation. *J Dermatol Surg Oncol* 11:321, 1985.)

Strip Harvesting Technique

For tumescence, sterile physiologic saline, administered with a 30–50-mL syringe, is injected into the subcutaneous tissue. Filling the area beneath the dermis increases the distance between the skin and the skull, and reduces risk of injury to underlying neurovascular structures. The infiltration of saline into the donor sites makes the donor skin more rigid, thereby reducing distortion when cutting strips of donor tissue, and, hence, reducing the chance of transecting hair follicles. The surgeon then matches a multibladed scalpel to the angle of the trimmed visible hair. The singularly most important aspect of strip harvesting is controlling the scalpel blades so that they remain parallel to the changing angle of the hair shafts throughout the cutting process. The hair of a healthy donor strip should be intact from the follicle root to the surface. Mastering the intricate technique of cutting parallel to the donor scalp yields an optimal strip of viable hairs, and is the surgeon's greatest challenge. The previously referenced instructional video by Arnold is a useful primer for the transplant surgeon who hopes to master the technique of strip harvesting.

Upon removal, the donor strips are cleansed of debris by gently rubbing between two pieces of saline-soaked gauze and then placing them in physiologic saline. Bleeding vessels are then cauterized, and the donor site is closed with sutures or staples. Staples and sutures are usually removed 7 days postoperatively.

Punch Technique

Conventional grafts harvested with motorized punches are removed gently, as pulling with force can damage the follicles and the dermal papillae. If necessary, the donor graft tissue is freed of its fibrous band attachment by cutting with scissors well below the dermal papillae. After their removal, the grafts are immediately placed in physiologic saline solution. Because the donor site skin is 0.5–1.0 mm thicker than the alopecic recipient skin, donor grafts need to be trimmed of excess fat. Trimming reduces cobblestoning, as does the cross-stitching of conventionally sized harvested grafts. Spicules of hair must be removed to prevent foreign body reaction (31). To camouflage the donor site, careful planning of graft spacing is necessary. Infiltration of anesthetics and large volumes of sterile, physiologic saline (8) into the donor sites makes the skin turgid and facilitates the accurate punching of grafts, in much the same way as it facilitates the cutting of strip grafts, reducing distortion and yielding an optimal number of grafts. To further optimize the quality of punched donor grafts, the motor-driven punches are resharpened for each procedure.

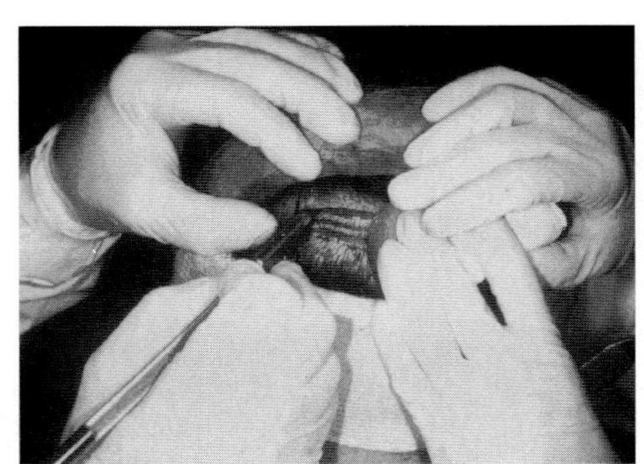
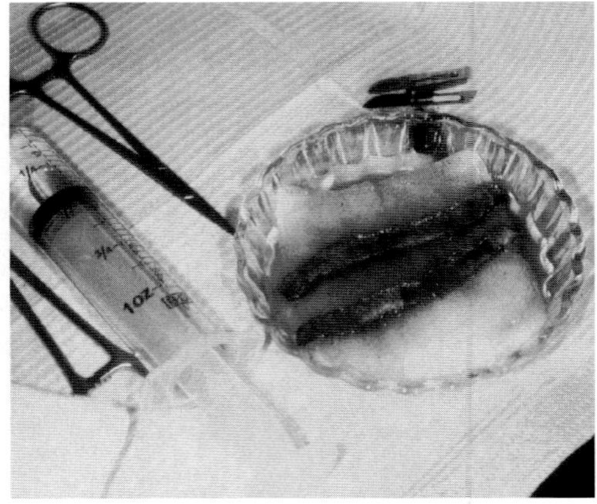

A,B

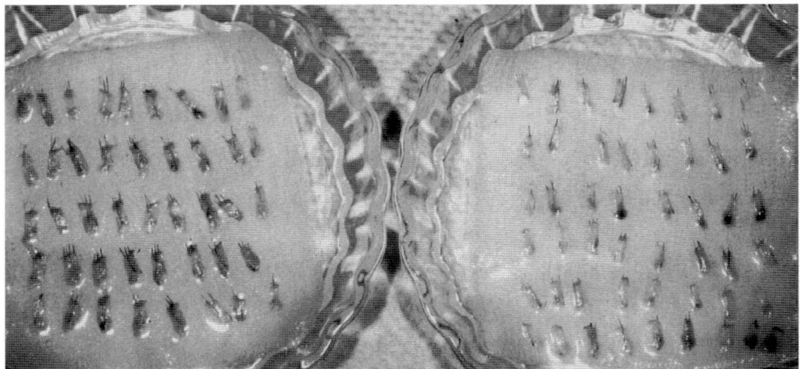

C

FIG. 4. (A) Strip harvesting with multibladed scalpel. **(B)** Harvested strips of donor tissue. **(C)** Mini and micro grafts prepared from harvested strips.

Preparation of Mini and Micro Grafts From Harvested Strips and Punches

A magnifier, a tongue blade soaked in saline as a cutting surface, Foerster forceps, and Personna surgical preparation blades are the instruments required for graft preparation (Arnold instructional video). The visible excess fat is trimmed from a harvested strip or punch as it interferes with the eventual insertion of the prepared graft into the recipient site.

Mini and micro grafts are prepared from punched donor tissue by meticulously cutting a circular 4.0–4.5-mm punch graft into quadrants (mini graft), and from there sectioning off a single hair graft (micro graft).

The preparation of mini and micro grafts from strip-harvested tissue necessitates align-ment of the Personna surgical preparation blade with the graft. The blade is placed between two hairs, and by pressing downward easily separates off a mini or micro graft. Lateral sawing motions are contraindicated when preparing the grafts, as this action dulls the blade and interferes with graft alignment (Fig. 4 and Arnold instructional video).

PLANTING THE GRAFTS

Punched Recipient Sites

Recipient sites for mini grafts containing 3–4 hairs are made with a 2.0-mm surgical punch. Care is taken to remove any fibrous tissue at the base of the recipient site to accommodate the thicker donor graft. Micro grafts containing one to two hairs may also be placed into 1.25-mm punch recipient sites. The recipient area can be grafted in three to four procedures without any grafts touching during any single procedure.

Slit Grafting

Tiny slit incisions (<2 mm), made with a no. 61 spear point-shaped blade, are used to create single hair micro graft recipient sites. Slits heal easily and are undetectable when placed just along the hairline. By concentrating on their scattered and seemingly randomized placement, the surgeon's goal is to mimic the natural growth of hair along the hairline. Typically, 120–150 hairline-placed micro grafts are used, and can be placed between mini and conventional grafts to create a more natural appearance. Rarely is any suturing of mini and micro graft recipient areas required.

LASER TECHNIQUE

Harvesting donor grafts for transplantation using the laser technique is performed in the same manner as described above. The laser is used solely to create recipient sites for single, micro, and mini hair grafts. Planning and distribution of grafts is also executed in the standard fashion. After oral or intravenous sedation is given, the cutaneous sensory nerves of the scalp are anesthetized by a regional block with 2% Xylocaine (Astra Merck, Wayne, PA) with 1:100,000 epinephrine. These nerves include the supratrochlear and supraorbital nerves in the forehead; the auriculotemporal nerve anterosuperior to the helix; and the lesser and greater occipital nerves

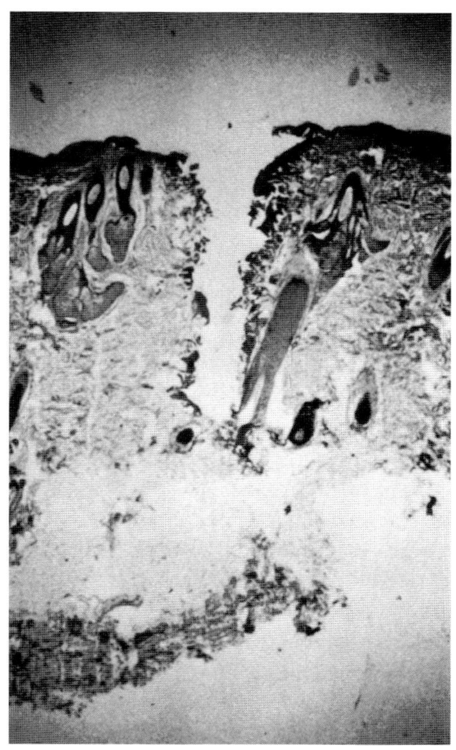

FIG. 5. Recipient laser site: 0.6-mm spot, 40 W, 0.1 second. Thermal damage: 40 μ. (Courtesy of M. Villanow, MD, Dusseldorf, Germany.)

posteriorly on the scalp. The recipient area of the scalp is then injected subcutaneously with 0.5% Xylocaine with 1:100,000 epinephrine.

The CO_2 laser is used in a single pulse mode with a duration of 0.1 second per pulse. The smallest scanning pulse diameter of the Sharplan SilkLase is 0.8–1.0 mm (Table 1). After ensuring proper laser safety for the operatory, all personnel, and the patient, a laser

TABLE 1. *Laser Specifications for SilkLase Flashscanner*

Focal length	80 mm
Scanning diameters	0.6–1.2 mm
Scanning duration	0.1 s
Spot size	0.6–1.2 mm
Instantaneous dwelling time	0.3 ms
Scanning pattern	Spiral

TABLE 2. *Transplantation Treatment Parameters*

Graft Type	Scanning Diameter (mm)	Laser Power Level (watts)	Single Pulse Duration (seconds)
Single hair	0.6	40	0.1
Micro graft	0.9	60	0.1
Mini graft	1.2	80	0.1

test is performed using a wet tongue blade. A test hole is then made in the patient's scalp to verify depth of penetration. If the hole is of insufficient depth (approximately 5 mm is desired), the scan time can be increased to 1.5 seconds (Fig. 5). The pattern of graft size and placement on the scalp follows the same principles as nonlaser transplantation. Laser settings and transplant parameters are outlined in Table 2.

The laser is best suited for single, micro, and mini hair grafts. Attempts at creating larger recipient holes with the laser have been found to create excessive heat and subsequent thermal damage to the surrounding scalp, which would interfere with graft survival. Minimal bleeding should be encountered in the lasered sites. Excess bleeding is usually controlled with pressure. A small amount of serous exude is routinely encountered in these sites, which is an indication that the transplanted graft will be nourished by imbibed fluid.

Placement of Hair Grafts

After preparing the recipient sites for their donor grafts, the most labor-intensive part of the hair transplant procedure follows, which is the actual placement of the grafts. Two nurse-assistants can spend up to 2 hours inserting up to 500 mini, micro, and conventional grafts. Foerster forceps are used to insert conventional and mini grafts into their individual openings, and Foerster micro forceps are used for micro graft insertion. Cotton-tip applicators, used to apply gentle pressure and to hold the graft in place, facilitate insertion. Single hair micro grafts can drop below the skin surface after insertion, and the 3-mm whisker of hair left in anticipation of this eventuality when the donor hair was trimmed in preparation for harvesting now proves to be fortuitous. The whisker of hair acts as a marker for each graft and provides leverage for the nurse-assistant to pull the graft level with the surface.

After hemostasis and cleansing are complete, an antibiotic ointment is applied. Conversing with the patient during the procedure always relieves anxiety. Proper draping, manual pressure, cotton applicators inserted into heavily bleeding holes, and bandaging minimize bleeding and help keep blood from the patient's view. When the recipient area is completely bald, the grafts can be taped down to facilitate bandaging and postoperative care. As much cleaning as is feasible is done after the grafts are set, which makes the postoperative care period easier for the patient. A light spray of hydrogen peroxide facilitates this cleanup procedure. If only a limited number of transplants are performed, it is possible for the patient to leave without a bandage. The donor site is prepared in such a way that the hair above camouflages the operative site. The recipient site can be let alone with just a thin layer of antibiotic ointment, and the surrounding hair can be styled over the site for cosmetic camouflage.

POSTOPERATIVE INSTRUCTIONS

Oral antibiotics, usually erythromycin or tetracycline (250 mg), are usually prescribed for a 7-day period postoperatively. The patient is instructed to apply a thin layer of antibiotic ointment to donor and recipient sites, twice a day for 10–14 days, to minimize dry crust formation and speed re-epithelization. Patients with mini and micro grafts are instructed to apply the antibiotic ointment the day following surgery and twice daily thereafter until the surgical sites are healed. A 1-week course of anti-inflammatory corticosteroids is also prescribed to reduce swelling. Analgesics to reduce discomfort (usually Tylenol with codeine or Lortab [UCB Pharma, Inc., Smyrna, GA]) are prescribed. No aspirin or alcoholic beverages should be taken for 48 hours after surgery; the aforementioned aspirin substitutes are permitted.

If bleeding occurs, patients are instructed to apply firm moderate pressure directly to the area with gauze or a clean handkerchief for 15 minutes and then to gradually release pressure. This usually stops bleeding. Strenuous physical activity is contraindicated on the first postoperative day and then only limited physical activity is allowed for the next 10 postoperative days. Edema or ecchymosis may develop at the recipient site in the first 24–48 hours after surgery and may last from 7 to 10 days. It may also spread to the forehead and eyelids; patients are instructed to sit up as much as possible and to sleep with the head elevated to reduce swelling.

Donor site suture removal takes place 7 days following surgery. Cross-stitch sutures placed over conventional grafts can be removed 3–5 days following surgery (32).

Great care should be taken when combing or brushing the hair near the site grafts. Shampooing may commence on the third postoperative day and should be very gentle until healing is complete. Patients may soak their entire scalp in the shower with just a gentle spray, shampooing very delicately and carefully. Dried and crusting blood can be removed by soaking with a 3% hydrogen peroxide solution.

Postoperative pain is rare; in fact, temporary hypoesthesia and paresthesia are not uncommon because sensory nerves are often severed. Patients should be reassured that these altered sensations are usually temporary and will normalize within 6 months. Patients should also be advised that any excessive swelling or pain, or any pulsation at the operative sites, should be brought promptly to the surgeon's attention. It may be desirable, although certainly not essential, for patients to return the day after surgery for a check-up. At this time, with the aid of a hydrogen peroxide spray, the operative sites can be cleansed and checked. The donor site rarely needs redressing on this visit, and the recipient site, if not concealable by hair styling, can have a small nonadherent antibiotic dressing applied. A hair prosthesis can be worn if the attachment sites are placed so as not to cover any donor grafts. Whenever possible, the length and styling of the hair is planned in advance to conceal the operative sites.

If for any reason a graft falls out, patients are instructed to handle it carefully and to cleanse it in saline or an 8-oz glass of tepid water plus a teaspoon of salt. They are further instructed to wrap the graft in a clean cloth saturated with the mildly salted water and to store it in the refrigerator for no more than 4 days. The graft can then be replaced within a 4-day period. If a graft cannot be saved, the site can be regrafted at the next transplant visit.

FOLLOW-UP CARE

The first site should be given a minimum of 1 month to heal before further grafting is undertaken. This allows for maximal vascularity and optimal hair growth, and prevents avascular necrosis. If performing follow-up transplants after 1 month and before 3 months (which is the interval when the hairs from previous grafts have been shed and before the new hairs begin to grow) care must be taken not to inadvertently remove the sometimes difficult-to-detect previous grafts that are temporarily free of hair (33). For best results, new hair growth should be evident about 3 months postoperatively before additional transplants are undertaken.

It is impossible to predict, with any degree of accuracy, the number of hairs in any given graft. The number is usually 8–15 for conventional grafts, 2–4 for mini grafts, and 1–2 for micro grafts. It is important to convey to the patient that the visible portion of the transplanted hairs will be shed within 1 month. Occasionally, one or two of the hairs are not shed and continue to grow. Permanent hair growth starts about 3–4 months after surgery, the length of a typical telogen period.

SEQUELAE

Cobblestoning or elevation of grafts can be treated by electrodessicating the elevations, by cutting them flat with a blade, or, rarely, by dermabrasion. Hyperpigmentation can be treated by bleaching, cryotherapy, or dermabrasion. Hypopigmentation is common, because the skin of the donor grafts has been relatively sun-protected, and the recipient areas can be quite tan with actinic alterations. Tanning is slow but will eventually blend these sites.

Occasional bacterial infection requires appropriate antibiotic treatment. Inflammation indicates the need to search for trapped hair spicules. Besides bleeding, other rarely seen

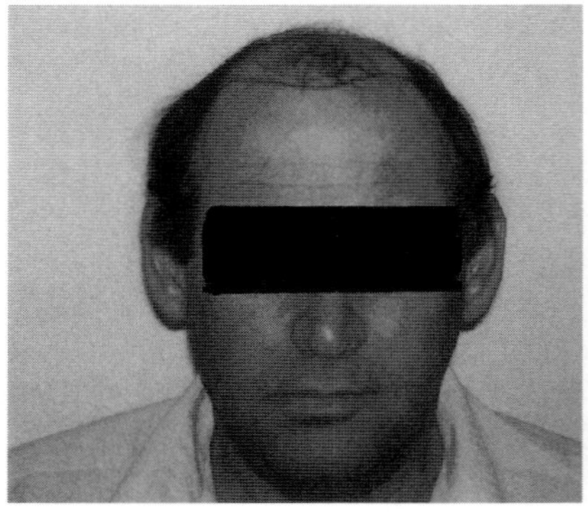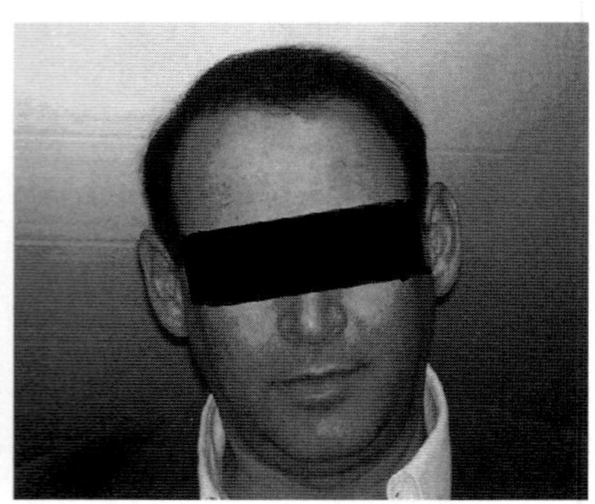

A,B

FIG. 6 (A) Before and **(B)** 6 months after laser-assisted hair transplantation. (Courtesy of B. Finkel, MD, and S. Golda, MD; Haifa, Israel.)

vascular problems are aneurysms, arteriovenous fistulas (34), and pyogenic granulomas. Avascular necrosis can occur if the grafts are too numerous and/or placed too close together, or if donor site suturing is too tight. The unavoidable transection of nerves can produce temporary hypesthesia, and as they regenerate, paresthesia. Rarely, a painful neuroma will develop; it can be treated with intralesional corticosteroid injections or excision.

Keloids, which occur rarely, can be treated with intralesional corticosteroids. If a keloid occurs in a recipient site, it usually interferes with hair growth, and may be a contraindication to further transplants.

The benefits of hair transplantation far outweigh the problems, making it a highly successful and gratifying procedure (Fig. 6).

ANCILLARY TECHNIQUES

Free scalp flaps were reported by Harri et al. (35) in 1974. Juri introduced flaps at the 1975 *International Congress of Plastic Surgeons in Paris* (36), and the technique was refined by others (37–40). Bald scalp reduction, first reported by Blanchard and Blanchard (40), has become, with contributions by others (41–46), one of the most enduring and valuable adjuncts to grafting. Kabaker and others (39,47) have demonstrated the usefulness of tissue expanders for bald scalp reduc-

tion. Frecht's method of scalp extension may duplicate the advantages of tissue expanders without the disadvantages (48).

Hair transplantation is a safe and efficacious method of redistributing scalp hair into a cosmetically acceptable pattern, and with application of the aforementioned complementary techniques, cosmetically optimal results are even more accessible to today's patient with AGA. Furthermore, the limiting factors of donor hair quantity and quality in hair restoration surgery may someday be overcome by hair follicle cloning, whereby the bald scalp can be populated by virtually unlimited numbers of test tube follicles (49). Until a safe and effective method of regrowing the miniaturized follicles of androgenetic pattern baldness (50) is perfected, hair transplantation will continue to be used. For the AGA patient and for the patient needing hair growth in areas of alopecic scars, surgical measures that are both finite and permanent are clearly the treatment of choice.

REFERENCES

1. Okuda S: Klinische und experimentelle Untersuchungen uber die Transplantation von lebenden Haaren. *Jpn J Dermatol* 40:537, 1939 (Japanese).
2. Okuda S: Clinical and experimental studies of transplantation of living hairs. *Jpn J Urol* 46:135–138, 1939 (Japanese).
3. Orentreich N: Autografts in alopecias and other selected dermatological conditions. *Ann NY Acad Sci* 83:463, 1959.

4. Kobori T, Montagna W, eds. *Biology and disease of the hair.* Baltimore: University Park Press, 1976.

5. Friederich HC: Indikation and Tecnik der Operativ-plastischen Behandlung des Haarverlustes. *Hautarzt* 21:197–202, 1970.

6. Orentreich N: Pathogenesis of alopecia. *J Soc Cosmet Chem* XI:479, 1960.

7. Orentreich N, Rizer RL: Medical treatment of androgenetic alopecia. In: Brown AC, Crounse RA, eds. *Hair, trace elements, and human illness. Part 4. Hirsutism and alopecia.* New York: Praeger, 1980:294–304.

8. Norwood OT, Shiell RC: *Hair transplant surgery,* 2nd ed. Springfield, IL: Charles C. Thomas, 1984.

9. Hamilton JB: Patterned loss of hair in man: Types and incidence. *Ann NY Acad Sci* 53:708–728, 1951.

10. Szasz TS, Robertson AM: The theory of the pathogenesis of ordinary human baldness. *Ama Arch Dermatol Syphilol* 61:34–48, 1950.

11. Frankel EB: Hair transplantation: Additional observations. *Cutis* 15:545, 1975.

12. Tezel J: Miniature drill expedites hair transplantation. *Cutis* 5:461, 1969.

13. Carreirao S, Lessa S: New technique for closing punch graft donor sites. *Plast Reconst Surg* 61:455–456, 1978.

14. Pierce HE. An improved method for closure of donor sites in hair transplantation. *J Dermatol Surg Oncol* 5: 475–476, 1979.

15. Vallis CP: Surgical treatment of receding hairline. *Plast Reconstr Surg* 33:247, 1964.

16. Grevelink JM, Brennick JB: Hair transplantation facilitated by flashscanner-enhanced carbon dioxide laser. *Operative Techniques in Otolaryngology* 5:278, 1994.

17. Villnow MM, Slatkine M, Strobele B, Mead D: Megasession hair transplantation with a CO_2 laser flashscanner technology. *Laser Med Surg* 13:259, 1995.

18. Green HA, Domankevitz MS, Nisioka NS: Pulsed carbon dioxide laser ablation of burned skin: In vitro and in vivo analysis. *Lasers Med Surg* 10:476, 1990.

19. Zweig AD, Meierhofer B, Muller OM et al: Lateral thermal damage along pulsed laser incisions. *Lasers Med Surg* 10:262, 1990.

20. Fitzpatrick RE, Goldman MP, Ruiz-Esparzra J: Clinical advantage of the CO_2 laser superpulsed mode. *J Dermatol Surg Oncol* 20:449, 1994.

21. Selmanowitz VJ, Orentreich N: Hair transplantation in blacks. *J Natl Med Assoc* 65:471, 1973.

22. Orentreich N: Hair problems. *J Am Med Wom Assoc* 21: 481, 1966.

23. Stough DB, Berger RA, Orentreich N: Surgical improvement of cicatricial alopecia of diverse etiology. *Arch Dermatol* 97:331, 1968.

24. Orentreich N: Hair transplants. In: Maddin S, ed. *Current dermatologic management.* St. Louis: CV Mosby, 13–20, 1970.

25. Ayres S: Hair transplantation. In: Epstein E: *Skin surgery,* 3rd ed. Springfield, IL: Charles C. Thomas, 1970.

26. Marritt E: Transplantation of single hairs from the scalp as eyelashes. *J Dermatol Surg Oncol* 6:271–273, 1980.

27. Nordstrom REA: "Micrografts" for improvement of the frontal hairline after hair transplantation. *Aesthetic Plast Surg* 97–101, 1981.

28. Marritt E: Single hair transplantation for hairline refinement: A practical solution. *J Dermatol Surg Oncol* 10:962–966, 1984.

29. Bradshaw W: Quarter-grafts: A technique for minigrafts. In: Unger WP, Nordstrom REA, eds. *Hair transplantation,* 2nd ed. New York: Marcel Dekker, 333–351, 1988.

30. Stough DB, Nelson BR: Incisional slit grafting. *J Dermatol Surg Oncol* 17:53–60, 1991.

31. Altchek DD, Pearlstein HH: Granulomatous reaction to autologous hairs incarcerated during hair transplantation. *J Dermatol Surg Oncol* 4:928, 1978.

32. Orentreich N, Orentreich D: Cross stitch suture technique for hair transplantation. *J Dermatol Surg Oncol* 10:12, 1984.

33. Orentreich N, Orentreich D: Androgenetic alopecia and its treatment. The physiology of hair growth. In: Unger WP, ed. *Hair transplantation,* 3rd ed., revised and expanded. New York: Marcel Dekker, 1995.

34. Sounder DE, Bercaw BL: Arteriovenous fistula secondary to hair transplantation. *N Engl J Med* 283:473, 1970.

35. Harri K, Obmori K, Obmori S: Hair transplantation with free scalp flaps. *Plast Reconstr Surg* 53:410, 1974.

36. Juri J: Use of parieto-occipital flaps in the surgical treatment of baldness. *Plast Reconstr Surg* 55:456, 1975.

37. Elliott RA: Lateral scalp flaps for instant results in male pattern baldness. *Plast Reconst Surg* 60:669, 1977.

38. Kabaker S: Experiences with parieto-occipital flaps in hair transplantation. *Laryngoscope* 88:73, 1978.

39. Fleming RW, Mayer TG: Short vs. long flaps in the treatment of male pattern baldness. *Arch Otolaryngol* 107:403, 1981.

40. Blanchard G, Blanchard B: La reduction tonsurale (detonsuration): Concept nouveau dans le traitement chirrurgical de la calvite. *Rev Chir Esth* 4:5, 1976.

41. Blanchard G, Blanchard B: Obliteration of alopecia by hair-lifting: A new concept and technique. *J Natl Med Assoc* 69:639, 1977.

42. Stough DB, Webster RC: *Esthetics and refinements in hair transplantation.* The International Hair Transplantation Symposium, Lucerne, Switzerland, February 1978.

43. Sparkuhl K: Scalp reduction: *Serial excision of the scalp with flap advancement.* The International Hair Transplant Symposium, Lucerne, Switzerland, February 1978.

44. Unger MG, Unger WP: Management of alopecia of the scalp by a combination of excisions and transplantation. *J Dermatol Surg Oncol* 4:670, 1978.

45. Bosley L, Hope CR, Montroy RE: Male pattern reduction (MPR) for surgical reduction of male pattern baldness. *Curr Ther Res* 25:281, 1979.

46. Alt TH: Scalp reduction as an adjunct to hair transplantation: Review of relevant literature and presentation of an improved technique. *J Dermatol Surg Oncol* 6:1011, 1980.

47. Kabaker S, Kridel R, Krugman N, Swenson R: Tissue expansion in the treatment of alopecia. *Arch Otolaryngol* 112:720, 1986.

48. Frecht P: Scalp extension. *J Dermatol Surg Oncol* 19:616–622, 1993.

49. Yang JS, Lavker RM, Sun T: Upper human hair follicle contains a sub population of keratinocytes with superior in vitro proliferative potential. *J Invest Dermatol* 101: 652–659, 1993.

50. Orentreich N, Durr NP: Biology of scalp hair growth. *Clin Plast Surg* 9:197–205, 1982.

Office-Based Surgery of the Head and Neck
Edited by Yosef P. Krespi, MD
Lippincott–Raven Publishers, Philadelphia © 1998

28

Laser-Assisted Hair Removal

Monica Elman, Michael Slatkine, Amir Waldman, and Zvi Rozenberg

The concept of using selective photothermolysis created by a pulsed laser for hair removal was first presented by Zaias in 1990 (1). The deep penetration of the laser beam into the skin (Fig. 1) enables scattered radiation to impinge hair shafts and follicles and be selectively absorbed by melanin. This is followed by thermal necrosis limited to the follicle zone owing to the short duration and limited energy of the pulsed laser source. Following the Zaias proposal, promising preliminary results of laser-assisted hair removal have been published by Grossman and Anderson (2) and by Goldberg (3). All authors report minimal pain. The procedures are fast and it is expected they will dramatically reduce both the time and the number of visits currently needed to achieve long-lasting depilation with electrolysis.

This chapter provides a brief overview of selective photothermolysis for hair removal with free-running pulsed lasers and summarizes an 18-month ongoing study with the Sharplan EpiTouch laser (Sharplan Lasers Inc., Allendale, NJ). The basic operating principles of laser-assisted hair removal are presented together with the treatment techniques and clinical results.

SELECTIVE PHOTOTHERMOLYSIS OF HAIR FOLLICLES

To obtain effective photothermolysis of the entire follicle, including the bulb and the bulge (a condition believed necessary for long-lasting hair removal), the laser radiation should penetrate at least 3 mm into the tissue, and be strongly absorbed by melanin and not by oxyhemoglobin. Figure 2 depicts the absorption spectrum of melanin and oxyhemoglobin. Red lasers are clearly the lasers of choice. They are currently popular in dermatology clinics in their Q-switch modes (20–30 nanoseconds time duration) for tattoo removal and the treatment of various pigmented lesions (4). However, because hair follicle diameter is typically in the 30 to 100 μm range, and thermal relaxation time is a few milliseconds, the lasers should be used in their free-running mode with sufficient energy for removal.

The energy density level necessary to coagulate a hair follicle depends on the hair shaft color, diameter, and depth. A prerequisite for follicle coagulation is Caucasian skin, because a dark epidermis does not allow the laser radiation to penetrate into the dermis. The temperature distribution along the hair follicle is expected to decrease with depth. It was theoretically analyzed with a statistical Monte-Carlo computer simulation of the scattering of a ruby laser beam in the vicinity of a hair shaft. The analysis leads to the following theoretical conclusions:

1. The temperature of an irradiated follicle is rapidly decreasing with hair shaft depth, as depicted in Figure 3.
2. Internal scattering of light in the skin leads to a minimal spot size of approximately 3–4 mm below which further beam size reduction above the tissue would not increase energy density inside the tissue.
3. The energy density necessary to fully coagulate (T~ 60°C) a follicle with a black hair shaft of 50 μ diameter and 3 mm

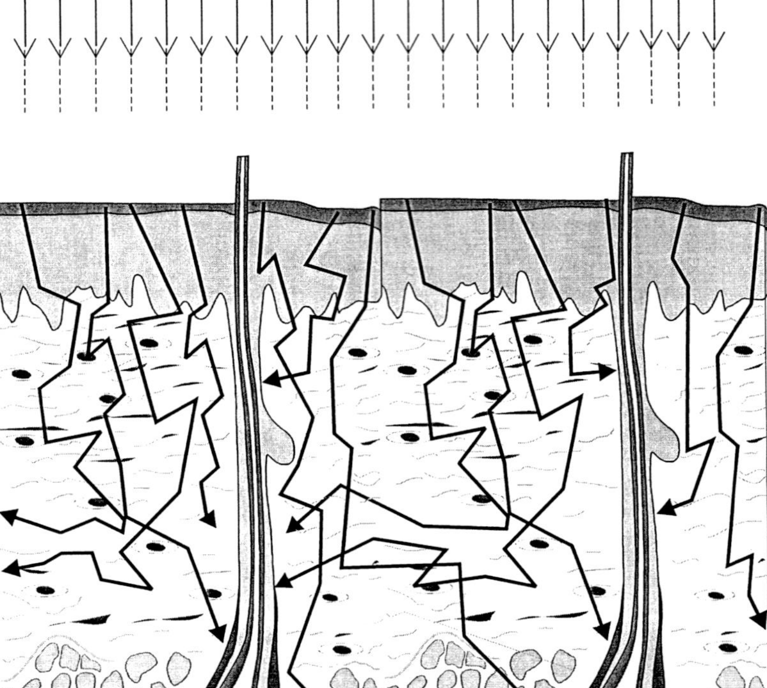

FIG. 1. Operating principle of laser-assisted hair removal.

depth is 20 J/cm^2 with a spot size of 5 mm. A lighter hair would necessitate higher energy densities.

4. The necessary energy density for the coagulation of a hair follicle is proportional to the hair shaft diameter, as long as the bulb and follicle thickness are proportionate to the hair shaft diameter. The thinner the hair, the lower the energy density level.

We have measured the diameter of hairs taken from the arm in a multitude of treated volunteers and found them to range mostly between 30 and 70 μ. Other hairs including bikini line hairs, which are an important tar-

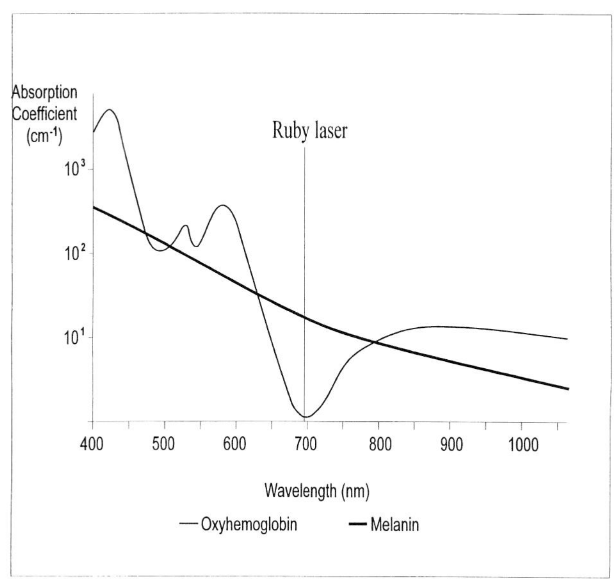

FIG. 2. Absorption spectrum of melanin and oxyhemoglobin.

get of laser-assisted hair removal, are usually thicker. As a result, a laser generating 20–40 J/cm² energy density with a spot size of 4–5 mm and a pulse duration of less than a few milliseconds is adequate for hair removal.

TREATMENT TECHNIQUE

A prerequisite for laser-assisted hair removal is Caucasian skin, since a dark epidermis does not allow laser radiation to penetrate into the dermis.

The treatment starts by shaving the hairs. In order to cool the skin, a transparent, room temperature, heat sink gel is applied to the treatment site during the procedure. Cooling the epidermis reduces immediate post-treatment inflammation and erythema considerably and also avoids possible epidermal damage in darker skin. A thin, patent-pending, laser-beam

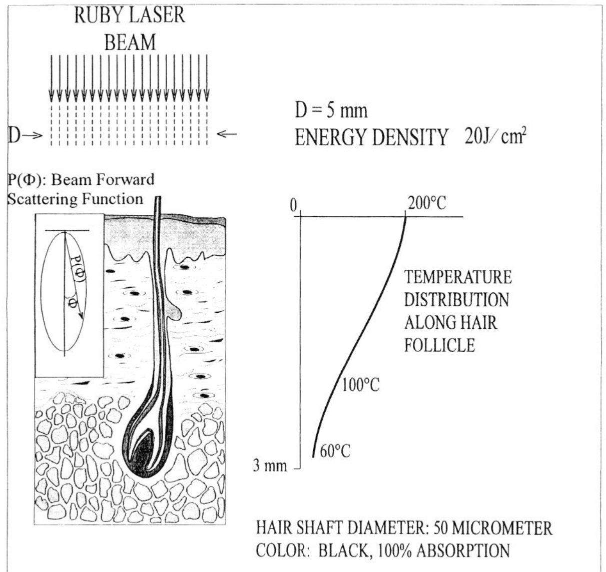

FIG. 3. Temperature distribution along a laser-irradiated hair follicle (computer simulation).

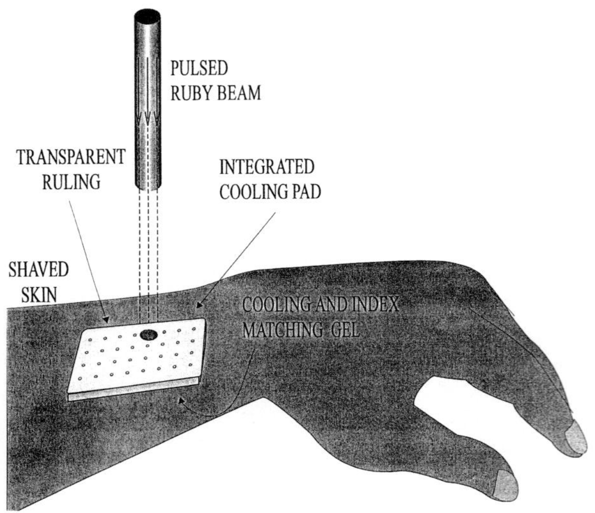

FIG. 4. Schematics of the laser hair removal technique.

aligning sheet is placed on top of the cooling gel to enable the proper positioning of the laser beam on the desired site before firing. This is necessary since the laser beam does not leave any visible marks on the skin. This also allows homogeneous coverage of the skin with the laser (see Fig. 4). The laser is operated at a 1-pulse-per-second repetition rate, thus covering a 12 cm^2 surface area in 1 minute. The laser energy is always kept at maximum level, while spot size is adjusted for proper fluence.

RESULTS

We have treated 150 patients on the arms, face, and bikini line with the EpiTouch laser set at 25–40 J/cm^2 energy density, 4–5 mm spot size (5). We have considered pigmented nevus and solar keratosis contraindications, as well as skin type IV and higher.

Figure 5 is a postoperative view of a 1 × 2-inch site 60 minutes after laser treatment, which lasted 60 seconds (1 pulse per second) with a cooling gel. Minimal redness is seen, which disappeared within 3–4 days. Postoperative results show 60% regrowth after 12 weeks, which necessitates more than one treatment as expected since only Anagen hairs are treated by the laser. Figure 6 shows the results of chin treatment after 3 months. Chin hair removal, as well as upper lip hair removal, needs 5–6 treatments, whereas bikini line hair removal needs 3–4 treatments.

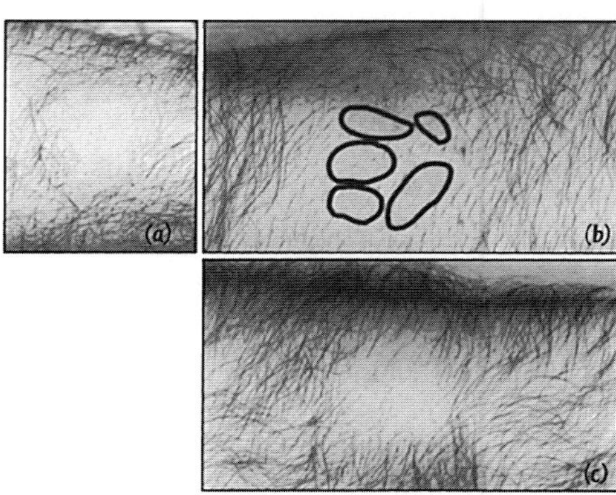

FIG. 5. Laser-assisted hair removal treatment. **(A)** One hour after treatment, **(B)** 12 weeks after treatment, **(C)** after 12 months; 9 months after second treatment.

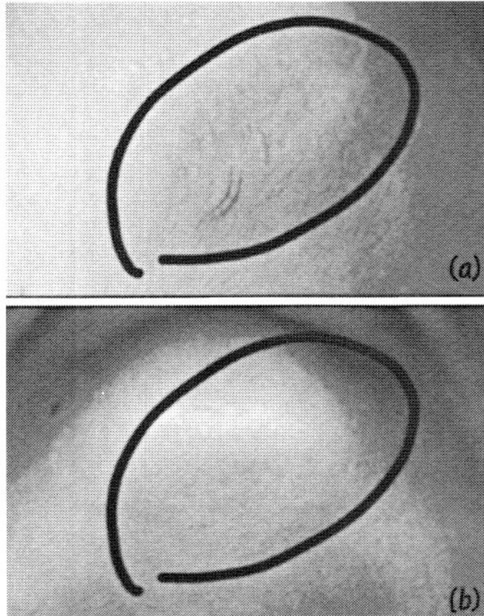

FIG. 6. Laser-assisted hair removal treatment on a woman's chin. **(A)** Before treatment, **(B)** 12 weeks after treatment.

CONCLUSION

Selective melanin-based photothermolysis with a free-running pulsed laser is a promising noninvasive technique for Anagen hair depilation. Additional studies will assess the extent of depilation long-lasting and its dependence on the hair growth cycle and hair and skin parameters. The laser depilation technique simultaneously hits many hair follicles and can operate at a repetition rate higher than one pulse per second. This is faster than conventional electrolysis, which also requires many patient visits, as opposed to an expected three to seven visits for laser depilation. Patients should be aware of multiple visits; necessity and permanency should not be promised.

REFERENCES

1. Zaias N: *Method of hair depilation.* US patent 5,059,192, October 1991.
2. Grossman M, Anderson R: *Laser targeted at hair follicles.* Presented at the Annual Conference of the American Society for Lasers in Medicine and Surgery, April 1995.
3. Goldberg D: *Topical solution assisted laser hair removal.* Presented at the Annual Conference of the American Society for Lasers in Medicine and Surgery, April 1995.
4. Lowe NJ et al: Q-switch ruby laser. *J Dermatol Surg Oncol* 20:307–311, 1994.
5. Elman M, Waldman A, Slatkine M, Rozenberg Z: *Laser-assisted hair removal: 1½ year experience.* Presented at the World Congress of Dermatology, Sydney, June 1997.

Guidelines

Office-Based Surgery of the Head and Neck
Edited by Yosef P. Krespi, MD
Lippincott–Raven Publishers, Philadelphia © 1998

Guidelines for Office-Based Laser Procedures

Yosef P. Krespi, MD

INTRODUCTION

Many laser procedures are safe and appropriate to perform in the office setting. High standards of practice, similar to those in the institutional setting, should be maintained to ensure quality of care for the surgical patient who undergoes an outpatient surgical procedure in an office-based surgical facility (1).

LASER PRIVILEGES

There mere acquisition of a skill is not the only criterion by which to measure qualifications. The office setting should not provide an opportunity for practice of inadequately trained personnel. Office staff must meet accepted standards of training and experience and should generally qualify for and hold privileges in an institutional setting (2,3). As new technology is introduced into the clinical setting, it is essential that all medical staff be appropriately educated and their skills assessed (4).

PATIENT AND PROCEDURE SELECTION

Prudent selection of both procedures and patients appropriate for office-based laser procedures is critical. Procedures that have intrinsic risk or require technology not available in the physician's office are more appropriately performed in an institutional setting.

In order to determine and apply proper indications for a procedure and to select the appropriate patients for applications of the technology, comprehensive knowledge of the disease process and experience in the management of patients with diseases that are treatable with the laser are essential. Prompt recognition and management of complications can only be achieved when the individual or team member is fully qualified in all aspects of the treatment of the disease (5).

PATIENT SAFETY

Patients should receive clear preprocedure instructions. Confirmation of important compliance issues such as NO status should be documented.

Conscious sedation used as an adjunct for office-based laser procedures must be conducted safely. There must be appropriate instrumentation and expertise in managing respiratory depression and cardiac arrest. Oximetry and automated blood pressure monitoring should be routinely employed; electronic cardiographic monitoring should be available. Oxygen, drugs, and equipment routinely used in cardiopulmonary resuscitation, including adequate suction, must be available.

The availability of emergency transport to an acute care facility willing to accept patients from the physician's office should be guaranteed.

The laser procedure should not be compromised by lack of equipment required to perform the proposed procedure.

All patients undergoing office-based laser procedures must be sufficiently recovered from the procedures and sedation prior to discharge. Following procedures requiring sedation, vital signs should be monitored and respiratory function and mental status should be assessed

---

Adapted from American Society for Laser Medicine and Surgery, Inc., April 1997.

in a manner similar to hospitalized patients. If sedation has been used, the patient must be accompanied by a reasonable adult at discharge. Written instructions regarding common complications, directions for returning for emergency evaluation, and caution as to continued functional impairment for many hours following conscious sedation are appropriate.

Periodic preventative maintenance and testing of bioelectrical equipment should be done by a qualified professional.

Standards protocols for both personnel and patient protection from infectious disease must be rigorously observed, including body fluid isolation, proper specimen handling, as well as proper instrumentation cleaning and disinfection (6).

RECORDS AND
QUALITY ASSURANCE

Each patient should have, at a minimum, a brief history and physical examination by the physician. Serious cardiopulmonary disease or other disease should be excluded by appropriate clinical and, if necessary, laboratory evaluation.

The patient chart should contain the clinical examination and evaluation, the justification for the procedure, the description of the treatment, and the patient's status on discharge. Informed consent for the procedure should be documented on the chart and be consistent with local professional standards and applicable state law.

Records should be maintained so that complications and problems can be identified and compliance with recommendations for clinical and laser treatment ensued (6).

ADDITIONAL RESOURCES

American College of Surgeons monograph *Guidelines for Office Endoscopic Services* (1991) and *Guidelines for Optimal Office-Based Surgery*.

REFERENCES

1. Accreditation of the office-based surgical facility. *Bulletin of the American College of Surgeons* 80 (8), 1995.
2. Standards of training for physicians for the use of lasers in medicine and surgery. American Society for Laser Medicine and Surgery, Inc., Nausau, WI, 1991.
3. American National Standards Institute (ANSI), 11 West 42nd Street, New York, NY 10036.
4. Statement on emerging surgical technologies and the evaluation of credentials. *Bulletin of the American College of Surgeons* 79 (6), 1995.
5. Statement on issues to be considered before a new surgical technology is applied to the care of patients. *Bulletin of the American College of Surgeons* 80 (9), 1995.
6. Guidelines for office-based surgery: Quality assurance. *Bulletin of the American College of Surgeons* 79 (10), 1994.

SUBJECT INDEX